Stress

To Piet Wiepkema

Stress
Conceptual and Biological Aspects

Frederick Toates

The Open University, Milton Keynes, UK

JOHN WILEY & SONS

Chichester · New York · Brisbane · Toronto · Singapore

Other Wiley Editorial Offices

John Wiley & Sons, Inc., 605 Third Avenue,
New York, NY 10158-0012, USA

Jacaranda Wiley Ltd, 33 Park Road, Milton,
Queensland 4064, Australia

John Wiley & Sons (Canada) Ltd, 22 Worcester Road,
Rexdale, Ontario M9W 1L1, Canada

John Wiley & Sons (SEA) Pte Ltd, 37 Jalan Pemimpin #5-04,
Block B, Union Industrial Building, Singapore 2057

British Library Cataloguing in Publication Data

A catalogue record for this book is available from the British Library

ISBN 0 471 96021 7

Typeset in 10/12pt Century Schoolbook by Dorwyn Ltd, Rowlands Castle,
Hants
Printed and bound in Great Britain by Bookcraft (Bath) Ltd, Midsomer
Norton, Avon
This book is printed on acid-free paper responsibly manufactured from
sustainable forestation, for which at least two trees are planted for each one
used for paper production.

Contents

Preface

Any attempt at a synthesis of stress research could only be undertaken by a masochist. The area is one of notorious conceptual difficulty, even by the standards of the behavioural sciences. Rightly or wrongly, I have elected to be that masochist.

Researchers into stress commonly look at an isolated phenomenon, such as the effects of corticosteroids on the immune system, stress-induced analgesia or the relationship between corticosteroids and avoidance learning. This specialization is of course inevitable for a subject as vast as stress. However, the fragmentation has a cost and that is a lack of an overview that can point to the relationships or potential relationships and interdependence between the phenomena. The number of articles devoted to stress rises exponentially yet we still lack an adequate definition of stress. Although this book cannot claim to provide an entirely satisfactory definition, what it aims to do is to provide an organizing framework, a tentative model, that can serve to synthesize the literature and perhaps lead to greater parsimony in this area. It is my belief that stress can be better understood by looking at the normal unstressed performance of the processes that are of interest in states of stress. Hence, an important part of the book consists of looking at basic behavioural processes.

If stress is like the *Times* crossword, I cannot claim to have given a solution. What I hope that I can honestly claim is to have filled in a few tentative overlapping clues so that others may fill in some of the remainder.

Of necessity, the review has had to be not just selective but massively selective; doubtless authors whose work has been omitted from discussion can provide perfectly good reason to argue that no synthesis could be complete without discussion of their work. Unfortunately, this is inevitable in a review of this nature. I make no claim to comprehensiveness. Results and theories have been selected on the grounds that they seemed to me to be the ones that most lent themselves to development of a theoretical synthesis.

Some of the experiments discussed in this study raise uncomfortable ethical issues. I would certainly not do them myself but must face the dilemma that their results seem to be of value. Some experiments would find it difficult to obtain acceptance from an ethical committee, such as that which monitors Open University research. Some would no longer be permitted at all in Britain. I do not know the answer to the moral dilemma that is posed by discussing such experiments, but I can merely acknowledge it. I sincerely hope that theoretical modelling might allow some experimentation to be circumvented.

Much of the work for this study was carried out while the author was a visitor at the Department of Ethology at the Swedish Agricultural University, Skara, Sweden. I am grateful to the university and to the Swedish National Research Council for a grant that made this stay possible. I am very grateful to Professor Piet Wiepkema of Wageningen Agricultural University for persuading me to take an interest in applied behavioural science in the first place and to Mike Stewart of the Open University for suggesting this book. The book has been greatly improved by the comments of Kent Berridge of the University of Michigan, Paul Brain of the University of Wales, Basiro Davey of the Open University, Per Jensen of the Swedish Agricultural University, Barry Keverne of Cambridge University, Piet Wiepkema of Wageningen Agricultural University and Fred Westbook of the Australian National University.

Frederick Toates
March 1995

Chapter 1

Introduction

1.1 CONCEPTUAL ISSUES IN STRESS RESEARCH

What is stress? On the one hand, the scientific study of stress has without doubt proven fruitful; we know a lot about what happens when animals are subject to situations generally termed stressful. The study of stress has served as a powerful stimulus to bring the otherwise rather disparate disciplines of ethology, psychobiology and immunology together in developing integrative theoretical models (Wiepkema and Van Adrichem, 1987). On a more popular level, books on how to combat stress abound and few can doubt the appropriateness of the term in an everyday context. The unambiguous signs of stress are all too clear. Rather like the common use of the words 'good' and 'evil', we seem to have little trouble in knowing what is meant when the term 'stress' is employed.

On the other hand, as a topic of scientific study, stress is paradoxical. The term is intrinsically problematic; like good and evil, trying to define it in a rigorous way generates inordinate difficulty. Extensive discussions have failed to deliver a scientific definition of when an animal is stressed. Unlike, say, studying feeding or drinking, stress poses profound conceptual problems of definition which have generated many pages of discussion. As in the case of the word 'drive' in psychology, with its similar inherent circularity of definition, some authors wish to banish the term 'stress' from academic discourse. For example, Rushen (1986) writes: 'Stress itself is one of those terms that we use to shield us from our ignorance. We would be better off without it. It survives because it is a convenient term to indicate the general topic under discussion. Attempts to provide such a vague concept with a precise physiological definition engender confusion and mis-understanding'.

Maybe it is sufficient justification for employing the term 'stress' that at least the title serves as a convenient organizing theme. However, there is a common feeling that use of the term can really only be justified as a scientific concept if it is able to meet the criterion of parsimony (Freeman, 1985). Does its use enable us to economize on words? At this point in time, from the number of papers devoted unsuccessfully to trying to define stress, one might doubt that it does.

Like 'drive', despite appeals for its banishment, 'stress' refuses to go away but simply reappears in new forms. Is the word 'stress' to be used to denote a particular class of stimuli, a set of behavioural responses or the state of the intermediate physiology? Is it to be used as a noun, a verb or an adjective? In practice, it tends to be used as all of these (Engel, 1985). Thus we have such expressions as to *stress* an animal, to cause *stress* and for an animal to exhibit a *stress* response. Not uncommonly, two uses are confounded in a single sentence, for example, '. . . stress induced in poultry as a result of hysteria or heat stress . . .' (Harvey *et al.*, 1984). As Jewell and Mylander (1988) so aptly express it: 'It seems as if stress, in addition to being itself and the result of itself, is also the cause of itself'.

Imagine the confusion if a comparable usage were to prevail in, say, feeding research, with a single term used to describe the stimulus of palatable food, the physiology of low blood glucose and fat deposits, and the behaviour of feeding. None the less, the confusion has not prevented an impressive body of data and theory from being generated in an area of research that we all term with some certainty 'stress'.

What then is stress? Under what circumstances is an animal stressed? The answer will probably depend upon the purpose behind the question and level of explanation offered. In the present study, the emphasis will be on behavioural definitions though we shall not ignore physiological indices. Chrousos *et al.* (1988) give the definition: '. . . stress is the recognition by the body of a stressor and therefore the state of threatened homeostasis; stressors are threats against homeostasis; and adaptive responses are the body's attempt to counteract the stressor and reestablish homeostasis'. Similarly, Sapolsky (1994, p. 7) defines a stressor as 'anything that throws your body out of homeostatic balance — for example, an injury, an illness, subjection to great heat or cold'. This seems unambiguous, apart from a few definitional problems as to exactly when the homeostatic state of reference prevails. However, it has the problem that almost anything likely to be encountered will constitute a stressor, including a sexual encounter or feeding (Woods, 1991). Although it can be salutary to be reminded of the features shared in common with a number of such challenges to

Table 1.1. Possible situations that might constitute stress

	Short-term stimulation	Long-term stimulation
Aversive stimulation	A	B
Pleasant stimulation	C	D

homeostasis (e.g. certain hormonal changes), as a definition of stress it raises problems. For example, prescriptions for the seemingly laudible aim of stress reduction would presumably need serious qualification when it concerned experience with such usually acceptable 'stressors' as feeding and orgasm.

In trying to provide a definition, some look at the stimulus/input side, some at the behavioural output and others at the intermediate physiology. Looking at the stimulus side, some of the possible criteria are summarized in Table 1.1.

To some authors, only the criterion summarized in cell B constitutes stress whereas, to others, cells A and B but not C and D represent stress. As just noted, some theorists would include cells C and D as candidates for defining stress. For instance, positively reinforcing sexual activity can induce symptoms similar to those induced by aversive stimuli (Duncan *et al.*, 1993). Vaginal stimulation in human females, reported as pleasant, can induce similar physiological responses (e.g. increases in blood pressure and respiration, an analgesic state) to aversive stimulation (Komisaruk and Whipple, 1986). But should such situations be termed stressful? They appear to constitute a deviation from homeostasis. Thus to some authors, all of the cells indicated can be associated with a state of stress. In such terms, even prolonged pleasant stimulation could be stressful if it is of a certain quality, e.g. involving a homeostatic deviation and/or powerful and unexpected stimulation. Presumably no serious researcher would wish to confine stress to cells C and D.

Defined in terms of cells A and B, stress is a state that can arise acutely and be countered by effective action. Long-term disturbance to homeostasis might then be given a stronger term such as *dis*stress or *chronic* stress. Another approach to defining stress (cell B only) is to see it as a more chronic state that arises only when defence mechanisms are either being chronically stretched or are actually failing. This is the line that will be adopted here. However, it is impossible to arbitrate on which of the possible criteria is superior. It is simply important that the reader keeps in mind the different definitions that are found in the literature.

Consider the following sample of situations in which, typically, an animal is described as stressed. When it is: (1) exposed to inescapable electric shock; (2) placed in the cage of a dominant animal with no possibility of escape; (3) able to obtain food and water only at the price of entering the territory of a rival and threatening animal; (4) placed in overcrowded conditions; (5) separated when infant from its caregiver and shows an alarm reaction; and (6) placed in a small barren environment and displays abnormal and apparently pointless rituals over long periods of time. What have these situations in common that could lead to the notion of stress? Is it something about the external events that impinge upon the animal, such as electric shock? Is it the animal's behaviour, such as ritualized pacing? Or is it the internal state of the animal, such as an elevated heart rate or the appearance of elevated levels of certain hormones (e.g. adrenaline and corticosteroids)? We shall argue that, in some respects, it can be all of these things, although in each case we will need to qualify our argument.

One potential, if not actual, use of the stress concept is in achieving parsimony of expression. Some researchers have taken a physiological perspective and have tied the definition of stress to the combination of elevated corticosteroid levels, loss of weight and loss of reproductive capacity. If certain consistent patterns of physiological and behavioural consequences follow from placing an animal in one of a number of different contexts, the term stress could be employed as a shorthand for the physiological and behavioural consequences. (Alternatively, one might want to use the term stress to refer just to the pattern of physiological changes.) In these terms, stress might be called an *intervening variable*, something that intervenes between certain stimuli and certain behavioural responses (a similar logic applies to the terms 'drive' and 'motivation' in psychology; Miller, 1959; Toates, 1986). Use of the term stress can potentially serve a function of parsimony if a number of changes in response can be assumed by specifying that a state of stress has been caused by a stimulus. Figure 1.1 illustrates this.

There are some broad classes of behavioural change that appear in a number of situations that are termed stressful. For example, Chrousos *et al*. (1988) suggest that stress can be associated with: (1) changes in alertness and attention span; (2) a decrease in reflex time; and (3) a suppression of feeding and sexual behaviour. However, in practice, as will be demonstrated in the present study, life is unfortunately not as simple as to permit one single term 'stress', to be used as an intervening variable without qualifications being added. Internal states that we would wish to characterize as stress differ according to the nature

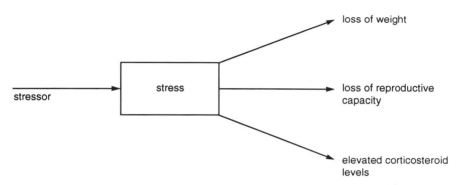

Figure 1.1. Potential parsimony of expression obtained by postulating a state of stress

of the situation in which the animal finds itself (Shavit and Martin, 1987); one all-embracing internal state of stress seems unattainable.

As represented in cells A and B, stress usually carries connotations of unpleasantness: the animal is in a situation that it would not be in, were it able to take appropriate action. So is stress synonymous with suffering? If this was so, we might then suffice with the one word 'suffering' and dispense with the problematic word 'stress'. It is true that there is considerable overlap between suffering and stress. A suffering animal might be described as a stressed animal. However, stress is probably best used to describe a particular kind of aversive state. Also it could be argued that, if defined in terms of the hormonal response, stress can appear at its maximum level in *anticipation* of suffering (Arthur, 1987; see Section 5.6). Furthermore, suffering, a word with conscious and subjective human overtones, is perhaps even more problematic than stress. There is a range of situations that seem mildly stressful by such indices as hormone changes but which might not be described as involving suffering. The following sections lead towards a development of a model of stress by first considering some possible criteria for defining stress. None of these gives a watertight definition but each can provide pointers as to when stress might be present.

1.2   CRITERIA OF STRESS

1.2.1   External Stimuli

It is logical to start with events that impinge upon the animal — sometimes termed the 'input'. Could these provide a definition of stress? Can we identify a number of external stimuli, such as electric shock, extremes of hot and cold, or the presence of a dominant animal, that by some common property invariably can be said to evoke stress? One sometimes terms such stimuli *stressors* and it can be useful to attempt to list them. However, attempts at such classification soon lead to the conclusion that stressors cannot be defined by their intrinsic physical properties but only by their effects upon the body. Thus, Rivier (1991a) defined stress as: '. . . any threat—real or perceived—which can alter homeostasis'. In reference to external stimuli, such definitions might provide some parsimony in that a wide range of stimuli and events which hitherto might be felt to have little in common, e.g. haemorrhage, a predator, bereavement and activation of the immune system by a foreign body, are brought under the same rubric. They have the capacity to effect some common hormonal changes (discussed later). However, as was noted earlier, interaction with positive and unavoided stimuli can sometimes exert a similar effect to a traditionally described stressor. Also unambiguously negative events can sometimes elicit rather different hormonal profiles.

As will be shown in Chapter 5, the capacity of a particular stimulus to evoke signs of stress, as indexed by changes in the physiology and behaviour of an animal, depends also upon factors other than its physical properties. For example, suppose two rats are subjected to identical electric shocks. The first animal can exert some control over the shocks; by manipulating a wheel it is able to terminate the shock. The second rat can do nothing to control the shocks. On examination, by criteria of pathology, the latter will reveal serious signs of stress whereas the former will either appear unstressed or will show less severe signs of stress. The difference cannot be attributed to differences in external stimulation as these are identical. Having a course of action available, sometimes known as a *coping strategy* (Section 1.3.10; also described in Chapter 5), has ameliorated the effect of shock in the first animal. For another example of the problems in using external stimuli as the definition, consider that novelty is a potent stimulus of hormonal changes described as stress-related (File and Peet, 1980). However, novelty is not a property of the external stimuli *per se*. The same stimuli when familiar would not have the same effect. Novelty is not an intrinsic property of the external world but a property of the animal in interaction with its environment.

Take another situation that complicates the picture still more if we rely upon external stimuli to provide a definition. An animal is trained in a Skinner box to press a lever to earn food. Then, after the behaviour is established, the food is removed from the apparatus so that when the rat presses the lever no food appears. This causes changes in the level of secretion of certain 'stress hormones', corticosteroids (described later), in the body, which we might term a stress response. The situation is usually described as one of *frustration*; rats will often try to escape from such an environment. However, it would be odd to describe *no food* as a stimulus. By the same token the rat received *no* water and *no* mate. The point is that 'no food' must be seen in context. The non-appearance of food might be described as a stressor in a context in which: (1) the animal is hungry and motivated to seek food and (2) has some *expectation* of food. As a general rule, events in the external world or their absence need to be placed into the context of the animal's current goals, expectations and strategies before we can attribute a role to them in arousing stress. These three examples illustrate that, before its stress evoking capacity can be described, the external situation needs to be qualified in terms of, respectively, the animal's control, familiarity and expectations.

However, provided the caution is borne in mind, for some purposes it can be convenient to label such things as electric shock as stressors. By analogy to the use of 'stressor', it is convenient to group bacteria and viruses together under the rubric 'pathogen', without implying that their presence invariably causes disease; immunological and other factors analogous to coping strategies also play an intervening part. To be cautious though, and as a reminder, I shall sometimes term such things as shock and loud noise *potential stressors*, implying that their power to evoke stress is not always seen.

1.2.2 Physiological States

1.2.2.1 Hormonal reactions

Attempts at integrative definitions, models and theories of stress usually place weight upon physiological states that occur at times when the animal encounters aversive stimulation. Confronted with a threat such as a predator or a rival, an animal commonly takes such action as running away or attack. Closely associated with this behaviour, fundamental reorganization of the animal's physiology occurs. For instance, behavioural effort requires a diversion of blood from such organs as the stomach to the muscles, so as to supply them with metabolic fuel (e.g. glucose, O_2).

From the angle of physiological indices, some hopes of an integrative perspective might be raised by noting two things. First, it has proven convenient to distinguish two major physiological systems that are commonly involved in the reaction to an emergency. One involves activation of a branch of the *autonomic nervous system* (ANS; the 'sympathetic' branch) and traditionally there has been a tendency to define stress in terms of such visceral responses as elevated heart rate that are mediated by this branch (Natelson *et al.*, 1987). (Later it will be argued that excess activity on the part of the other ANS branch, the parasympathetic, is also associated with stress.) The other system has the daunting name of the hypothalamic–pituitary–adrenocortical (HPA) system (the significance of this term will be described in the next chapter) involving elevated levels of hormones: adrenocorticotrophic hormone (ACTH) and corticosteroids. Both of these systems are commonly activated by certain stimuli, e.g. a haemorrhage, surgery, a predator or electric shock. Secondly, a diverse range of stimuli apparently having little else in common can serve to activate these two systems. For example, both the physical trauma of haemorrhage and the psychological challenge of public speaking can do so (Kuchel, 1991). Thus, a reaction by both these systems is used as a pointer to a state of stress. From this perspective, the hormones that are part of these systems, e.g. adrenaline (part of the ANS) and ACTH and corticosteroids (part of the pituitary–adrenocortical system), are sometimes termed the 'stress hormones' (e.g. Dantzer, 1991). In the classic writings of Hans Selye (e.g. Selye, 1973) an elevation in corticosteroids is synonymous with stress (see also discussion in Rushen, 1986). Thus, in such terms, presumably one would not say that stress *causes* elevated corticosteroid levels as stress *is* the elevated level.

Selye (1973) referred to a syndrome of physiological changes that certain stimuli induce as the *general adaptation syndrome*. This syndrome consists of specific physiological changes (e.g. increased secretion of corticosteroids) but is non-specific in the sense that a diverse range of stimuli (e.g. cold, electric shock) are able to trigger the same physiological response. Thereby, Selye was able to define a class of stimuli as stressors: those stimuli having the capacity to trigger this syndrome. In Selye's terms, stressors were not necessarily negative things. Novelty, which would seem to fit neither a positive or negative label, can be more potent a stimulus for corticosteroid secretion than electric shock. A sudden pleasant event might evoke the same reaction as a negative one. In a similar vein to Selye, Rivier (1989) shows such things as toxins, infection, exercise, emotions, pain and sleep all as examples of stressors in that they have inputs that converge upon the hypothalamus and, acting through intermediate stages, promote excitation of corticosteroid secretion. According to Selye, seen as a stressor, 'a passionate kiss' might qualify equally well as electrical shock.

Corticosteroid levels are elevated during coitus and physical exercise in humans and at the time of food delivery, which could hardly be considered aversive events (see Rushen, 1986). Thus, in Selye's terms, all four cells of Table 1.1 are compatible with a state of stress. In Selye's model, the stimuli were not defined as a group by their intrinsic qualities but by their effects upon the body. Thus, in such terms, stress is neither something that can be, nor should be, always avoided. In a tradition related to that of Selye, stress was defined by Allen *et al.* (1973) as: '. . . a collection of diverse stimuli which damage or potentially damage the organism and have in common an ability to stimulate ACTH secretion. This results in increased glucocorticoid secretion which enables the organism to better adapt to potential or actual life-threatening challenges'.

However, to most of us, the term stress usually implies negative events and that is the use to which it will be put here. The present author has difficulty with the notion that a kiss can usefully be described as a stressor. Given such a reservation, one possibility is to see elevated corticosteroids as being a *necessary* but not *sufficient* condition to define the existence of stress. So stress might be defined in terms of being in a situation that the animal will attempt to avoid, associated with an elevated corticosteroid level. This is near to the logic that will be adopted here. If the context is taken into account, such an elevated response can be a useful index of stress. For example, in applied ethology, Broom (1991), in considering elevated corticosteroid secretion of domestic animals on being handled, argues that: 'a greater response indicates poorer welfare than a smaller response'.

Just as elevated hormonal levels are used as an index of stress, so it is sometimes argued that coping with stress can be defined objectively in terms of hormonal responses, e.g. attainment of a stable corticosteroid secretion rate (e.g. Benus, 1988). Benus notes that, at the start of a shock avoidance experiment, rats show a greatly elevated level of plasma corticosteroid but after they have learned a strategy that avoids shocks, their corticosteroid level falls to normal. In such terms, the rat would be described as stressed at the start of the experiment but not after learning the avoidance strategy, which would seem not to violate any common-sense notions of language.

Freeman (1985) argues that, whereas a vast range of threatening and potentially threatening situations are associated with a corticosteroid response, there are some life-threatening situations that are not. To Freeman, this undermines the theoretical parsimony of 'stress'. In the present study, the existence of elevated corticosteroids will be taken as evidence suggestive of stress but not necessarily the defining condition. Thus the stress concept will not be seen as undermined but in need of qualification. A further caution is needed in any attempt to equate stressors, the corticosteroid response and suffering. Typically, such things as electric shock are called stressors and by common intuition one might suppose that suffering could be associated with protracted exposure to them. However, as Arthur (1987) notes, anticipation of such stressors commonly provokes a greater corticosteroid response than confrontation with them. So using a corticosteroid index, one would end with a paradoxical situation of there being a greater stress at a time when the stressor has not yet arrived. As Arthur notes, in defining physiological stress in terms of the corticosteroid response: 'Physiological stress seems to be more closely related to the intention of the organism to be vigilant and to be ready to take corrective action than to distress and suffering'.

Concerning the ANS, difficulties also arise in trying to associate stress with a physiological index. In the context of the sympathetic nervous system (SNS), McCarty (1983) considers a stressful stimulus to be: '. . . any external event which precipitates a significant activation of the sympathetic–adrenal medullary system and a measurable change in behaviour'. Such a definition thereby excludes physiological challenges that do not involve behaviour. Considered in a broader context, there might be a predominant parasympathetic reaction in a situation that by common intuition one would describe as stressful. Conversely, in humans, Frankenhaeuser (1976) reports a high rate of adrenaline secretion accompanying such emotions as joy and excitement, as well as anger and fear. Giving food at the end of a period of deprivation can be associated with higher levels of plasma noradrenaline than deprivation itself, whereas by common-sense reasoning the latter might be thought of as more stressful than the former (Ingram *et al.*, 1980). As argued earlier, in the terms developed here, for a hormonal change to be a useful index of stress, we would need to qualify it within a context (e.g. an assumed associated negative emotion). The alternative of simply using the hormonal response might be to include too much under the stress heading or be misleading.

In spite of some anomalies and the need for qualifications, the assumption that elevated corticosteroids and adrenaline secretion are an index of stress has proven useful and is widely made in the scientific literature. By the same criterion, a reduction in the levels of corticosteroids and free fatty acids (an index of SNS activity) is commonly interpreted as being synonymous with a reduction in stress. For example, a 'protective effect' of low doses of alcohol is possibly indexed by a reduction in these two reactions to a stressor (Brick and Pohorecky,

1987; Levenson, 1987; Pohorecky and Brick, 1987). Similarly, File and Peet (1980) speak of the efficacy of benzodiazepines in reducing stress, based upon their effect of reducing the corticosteroid response.

Closely connected with issues of definition in terms of physiology, one finds in the literature arguments of the kind—Can a reliable and sensitive *index* of stress be found (Natelson *et al.*, 1987)? Quite apart from the practical problems of actually finding such an index, as just described, the question raises some fundamental issues as to what the concept of stress is really all about. It plunges us straight into the dilemmas and circular arguments that have always plagued this area. In searching for an index, Natelson *et al.* subjected rats to electric shocks of increasing intensity and observed changes in their hormonal state. According to these authors, a reliable index would be, say, a hormone that shows a given increase in its rate of release each time a shock of given magnitude is applied. To be a sensitive index, the same hormone's rate of secretion would need to increase as shock intensity is increased.

Logically, if hormone activity is to be a useful index of some stress state within the animal, then this state should have some significance for the animal's behaviour. One might expect some measure of 'stressed' behaviour to change in concert with the hormonal index of stress. In rats subjected to electric shocks, plasma noradrenaline levels seem to provide a good physiological measure and such behaviours as moving around, rearing and vocalization correlate with it (Natelson *et al.*, 1987). However, the concept of using the noradrenaline response to shock as an index of stress poses a number of problems. Should one preclude less dramatic, but longer-acting, aversive stimuli as true causes of stress? These tend to provoke activity on the part of the corticosteroids. Corticosteroids are slower to respond to the application of potential stressors than are the catecholamines, such as noradrenaline. They have a short plasma half-life and furthermore there is a powerful endogenous rhythm in their secretion, quite unrelated to stressors. These are grave problems with using corticosteroids as an index, but surely this does not make chronic stressors any less stressful. In the present study, elevated levels of either plasma corticosteroids or noradrenaline or both will, considered in context, be seen as indices of stress.

Another problem raised by the research of Natelson *et al.* (1987) is what to conclude when the correlation between two possible indices of stress starts to break down. For instance, motor behaviour sometimes shows some habituation with repeated presentation of a stressor whereas the hormonal response remains at full strength. The problem is summed up by the comment of Natelson *et al.*: 'What is not known is whether this happened because behaviour is a more sensitive index of stress than the hormones and whether the stimulus was actually less stressful after being repeatedly delivered'.

This should urge some caution as to whether there really is some entity *stress* that can be indexed in various possible ways. While not disregarding such caution, the present study will use stress to refer to a state of the central nervous system (CNS) which commonly has certain associated hormonal states that can be used as pointers to the CNS state.

1.2.2.2 Brain states

Is it possible to define stress in terms of a characteristic state of the brain's neurophysiology? Hennessy and Levine (1979) closely associate stress with *arousal* noting the common basis of both reactions in: (1) absolute and relative novelty; (2) uncertainty; and (3) stimulus change. Such arousal or 'activation' can be measured by looking at the brain's gross electrical activity and noting a characteristic arousal profile. In rats, Endröczi (1972, p. 88) noted that signs of EEG arousal were followed shortly afterwards by an elevation of ACTH output, although he was cautious about inferring a causal sequence. Ursin (1988) assumes that the stress response is identical to the activation response. In his terms, activation arises when the brain registers disparity between a variable and one of its so-called 'set-values' (meaning much the same as reference value. See Section 1.3). Ursin argues in the following way, implying that activation forms part of a negative feedback control system: 'Activation will sustain itself until activation affects mechanisms that serve to solve the underlying discrepancy, by changing the actual values, or the set values, or shifting to other motivational systems. Eventually activation turns off activation'.

However, perhaps the animal is moved to obtain an arousal or activation level of some intermediate value rather than a low level. Hennessy and Levine (1979) note that some animals will work to increase sensory stimulation and speak of 'the tendency of an organism to maintain an optimal level of arousal'. In such terms, an arousal model would fit the common assumption that stress might arise from too little sensory stimulation (e.g. the boredom and pacing of some caged animals) as well as from too much. As Hennessy and Levine (1979) note, it would be interesting to know whether, in cases of understimulation, increasing stimulation can be associated with change in pituitary–adrenal activity. In an experiment on humans, it was found that both understimulation (boredom) and overstimulation were associated with higher excretion rates of adrenaline and noradrenaline, as compared with when performing work at a comfortable rate (Frankenhaeuser, 1976).

Arousal would seem to suffer from some of the same problems as using corticosteroid level as a measure of stress: almost anything of significance that happens to an animal will be drawn under the stress rubric. In the present study, in assuming that characteristic brain states constitute a state of stress, arousal is one possible pointer but it will not necessarily provide an exclusive definition. However, in the theoretical model that will be developed here, a protracted abnormally high state of arousal would certainly be strongly suggestive of a state of stress.

Recently, an interesting idea was advanced by Minor *et al.* (1994a,b). They suggested that stress can be characterized by a state of disruption of the metabolic homeostasis of the brain. As an intervening variable, this state would appear to offer some potential as it enables a number of behavioural variables to be predicted (e.g. loss of interest in incentive objects such as food and sex and a state of behavioural helplessness in the face of aversive stimuli). It might serve as an intervening variable for the state of passive stress described later but it is uncertain whether it might also label states of active stress.

1.2.3 Behaviour

As the third in the triad, input, physiological system and output, we have the output, behaviour. An animal that is described as under stress might be expected to behave in a certain way. The applied ethology literature assumes a number of different behavioural indicators of stress (Hart, 1988; Mason, 1991). For instance, the stressed animal might make repeated attempts to escape from its situation. It might consistently take evasive action when confronted with a rival. Or it might go into a corner and sit apathetically, ignoring such needs as food and water. It might pace up and down in a ritualistic fashion or engage in bizarre behaviours such as ritualized air sucking. It is clear that there is no one behaviour that can be used as an indicator of stress and it will be argued later that such diverse behaviours as active resisting and apathetic withdrawal can equally be considered as indicative of stress.

In an applied setting (e.g. animal husbandry), caution is needed in using abnormal behaviour as an index of stress and thereby implementing intervention. Any behaviour needs to be seen in the context of:

(1) what the animal achieves (or potentially achieves) by this behaviour, in terms of both the external environment and its internal state and (2) what would happen if the animal was prevented from behaving in this way. Bizarre behaviour might be indicative of stress, but the animal might be still more stressed if it was kept in a similar environment, but failed to 'discover' such behaviour or is prevented from showing it (Mason, 1991).

To refer back to Section 1.2.1, animals are described as having *coping strategies* available for dealing with potential stressors. The degree to which an animal would be described as stressed varies inversely with the extent to which it has available a coping strategy for dealing with the situation. Thus behaviour would need to be interpreted in terms of its effect upon the animal's environment and physiology.

1.2.4   Disease

One possible index of stress is the presence of illness and/or diseased tissue. Indeed, the pioneer of stress research, Selye (1973) saw the defining characteristic of stress as being a 'syndrome', a combination of: (1) an enlarged adrenal cortex; (2) shrinkage of lymphatic structures; and (3) ulceration in the stomach and upper gut. The value of a unifying concept of stress was suggested by Selye's assumption that elevated levels of corticosteroids were, at least in part, responsible for (2) and (3).

An animal exposed to uncontrollable electric shock will display damage to the wall of the stomach, which has sometimes been attributed to elevated levels of corticosteroids (Weiss, 1971). A chronically stressed animal will typically show decreased activity of the immune system and tumour rejection would be less. Therefore, we might assess the degree of stress by the index of pathology. Using the criterion of organic pathology, certain situations that are perhaps not obviously stressful to a human observer would be labelled so. For example, suppose rats are maintained on a schedule of 23 h food deprivation/1 h feeding in an apparatus that gives access to a running wheel. A significant number of animals will engage in extensive running in the wheel. The degree to which this situation induces gastric ulcers correlates positively with the amount of activity shown in the wheel (Paré, 1976).

However, as always in stress research, an irritatingly high level of caution is in order. Thus, Freeman (1985) notes that whereas traditionally defined stressors of poultry increase susceptibility to viruses they can *decrease* the risks on exposure to bacteria. An animal might be stressed by criteria of hormonal profile but no organ pathology yet identifiable. Conversely, the immune system might be compromised by various means not all of which we could usefully attribute the label 'stress'. Pathology is perhaps best seen as a guideline for the presence of stress in the context of knowing something about the kind of situations to which the animal has been exposed. Stress is a factor among many others that can bias towards pathology but it is wrong to assume necessarily a neat one-to-one relation between the two. Of a group of people exposed to the same stressful situation only a percentage will show signs of pathology (Weiner, 1992).

In applied ethology (Chapter 9), the concept of stress sometimes refers to warning signs of impending pathology that can trigger environmental intervention by humans. This leads Moberg (1985) to propose that: '. . . a prepathological state can be used as an indicator of stress and risk to the animal's well-being'.

For example, the immune system might be so suppressed or the animal's metabolism might have been so altered that normal growth is not possible. Moberg argues that stress research should take the direction of trying to define such prepathological states. However, Moberg (1985) argues that there is not a single biological response, such as secretion of corticosteroids, increased heart rate or a particular response that can provide an index of stress.

In animal husbandry, stress is of crucial economic value. A chronic elevation of corticosteroids is associated with depressed growth. This arises from the effect of corticosteroids on decreasing amino acid incorporation into body tissues and mobilization of energy reserves (Hemsworth and Barnett, 1987).

1.3   TOWARDS A THEORETICAL MODEL OF STRESS

1.3.1   Introduction

This section will attempt to provide a perspective that can offer hope of synthesis. The starting point of the discussion is the original adaptive function of those systems that appear to have excessive demands placed upon them in the stressed animal. In developing this perspective, it is necessary to discuss the emergence in evolution of emotion, motivation, learning, cognition and goal-directed behaviour. The possible criteria of stress described in Section 1.2 will be employed here but not in any exclusive sense. They will be considered as useful pointers within the framework developed.

The logic that will be developed is that stress is characterized by a stretching of CNS states to beyond their adaptive range of functioning. One assumes that the processes we observe to be underlying stress today have conferred a greater advantage than disadvantage during their evolutionary origins. However, in some species as observed today and particularly with domestication, the balance might have tipped to the side of these processes now being a net disadvantage. For example, the flight option is often not one available to a domestic animal yet it might be repeatedly placed in a situation for which, in evolutionary terms, flight would be the appropriate response. In order to develop such a logic, it will be necessary to consider the part that such states normally play in the control of behaviour, the evolutionary factors lying behind their emergence and a comparison between species in how behaviour is controlled. The states that are proposed are those described in such terms as motivation and affect. One useful starting point might be to consider briefly how things might have been otherwise: could one imagine an animal organized in such a way that such central states (having a capacity to be stressed) never evolved?

1.3.2   Hard and Soft Wiring

To put it metaphorically, evolution is presented with something of a dilemma between two possible solutions to the problem of how to organize behaviour. On the one hand, there is hard-wired, low-cost, reflexive processing whose locus of organization can be local and relatively peripheral, but which cannot offer flexibility. On the other hand, there are non-hard-wired processes that are centrally organized and offer flexibility but at a relatively high cost in terms of processing requirements (cf. Mayr, 1974; Epstein, 1982; Toates, 1994b, 1995a,b).

As a thought exercise, it is possible to envisage a very simple animal that consists of nothing more than a series of reflexes with mutual inhibition between them; although even here the need for negative feedback very soon becomes evident (Powers, 1973; Toates, 1994a). Excitation of one reflex might then simply inhibit what would normally be any mechanically incompatible reflexes. Such an animal would be drawn reflectively towards, say, sugar solutions and repelled reflexively by excessive heat. There would be a prescriptive solution to any problem. Such low-cost processing corresponds approximately (although not entirely; Toates, 1994a,b, 1995a,b) to the stimulus–response organization beloved of the early behaviourists (see Bolles, 1979). In such terms, the animal comes into the world with a series of largely preformed solutions (or 'procedures') that specify what to do.

Some will be fixed in strength, whereas learning would consist of a modification of the strength of other connections. In the words of Hirsh (1974), learning would be 'on the performance line'. Such is the simplest form of animal that one could imagine and it is doubtful whether anything, with the possible exception of the most basic invertebrates, corresponds closely to this.

Given such a basic design as a starting point (if only in the imagination of the theorist), it is clear that, to exploit a broader range of environments, there would be an advantage in performing processing that is at a locus somewhat removed from these links between input and output. For example, the wiring might soon get unwieldy if, as nervous system complexity increased, each afferent input, on triggering a response, still had responsibility for inhibiting any incompatible motor outputs. There would seem to be an advantage in a more central process of selective potentiation of reflexes that serve a given end-point and depotentiation of reflexes that do not serve it (Gallistel, 1980). In concert with such central behavioural control, endocrine systems that, by their actions on the physiology of the body, help the animal to meet the end-point can be excited or inhibited. For example, the endocrine profile of submission is rather different from that accompanying attack or copulation. Such systems are the focus of so much interest in the area of stress.

Invertebrates generally are relatively short-lived and, although there are some striking specialized exceptions, their opportunities for learning are somewhat limited. They tend to place more weight upon low-cost processing and have a relatively large prescribed set of reactions to deal with situations (Eisemann et al., 1984). However, there is evidence for more central processing even in invertebrates. For example, there is modulation of reflexes by processes outside the specific organization of the reflex itself, described by Harris-Warrick and Flamm (1986) as their 'sculpting'. There is evidence in invertebrates of the rudiments of the more complex systems seen in vertebrates. For example, a similar range of neuromodulators are involved in invertebrate reactions to aversive stimuli as are described in vertebrate stress reactions (Kavaliers, 1988, 1989). There is also evidence for functional co-ordination. For example, aversive stimuli induce opioid- and non-opioid-based analgesia in both invertebrates and vertebrates (Kavaliers, 1987).

Given the evolution of a facility to perform processing at a site removed from the more direct input–output links that exist, there would appear to be a strong pressure to elaborate this off-line processing. It will be argued here that such things as motivation, affect and cognition correspond to off-line processing and can only be understood in terms of an integrated package of processes that occupy a high level in a hierarchy of behavioural control (cf. Powers, 1973; Gallistel, 1980; Roitblat, 1991; Toates, 1994a,b, 1995a,b). By 'high' is meant relatively far from motor output. Lower levels get nearer to motor output, with the lowest level being individual motor neurons.

In such terms, flexibility is to be gained by storing information off the performance line, which can then be utilized according to circumstances. So given the 'dilemma' of evolution just described, what is the optimal design solution? This will depend upon species, environment, behaviour and experience. For invertebrates in a constant environment, with minimal interspecific social contact and a short life-span, cheap hard-wired processes might well suffice though they would probably need a facility for negative feedback. Vertebrates by contrast are relatively heavily off-line in their processing. Even for animals that employ more flexible systems, processing of information that can evoke a constant reaction from generation to generation can afford to be fairly hard-wired. Also it appears that even for behaviours initially organized in a more flexible way, with repetition of a given behaviour in a stable environment, more responsibility is devolved to the lower cost processes (Toates, 1994a,b, 1995a,b). This phenomenon is generally referred to as the automatization of behaviour (Kimble and Perlmuter, 1970) and for a number of reasons is relevant to the study of stress. There is evidence that behaviour initially carried out with emotion (e.g. shock avoidance) will, when highly accomplished as a result of repetition, be performed in a relatively emotionless way (Kimble and Perlmuter, 1970; Wiepkema, 1987; see Section 1.2.2.1).

The relation between the performance of behaviour in a flexible way and its subsequent performance in a more automatic way is a challenging one for theories of stress. It suggests that with repetition the animal is switching from a mode of control for which the notion of stress might be applied to a mode where stress is inappropriate. The hormonal indices suggest that this is a reasonable assumption (Section 1.2.2.1). However, it might be dangerous to assume simply that any animal showing evidence of 'autopilot control' is unstressed. Otherwise the logic would run counter to the common assumption that stereotypies are an index of stress (see Chapter 9). A possible resolution is that the behaviour that has become automatized is itself not associated with a stress reaction but other aspects of the environment might well be still stressful.

It is proposed here that flexibility comes at an inevitable cost and that is the possibility of stress. For fixed input–output connections, the notion of stress seems redundant. However, where processes of flexible strategy and choice are available, there is the possibility that the flexible strategies will fail over periods of time and that will be the index of stress as defined here. Flexible strategies require central monitors of their efficacy and the argument will be developed that stress represents a state of maladaptive stretching of these central processes.

1.3.3 Central States

The argument advanced here is that the evolution of soft-wired systems must be accompanied by that of central states. The advantage in evolving such central states is not difficult to appreciate from looking at some of the now rather well-worked out invertebrate examples (e.g. Walters *et al.*, 1981). For instance, in response to localized tissue damage, *Aplysia* takes some local actions: withdrawal of a particular body region and a release of mucus. However, there are also some reactions that are best described as 'central' in their locus of control and not specific to a particular site of stimulation. These include ink release, gill withdrawal and cardiovascular changes. This is suggestive of a central state that might be the precursor of something similar to pain and/or fear states in vertebrates. It would presumably be a parsimonious biological design to have tissue damage from whatever site or cues predictive of such damage stimulate a central state and then the central state influence each of these outputs (see Figure 1.2). The

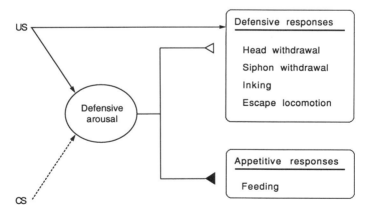

Figure 1.2. Model of the role of a central state. Note the potentiation of a set of functionally related reflexes and inhibition of another set. Note also the facility for classical conditioning to occur. US = unconditional stimulus; CS = conditional stimulus. (Reprinted from Walters *et al.*, *Science*, **211**, 504–506. Copyright 1981 American Association for the Advancement of Science)

cost of at least one extra synapse might well be offset by avoiding the extra neural machinery that would be involved in each site of skin stimulation making contact with each effector. Having such a central state provides the facility for conditioning (Walters *et al.*, 1981). Neutral stimuli paired with noxious stimuli can come to prime the system to respond more readily and strongly to the unconditional stimulus (UCS). They need not create a particular response themselves but just increase the efficacy of the UCS.

In *Aplysia*, food stimuli excite a group of what might be termed appetitive reflexes but depress a group of defensive reflexes (Hawkins and Advokat, 1977). Conversely, a noxious stimulus depresses the appetitive reflexes and excites the defensive. As the authors note, in constructing a diagram from arrows and boxes to represent the flow of information in the animal: '. . . boxes represent the traditional concept of motivational state, that is, intervening variables hypothesized to account for coincident variations in the strength of many related behaviours'.

1.3.4 Habituation and Associative Learning

The evolutionary advantage of being able to change behaviour in the light of experience is clear. Perhaps the simplest example is habituation and sensitization. But even here, with the wisdom of hindsight and looking at some real systems, as soon as we consider this issue, so that of central states should also concern us. For example, Groves and Thompson (1970) refer to a 'state' system that is off the direct stimulus–response (S–R) linkage but whose state plays a part in the magnitude of sensitization seen. A propensity to habituate to a repeated stimulus seems to need a safeguard mechanism to allow dishabituation at times when noxious or intense stimuli have been applied. In experiments on *Aplysia*, Castellucci *et al.* (1970) note that dishabituation can be produced by a strong stimulus applied to most parts of the animal's body surface. This suggests a common route by which the effects of a large number of such stimuli can be funnelled into a central state, which can then serve to dishabituate.

The common implicit assumption within accounts of this phenomenon is that habituation proceeds provided that nothing of 'particular significance' (Thompson, 1975) happens shortly after the stimulus is applied. If this is not the case, then dishabituation can be observed. But the notion of 'significance' would seem to imply some central state that serves as arbiter and frame of reference of the state of the world. One might suggest that this is the evolutionary precursor of a process of affect. In other words, there needs to be a monitor of the efficacy of action.

Associative learning enables the animal to exploit regularities in the environment and then change behaviour in response to environmental change. In terms of a basic design, learning might take the form of simple associations, for example, a stimulus regularly paired with excessive heat might come to evoke a withdrawal response, an S–R association. However, learning of the cognitive kind employing representations of the world (Dickinson, 1980) is, in the terms developed here, off-line. It implies a top-down control in a hierarchy.

1.3.5 Cognition

Despite some articulate objections from ethology's old-guard conservatives (e.g. Kennedy, 1992), in keeping with a number of authors, the argument will assume that animals show goal-direction, have cognitive capacities and that they construct cognitive representations of their environment which involve comparison between actual and expected states of the world (O'Keefe and Nadel, 1978; Toates, 1983; Ursin, 1988; Cabib and Puglisi-Allegra, 1990; Grossman, 1991). Animals are assumed to form predictions about the world, e.g. that one event predicts another (Dickinson, 1980). Based upon such a prediction the animal can take adaptive action, for example, a warning sound heralding a predator can be the cue to freeze. Animals also construct expectations about their actions, that behaving in a certain way yields a certain outcome (Bolles, 1972; Ursin, 1988). For example, an animal can learn that pressing a lever yields food or terminates a loud noise. Behaviour can usefully be described as goal-directed, meaning that it has some end-point towards which it is directed by flexible means (Toates, 1986, 1994a, 1995a). Cognition in the context of constructing expectations about the world allows the facility for the animal to react to what is expected but is *not* present in the world (Toates, 1995b). Specification of behaviour simply on the basis of stimuli present would not allow this facility. In the context of stress, this cognitive capacity is important in that processes of negative affect and emotion seem to be able to be stimulated by such expectations when they fail to be realized.

1.3.6 Pain: An Example to Illustrate the Argument

The value of a combination of both hard-wired local organization and the flexibility offered by a central monitor can perhaps be seen most clearly in the case of pain. Escape from tissue damage, whether real or incipient, can be organized to some extent at a local level in the form of a series of hard-wired protective withdrawal reflexes triggered by stimulation at each local site. This provides a rapid solution to a local noxious stimulus. However, there are serious limitations on what can be solved by such a mechanism. For a start, it cannot provide solutions for tissue damage arising internally, e.g. to be met by favouring a site of injury, rest and recuperation. It cannot provide the facility for creative solutions to the problem such as whole body contortions that minimize nociceptive input. It does not allow flexible pre-emptive action to avoid, for example, locations associated in the past with tissue damage. All of these advantages to survival require a central affect state such that the animal is motivated to act in a way that returns the level of this state to that associated with no tissue damage. Tissue damage, no matter where it arises, will trigger this central state and the state will play a part in any behaviour that corrects the state. The state will act as a frame of reference for learning and avoidance actions. For an example of the flexibility that central states offer, rats in arthritic pain learn to consume water containing analgesic substances (Colpaert et al., 1980).

The use of the example of pain can illuminate the present discussion and point to the (albeit tentative; Bateson, 1991) conclusion that insects do not experience pain and, by a logical extrapolation, are not usefully described as experiencing stress. Eisemann et al. (1984) pose the question—'Do insects feel pain?'. They note that insects which have suffered injury do not favour the injured limb by, for example, limping. Neither is there evidence that injury leads to a decline in feeding or mating tendency. Even severe injury or loss of whole body parts appears not to influence other aspects of behaviour. By contrast, reorganization of behaviour (e.g. suppression of appetitive behaviour) as a result of tissue damage or its threat is one of the powerful arguments for the existence of affective states in vertebrates (but see Bateson, 1991, for a caution). However, as noted earlier, some invertebrates (e.g. Aplysia) do show evidence of central states.

1.3.7 Positive Affect and the Organization of Behaviour

By a similar logic to that concerning negative affect, one needs to postulate positive affect systems. Such systems are presumably seen most clearly in the processes proposed to underlie vertebrate actions (Young, 1966; Berridge and Grill, 1984; Toates, 1986, 1988, 1995b; Berridge et al., 1989; Berridge and Valenstein, 1991; Cabanac, 1992).

Theorists postulate an affect process that monitors, say, the ingestion of nutrients. The role attributed to such a process is that of keeping the animal going on a consummatory task for as long as it is advantageous for it to do so. In its evolutionary origins, the triggering of such affect would be tuned to maintaining homeostatic balance. Affect can also serve as part of a memory of past encounters. Such a memory can then be recruited to play a part in current behaviour. For example, it is argued that the decision by *ad libitum* fed rats to traverse a very cold environment to feed on a tasty morsel (Cabanac and Johnson, 1983) is based in part upon a memory of the affect of past encounters with such tasty food. The relationship between affect and motivation is one of some controversy (Robinson and Berridge, 1993; Wise, 1994), but it might be argued logically that there are somewhat distinct (although doubtless interacting) affect and motivation processes within the CNS.

1.3.8 Bringing the Bits Together: The Application to Stress

A central assumption for developing the present model of stress is that motivation is to be seen as a process for co-ordination of the animal's actions in a given direction. This involves a goal direction, co-ordination of functionally related reflexes and the production of appropriate hormonal changes. Certain responses will be sensitized in the context of a certain motivational state; e.g. freezing in frightened rats under certain conditions (Fanselow and Lester, 1988) and lordosis in sexually receptive female rats (Pfaff, 1980). They will have a high probability of occurrence in this state. Presumably, it represents a good evolutionary design to specify by hard-wiring certain responses that can almost invariably be recruited in meeting an end-point. It can be argued that such organization involves relatively low cost (Toates, 1995a). Conversely, other aspects of behaviour reveal the flexibility that motivation allows; novel behaviour can be exhibited in meeting an end-point.

In such terms, just as motivation is revealed in a functionally coherent way, so might there be a pattern to the aberration of adaptive motivation/behaviour as revealed in stress. In the terms developed here, stress is something intrinsically related to the flexibility of behaviour involving central motivation and affect systems. On confrontation with a stressor, motivation can play an adaptive part in either active or passive strategies. In stress, there will be seen different packages of effects corresponding to failed active or passive strategies. The suggestion that will be developed here is that stress can be defined as a stretching of such processes of motivation, affect and flexibility to beyond their adaptive range. For instance, a perfectly adaptive process of fear with associated affect monitor can become distorted in a small environment under conditions of chronic crowding. Such a situation might lead to a chronic state of activation in a negative affect circuit. If the animal's reaction is one of passivity then something like human depression might be seen. Thus, animal welfare investigators might profitably look at the human condition of depression with its psychological and biochemical aspects (Willner, 1985) and extrapolate to non-humans. On the side of activity, fruitless attempts to gain mastery in a situation might similarly lead to extended and ultimately maladaptive triggering of negative affect circuitry. Such processes can only make sense in the context of understanding cognition, affect and motivation (Toates, 1994a,b, 1995a,b).

1.3.9   A Feedback Control Model of Stress

The analysis of stress presented here will emphasize the processes corresponding to aggressive and fear motivation, presumably their associated behaviours are those most closely linked to stress. However, other systems such as feeding and sexual motivation might also play a part in generating stress if they organize goal-directed behaviour that is frustrated for extended periods of time. The logic of this approach is the perspective that stress represents a stretching of adaptive mechanisms of coping with the world beyond a normal, non-pathological, range (Panksepp, 1990). Following this perspective, an understanding of stress will most likely not be achieved by looking for 'stress mechanisms' as such but rather by looking at the bases of the emotional responses associated with, for example, aggression and fear and how these bases perform under conditions termed stress.

Behaviour motivated by aggression and fear serves to protect the physical integrity of an animal, among other functions. When we come to try to explain the processes, there are a number of different explanatory languages that can be employed; one of these uses cognitive terms such as goal and expectation (Archer, 1988) and this will be the approach adopted here. Also in the terms developed earlier in this section, the behaviours seen in aggression and fear will be closely associated with central motivational and affect states. These states will potentiate functionally related sets of reflexes, guide goal pursuit and help monitor the efficacy of actions. These states will be richly influenced by conditional stimuli that in the past heralded events for which a fear or attack reaction was appropriate (e.g. Hollis, 1984).

In a comprehensive survey, Archer (1976, 1988) explains the basis of aggression and fear by considering the animal to incorporate *reference values* (sometimes termed *set-points*) on the state of the world. In an applied ethology context, Wiepkema (1987) employs a similar logic in using the term *Sollwert* for reference value. In such terms, consider the way that the animal's world actually is (termed *Istwert*), which might, or might not, correspond to the animal's reference values. If the actual state of the world departs significantly from the reference values, then there is a tendency for behaviour to be initiated in such a way as to move the state of the world or the animal's relationship to the world towards the reference values. One should not ignore the intrinsic problems with this approach and Archer does not attempt to ignore them. For instance, some intrusions (e.g. a rival animal or a particular configuration) will be particularly likely to trigger behaviour. The behaviours associated with fear and aggression are two such that are especially likely to be recruited. Positive emotion would be experienced in the event of an *Istwert* coming nearer to a *Sollwert*, whereas negative emotion would be experienced if the action moves them apart. In such terms, emotion can be seen as a monitor of the efficacy of actions (Simonov, 1986; Toates, 1988).

Take, for example, when an intruder enters an animal's territorial space. This could be described as causing a departure from the resident animal's reference values. Aggression is recruited and the animal acts in such a way as to drive the intruder out. Physiological changes occur: adrenaline is secreted into the bloodstream at a high rate, heart rate accelerates and blood vessels change diameter. When the intruder has left, the behavioural and physiological systems return to equilibrium. In the case of fear, rather than changing the external world, the animal changes its own relationship to the world. For example, it dives for cover and hence gets itself away from an intrusion.

In Wiepkema's model, a stress reaction is associated not only with disparity between *Sollwert* and *Istwert* but also with the animal's perception of the probability of being able to reduce the disparity (a similar logic being argued by Simonov, 1986). Thus, for example, in a protracted fight between two adult male rats over a 1 h period, both subsequent winner and loser showed drastic elevations of corticosteroid level for the first half (Schuurman, 1981). However, in the second half, the future winner showed a return towards normal levels of corticosteroids. This suggests that the perception of victory (in Wiepkema's terms, estimation of a high probability of correction of disparity) can also influence input to the corticosteroid system. In other words, a trigger to the corticosteroid system is based upon an *assessment* of the future probability of restoring equilibrium. Where uncertainty is involved (as in involvement in a fight with uncertain outcome) there is activation of corticosteroids. Where an outcome corresponding to elimination of disparity can be predicted, then there seems to be a suppression of activation. It will be argued that protracted disparity between *Sollwert* and *Istwert* necessarily involves uncertainty as to outcome and is synonymous with stress. Evidence will later be given of where cues for action are present but in an uncertain context and this triggers the corticosteroid system (Section 5.6).

A model involving *Sollwert* and *Istwert* is one of negative feedback, as illustrated in Figure 1.3. In a metaphorical sense, the term 'reference value' refers to how the animal's world 'should be'. To some, this raises profound philosophical issues but to others such issues can be answered by the assumption that motivational systems incorporating reference values have been shaped by evolution. Those animals that defended appropriate reference values survived to see another day and passed on their genes. Even noxious stimulation such as electric shock can to some extent be viewed in these terms. A way of closing the feedback loop (in other words, the possession of a coping strategy for terminating the shock; see later) will greatly affect the reaction of the so-called stress hormones. The physical stimulus is placed in a context that relates to control. The notion of control, the ability of an animal to exert agency over the world, will be a central one in the chapters that follow. It will be used in the sense that an animal having control can, by its action, affect the strength or duration of the potential stressors that impinge upon it. Although this is the sense adopted here, it is worth noting that the word control is used in a variety of senses in the literature and, taking all of them into account, its definition can prove as problematic as that of stress itself (Phillips, 1989).

In a similar vein to Archer (1979), I shall argue that the term 'stress' can be usefully employed to describe a state of brain and behaviour that arises from a failed effort over time of such negative feedback systems to bring their environment into alignment with their reference values. Control has failed. In an animal's evolutionary history, certain actions have tended to cause certain effects, specifically reference values have been attained. This represents the adaptive value of the motivational system and is illustrated in Figure 1.3. It will be argued that in the case of stress, action is initiated, but rather than restoring equilibrium, the action fails to have the consequence that it has served in its evolutionary origins. The action taken would normally be both behavioural and physiological (e.g. hormonal). In the language of feedback theory, stress consists in the negative feedback system going on to *open-loop* indicated by the dotted line in Figure 1.3d breaking the

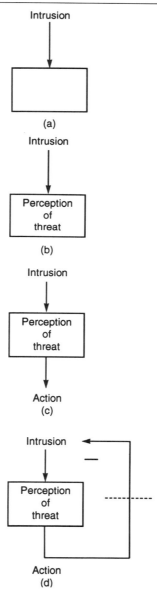

Figure 1.3. Representation of aggression and fear. (a) An intrusion occurs into the environment of an animal, (b) the animal perceives the intrusion as a threat (with assessment of abilities to effect action), (c) action consisting of behaviour and physiological activation occurs (which depends partly upon assessment) and (d) the action serves to correct the intrusion and return the system to the *status quo*. (Based upon Toates, 1992)

feedback loop (a similar line of reasoning is to be found in Ursin (1988) and in the Russian literature (Sudakov, 1980)).

The discussion so far has been moving towards a *systems view* of stress. By this term, I mean a view of the whole system of animal and environment. According to such a perspective, an animal has certain needs and goals (Toates, 1986; Ursin, 1988). Behaviour reflects its current needs, goals and knowledge of the environment, acquired in part through experience. Its physiological reactions will also depend upon this complex of information. Events in the environment impinge upon the animal's sense organs and some of these might be termed potential stressors. The animal will interpret these events in terms of their significance and the facility to effect action and might perform a response. This response might then change the animal's relation to the external world. In such terms, the adaptive significance of the behaviour and physiological changes can be understood. Both serve the same end: to maintain the integrity of the body (Archer, 1979). At a time of active behaviour (e.g. fight or flight), physiological changes provide the metabolism necessary for exertion. On the other hand, if a passive strategy is adopted, heart rate might be lowered (discussion in Chapter 6).

If the animal's attempts, whether active or passive, fail over a protracted period of time, it will be said to be in a *state of stress*. There will normally be elevated activation of corticosteroids but probably no other unambiguous physiological index of this state, as the physiology will reflect the nature of the failed attempts at control (cf. Shavit and Martin, 1987). For example, if the animal is trying an active strategy of attack or fleeing and is failing, the physiological state will probably be different from when it is unsuccessfully attempting to avoid aversive stimuli by freezing. However, the present approach will consider both to be examples of stress. (Thus there is no single intervening variable corresponding to stress that will make simple transformations from any input to any output.)

Failure to bring the world into alignment with reference values will be associated with activation of hormonal systems. As will be discussed in Chapter 5, the corticosteroid system will also be activated when the outcome of an action is less desirable than expected on the basis of past experience. For example, a rat that has been used to earning pellets of one kind in a Skinner box for lever-pressing will show corticosteroid activation if inferior pellets arrive.

Such a concept of stress ties the notion to a particular kind of malfunction. It is not synonymous with *any* challenge to homeostasis. Thus, as Fraser and Broom (1990, p. 261) point out: 'Slow growth could be due entirely to lack of food in an individual whose metabolic functioning was efficient. It adds little explanation to say that such a starved animal is under stress'. However, if the same low growth were due to an elevation of corticosteroids as a result of the animal being permanently in the vicinity of a dominant and aggressive conspecific, we would want to evoke the notion of stress. It would also make sense to evoke the notion of stress if the metabolic imbalance was caused by a protracted failure to get to food as a result of competition.

1.3.10 Coping

The term 'coping' is a commonly used but somewhat ambiguous one in the literature. In a similar approach to that developed here, Fraser and Broom (1990, p. 259) argue: 'When regulatory systems are operating but are not coping with environmental conditions then the word stress should be used'. Similarly, Archer (1979) defines stress as: '. . . the prolonged inability to remove a source of potential danger, leading to activation of systems for coping with danger beyond their range of maximal efficiency'.

It is sometimes asked whether a response enables the animal to cope with a stressor or whether the response is reinforcing (e.g. Mason, 1991). In some cases, coping and reinforcing can be defined such that these expressions are virtually synonymous. Thus, for example, if an animal can learn to terminate a loud sound by performing an instrumental response this is an unambiguous case of reinforcement. It could also be termed a coping response. In other situations, coping is used to mean a consequence that is beneficial in some way to the animal's physiology. The benefit might be in terms of reduced ulceration or corticosteroid levels. But the usage does not necessarily imply that a behaviour could be learned by means of the consequence being contingent upon the behaviour, the definition of reinforcement.

In some cases, coping is used in the sense that an animal might be said to be coping with dehydration by drinking, i.e. an alleviation of a physiological deviation from normal. A disturbance to homeostasis can be met by both extrinsic (e.g. drinking) and intrinsic (e.g. renal) controls. By analogy, some authors refer to intrinsic (hormonal) and extrinsic (behavioural) coping and argue that the extrinsic might be necessary if the intrinsic fails (e.g. Barnett *et al.*, 1985). The present model will attempt to give a rational account of what might be meant by coping.

The model of stress that will be developed is essentially based upon psychobiological principles and is intended primarily to produce a synthesis of the animal literature. However, it is entirely compatible with contemporary theories of human stress that address such things as cognitive demands and coping skills. For example, Bandura *et al.* (1988) refer to psychological stress as being: '. . . the result of a relational condition in which perceived environmental demands strain or exceed perceived coping capabilities in domains of personal import'.

1.3.11   Stress and Fitness

To try to gain some objective measure of whether an animal is coping, Fraser and Broom (1990) appeal to the ethological concept of *fitness*, expressed in terms of long-term reproductive capability (not to be confused with the lay health-related use of the term). The individual who is not coping is showing a reduction in fitness. Although the literal meaning of the word fitness, in terms of reproductive success, creates some anomalies if used in an applied setting (Jensen, 1995), none the less with some caution it might prove helpful. Thus, assuming all other things to be equal, an animal showing a chronically elevated level of secretion of corticosteroids will thereby have a reduction in fitness, e.g. growth will be stunted, the risk of infection or tumour development is greater and reproductive capacity is lowered. In such terms, Fraser and Broom define stress as: '. . . an environmental effect on an individual which over-taxes its control systems and reduces its fitness'.

This definition ties stress to detrimental effects; for example, a transient elevation of corticosteroids accompanying mating or seeing off a rival in a contest for a mate would not be seen as stress. In promoting their definition, Fraser and Broom (p. 259) sanitize the vocabulary, ruling out such dichotomies as 'good stress and bad stress or overstress and under-stress'. For example, one domestic environment can usefully be compared with another in terms of fitness. However, although it serves a vital role, the present author must boringly repeat the message: as with other indices, the concept of fitness must be used with some caution. For instance, simply, capturing a wild animal and placing it with conspecifics might increase its fitness by the factor that it might otherwise have been exposed to predation but this might not lower its stress level.

1.4   CONCLUDING REMARKS

A watertight definition of stress has not emerged from the hundreds of thousands of articles available on the subject in the scientific literature and it will probably not emerge here! However, it is to be hoped that what will be clarified are a number of different criteria of stress within which correlations to some degree can be seen. One possible definition is in terms of hormonal profile, most usually elevated activity in the HPA axis. However, this would bring under the definition of stressor a wide variety of very different stimuli some with positive connotations.

According to the analysis proposed here, four criteria of stress will be described: (1) a behavioural system is on open-loop for a considerable period of time; (2) there is normally excessive activity in a neurohormonal control system (either of the two systems, sympathetic catecholamine and corticosteroid or both, are normally what is discussed but the parasympathetic branch of the ANS is also a candidate and will be discussed later); (3) the animal is prone to classes of pathology (e.g. gastric ulceration, depression, hypertension); and (4) bizarre behaviour is shown (e.g. stereotypies). In some cases, we can say an animal is stressed according to all four criteria. In other cases, fewer than these four will be present. According to the argument proposed here, criterion (1) will always be evident whereas 2–4 commonly will be so. Hence, criterion 1 will be emphasized as the defining feature of stress, which will be seen as: (a) *a protracted failure of the animal to maintain alignment between its reference values and the actual state of the world* and (b) *the absence of an assessment of near-future realignment.* This will create a rather different demarcation from a definition that relies upon the HPA axis though there will be considerable overlap. Stress is something with a certain time course to it. For instance, over time there are increases in (1) hormonal levels, (2) frequency of stereotypies and (3) bodily indices of pathology. In later chapters, evidence will be presented that the trigger to the HPA system is the *perception of the probability that in the near future action will need to be taken.* If subsequent events allow such action to be taken with successful outcome, the HPA system is inhibited. Also if the animal can anticipate that the demands of the situation can soon be met there might be such inhibition. If not, and the challenge is interpreted as 'open-ended', the roots of stress are apparent.

In order to move towards a better theoretical perspective on stress and to justify the definition proposed, it will first be necessary to look at some of the neurophysiology, endocrinology and biochemistry of stress (Chapters 2 and 3). Chapter 4 looks briefly at the relevance of the immune system to discussions of stress. The term stress will be used to describe the state of protracted and ineffective recruitment of behavioural coping strategies. However, to understand the state of stress, the normal and effective functioning of these behavioural processes will first be examined. This will be the focus of Chapters 5 and 6.

We might have to live with not having a completely watertight definition of stress. We can strive to define stress as best we can while accepting this. To some extent, the lack of an absolutely precise definition does not matter too much; at the very least, the term 'stress' is a convenient chapter heading that brings a number of diverse phenomena together. The practical utility of this research, both in terms of human health and animal welfare, is beyond doubt and will be described later.

Chapter 2

Neuronal and Hormonal Controls

2.1 INTRODUCTION

Chapter 2 will begin to give synthesis between the theoretical ideas developed in Chapter 1 and data on the biological processes underlying stress. The focus here will be on the two principal neurohormonal axes involved in stress, introduced in Chapter 1. Chapter 3 will look at some of the neurochemistry that seems to be most relevant.

In states described as stress, characteristic changes in the activity of the nervous system and changes in the rate of release of hormones both centrally at the brain and in the periphery are seen. These neural and hormonal events are intimately connected; hormones influence, and are influenced by, the nervous system. Therefore, any division between the nervous system (neurophysiology of stress) and hormones (endocrinology of stress) is bound to be arbitrary. Indeed, a given substance can act within the central nervous system (CNS) as a neurotransmitter (Chapter 3) and more peripherally as a hormone (this chapter). Further interactions, between both these systems and the immune system, form the topic of Chapter 4. The neurophysiology and endocrinology of stress is a vast topic and it is impossible to cover it here. Chapters 2–4 can hope merely to describe some of the major pathways involved in stress. There are other pathways but space does not permit their inclusion. The reader wishing for a more detailed account should consult such references as Kuchel (1991) and Van de Kar et al. (1991).

A hormone is a chemical that is released into the bloodstream at one site and which exerts an influence at a more distant site. It is subsequently inactivated in some way, i.e. removed from the bloodstream. In some cases, a hormone will cause the release of a second hormone, which might in turn cause the release of a third hormone. Where such sequences of hormone actions occur, we sometimes refer to the sequence of effects as a *hormonal axis*. In a more general sense, whether dealing with neurons or hormones in a pathway, the term 'axis' can be employed to mean a sequence of causation in a specific pathway, A, B, C, etc. Activity at A affects activity at B which in turn affects C, and so on.

There are two axes that are most clearly implicated in stress. These are the *sympathetic–adrenal–medullary axis* (SAM) and the *hypothalamic–pituitary–adrenocortical axis (HPA)*. In emphasizing these two axes, the present study is taking the classical approach to stress. However, pursuing this line should not be allowed to detract from the fact that a wide range of different hormones are involved in stress (Weiner, 1992, p. 196). Also, as will be described later, the parasympathetic nervous system (PNS) plays an important part in stress.

As is implied by the names SAM and HPA, the adrenal gland forms part of both of these axes. In this context, often the term 'gland' is simply used in the singular, relating more to function than to specific anatomy. In fact, there are two such glands (see Figure 2.1). The adrenal glands are located at the kidneys and each is made up of two distinct components or 'endocrine organs': the *adrenal medulla* (forming part of the SAM axis) and the *adrenal cortex* (forming part of the HPA axis).

We shall need to describe each of the two axes. The first axis is dealt with in the broader context of the autonomic nervous system, of which it forms a part.

2.2 THE AUTONOMIC NERVOUS SYSTEM

2.2.1 General

The division of the nervous system having responsibility for control of the body's visceral functions (e.g. gut motility, arterial pressure) is known as the autonomic nervous system (ANS) (see Ganong, 1975; Guyton, 1991). As its name implies, it is a somewhat self-governing part of the nervous system in that, to some extent, it can carry on these functions even in the absence of outside influence, e.g. our conscious intervention. However, the ANS also receives inputs from regions of the CNS concerned primarily with decision making, motivation and emotion.

The ANS is composed of two branches: the sympathetic and parasympathetic; their fibres extend to the various organs (e.g. heart, adrenal gland) whose activity the system governs. The actions of the two branches are, in some respects, antagonistic to each other. Often

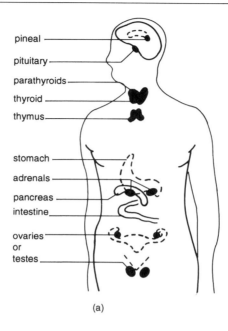

(a)

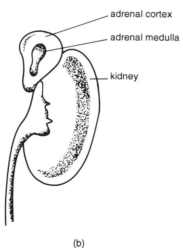

(b)

Figure 2.1. The adrenal glands (a) shown in relation to the rest of the body (Reproduced with permission from Gray, J.A. *The Psychology of Fear and Stress*. Cambridge University Press, 1987, p. 56, figure 5.2) and (b) a single gland showing adrenal medulla and cortex (Reproduced with permission from Archer, J. *Animals under Stress*. Edward Arnold. Copyright Williams & Wilkins 1979, figure 4.2b)

activity in one branch will excite a given organ, while activity in the other branch will inhibit it.

Consider the pathways of neurons that run from the brain to those organs that are controlled by the ANS. The neurons in part of both ANS branches employ acetylcholine as their transmitter substance, and these neurons are therefore described as *cholinergic*. However, the transmitter substance employed by those neurons that are at the end of the pathway outwards are perhaps of greatest interest in studying stress. Such neurons innervate the heart, gut, sweat glands, and so on. In the case of the parasympathetic branch, this transmitter is also acetylcholine. A few of such terminal neurons in the sympathetic branch also employ acetylcholine, for example, at the adrenal medulla (Forsyth, 1974). However, the vast majority employ noradrenaline, also termed 'norepinephrine', and are described by the adjective *noradrenergic*.

The difference in effect arising from activation of the sympathetic and parasympathetic branches is due, in important part, to the different properties of the two transmitter substances, acetylcholine and noradrenaline, considered in terms of their effects upon the end organs. For some purposes, one can speak of a parasympathetic effect and a cholinergic effect as being synonymous, as can one use sympathetic and noradrenergic to some extent synonymously. Also as a simplification, we shall speak in such global terms as 'sympathetic activation', although we need to remember that such an analysis can disguise local differences in sympathetic activity at particular targets in response to local demands (Weiner, 1992, p. 198).

2.2.2 Action of the Sympathetic Branch

The sympathetic branch of the ANS, usually known as the sympathetic nervous system (SNS), initiates a number of physiological changes that prepare the body for, as W. B. Cannon put it, 'fight or flight'. Typically, an event such as electric shock or confronting an animal with a rival would activate the SNS. As a result of its activity, cardiac output is increased. There is constriction of arterioles in the skin and gut, among other places, and as a result blood is diverted from the stomach and intestine to the muscles that are involved in escape (the 'voluntary muscles'). Cardiac activity, among other things, is increased and, at skeletal muscle, sympathetic activity causes vasodilation of arterioles (see Vander *et al.*, 1994, p. 436 for details; Veith, 1991).

Sympathetic activation is mediated via what are sometimes termed direct and indirect pathways. The direct pathway describes neurons that terminate on target organs and release noradrenaline. The indirect pathway refers to the release of adrenaline and noradrenaline from the adrenal medulla. These are carried in the bloodstream and broadcast generally to affect a variety of target organs. Again as a simplification, it is often useful to think of a global activation of the sympathetic system involving parallel release of adrenaline and noradrenaline. For our purposes, this will be the working assumption made here. However, at times, the mode of control departs from this (Weiner, 1992, p. 200), as will be discussed later. Also different local parts of the system can be activated individually according to local conditions (Veith, 1991).

One effect of adrenaline is to increase the supply of glucose to the muscles. This is achieved in part by a direct effect of adrenaline in increasing the rate of glucose production at the liver and thereby increasing the plasma glucose concentration (Taborsky and Porte, 1991). However, the more important means of stimulating glucose production is mediated via its effect on inhibiting the secretion of insulin and sensitizing the role of glucagon. Noradrenaline also plays a part in glucose production, mainly in its capacity as a local neurotransmitter at the terminals of sympathetic neurons supplying the liver (Taborsky and Porte, 1991). In rats, following the start of a fight, the effect of catecholamines in elevating carbohydrate metabolism is seen very rapidly (Haller, 1993).

In conditions described as fear or anger the whole of the SNS tends to be activated. Activation of the SNS causes release of noradrenaline at the nerve terminals which contact blood vessels and heart muscle etc. In addition to noradrenaline, a fraction of such noradrenergic neurons also contain and release another transmitter, known as neuropeptide Y (NPY) (Morley, 1989; Weiner, 1992, p. 240). NPY is released also at the adrenal medulla (described in Section 2.2.4). In the periphery, NPY serves the function of helping to constrict blood vessels.

Within the brain corticotrophin-releasing factor (CRF; see Chapter 3), acting as a neurotransmitter, plays a prominent part in activation of the sympathetic branch of the ANS. Intraventricular infusion of CRF is followed by a rise in plasma adrenaline and noradrenaline levels (Koob *et al.*, 1988).

2.2.3 Action of the Parasympathetic Branch

Traditionally, in the minds of scientists, whereas the sympathetic branch of the ANS was associated with activity and emotional arousal, the parasympathetic branch was felt to be associated more with quiescence and 'day-to-day living' (Ganong, 1975; Sapolsky, 1992). For instance, parasympathetic activity promotes the digestion and absorption of food from the alimentary tract. Saliva is secreted in the mouth. Acid, pepsinogen, mucus and gastrin are secreted by the stomach.

A reciprocal antagonism between the sympathetic and parasympathetic branches has been normally assumed (e.g. Sapolsky, 1994, p. 24). For example, whereas sympathetic stimulation increases the heart's pumping activity, parasympathetic activity decreases it. However, as Section 2.5 discusses, this rather simple view of antagonism between the two autonomic branches needs careful qualification. Intense emotion can sometimes be associated with parasympathetic activity (Vingerhoets, 1985), in addition to sympathetic activation. In states of extreme fear, diarrhoea, urinary incontinence and fainting can be observed, reactions which are manifestations of elevated parasympathetic activity (reviewed by Vingerhoets, 1985).

2.2.4   Control within the sympathetic–adrenal–medullary axis

2.2.4.1   Release of adrenal–medullary hormones

In response to activity in the SNS, the adrenal medulla secretes into the bloodstream hormones, *adrenaline* and, usually to a lesser extent, *noradrenaline*. Such activity can arise from confrontation with a stressor. However, other factors can also increase secretion of these hormones, e.g. hard physical exercise. Although situations that elevate one of these hormones usually elevate both, there is not invariably a unitary action of the SNS. Thus, whereas hard physical exercise is particularly effective in elevating noradrenaline levels, public speaking has a more dramatic effect upon adrenaline levels (Dimsdale and Moss, 1980). There is some suggestion in the literature that noradrenaline secretion is associated with goal-directed activities, in this context the fight aspect of fight or flight. In these terms, adrenaline is associated with both active fear responses and helplessness (see Henry, 1980). In most mammalian species, adrenaline is the major catecholamine produced by the adrenal medulla. In such a case, plasma noradrenaline level reflects activity in neurons of the sympathetic system whereas adrenaline is a reflection of adrenal medulla secretion. However, there are species differences and in some cases noradrenaline is the major adrenal catecholamine (Axelrod and Reisine, 1984).

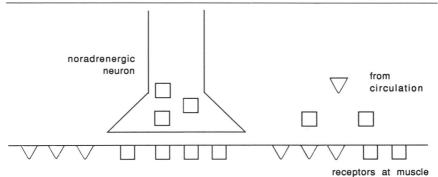

Figure 2.2. Action of sympathetic branch of the autonomic nervous system. Receptors receive noradrenaline (□) from noradrenergic neurons and adrenaline (∇) and noradrenaline of adrenal origin

2.2.4.2 Effects of adrenaline and noradrenaline

Noradrenaline and adrenaline released from the adrenal medulla can exert similar effects to that of adrenergic neural activity, often serving to reinforce to some extent that effect (see Ganong, 1975). They increase the frequency and strength of heart contractions, as well as dilating coronary blood vessels. Hence, activity on the part of the SNS can exert two complementary effects upon the organs that it innervates: (1) a direct neural effect of noradrenaline released from nerve terminals and (2) the hormonal effect of noradrenaline and adrenaline secreted by the adrenal medulla. This is shown in Figure 2.2.

Noradrenaline causes a constriction of blood vessels in a range of organs, and, conversely, adrenaline dilates the blood vessels of the skeletal muscles (Vander *et al.*, 1994, p. 436).

In addition to their capacity to elicit vasoconstriction or vasodilation (according to target vessel) and to reinforce the effects of neural activity, adrenal–medullary hormones help to mobilize free fatty acids and promote glycogenolysis in the liver and skeletal muscles. The state of high adrenaline level associated with a high concentration of fatty acids and a low insulin level is one in which there is a bias in favour of the brain as far as glucose availability is concerned (Smith, 1973). In this way, the effects of adrenomedullary secretions can be viewed in terms of an 'emergency function'.

2.2.5 Action of Both Branches

What has been termed the *doctrine of autonomic reciprocity* involves three related principles (Berntson *et al.* 1991). These are: (1) there is a

dual, sympathetic and parasympathetic, innervation of target organs;
(2) there is a functional antagonism between the branches; and (3) there
is a reciprocal control in that excitation of one branch is associated with
inhibition of the other branch. In this view, control would shift between
dominance of the sympathetic, through neutrality to dominance of the
parasympathetic. As was suggested in Section 2.2.3, the assumption of
an invariable reciprocal control is not always an accurate one, although
the ANS might well usually act in this mode (Berntson *et al.*, 1991).
Thus, parallel sympathetic and parasympathetic activation can sometimes be seen, for example in association with feeding (Steffens *et al.*,
1986). As another example, intense fear can induce a sympathetically
mediated increased heart rate and blood pressure accompanied by parasympathetically mediated bowel and bladder emptying. At even a single
organ (e.g. the heart), a conditioned stimulus paired with shock can
acquire the ability to trigger both sympathetic and parasympathetic
reactions (see Berntson *et al.*, 1991).

When a rat is confronted by a rival and is putting into effect a fight or
flight reaction, the sympathetic activity tends to be dominant. However,
confronted by a caged rival, for which immobility is the response, increased sympathetic activity but a *decrease* in heart rate is sometimes
seen (Bohus *et al.*, 1987b). Forced immobilization is associated with both
sympathetic and parasympathetic activation (Henry *et al.*, 1986). In a
variety of situations of inactivity, sympathetic excitation of the heart
appears to be cancelled by a parallel parasympathetically mediated inhibition, such that cardiac deceleration is seen (Obrist *et al.*, 1974b).

Two distinct pathways have been located in the hypothalamus of
rabbits, whose electrical stimulation elicits, respectively: (1) hind-limb
thumping, increased heart rate and blood pressure or (2) tonic immobility, raising of the ears, increased blood pressure accompanied by a
decrease in heart rate (Schneiderman and McCabe, 1985). Pattern 1
was described as the 'active coping (defense reaction)' and pattern 2 as
the 'vigilance (attentional)' pattern. A similar distinction in cardiac
performance was described in humans, comparing situations in which
active coping or passive coping (involving increased vigilance) occurs.

2.3 THE HYPOTHALAMIC–PITUITARY–ADRENOCORTICAL AXIS

2.3.1 Introduction

At the adrenal cortex, a group of hormones alternatively known as
corticosteroids or *glucocorticoids* is synthesized, stored and released.

In the blood, they exist bound to proteins (Daughaday, 1967). Their concentration in the blood depends upon the difference between their rate of release and rate of inactivation (Yates and Urquhart, 1962). There are various hormones under the general heading of cortico-steroids and in this respect there are some important species differences. In rats, the major corticosteroid is corticosterone (Bohus and de Kloet, 1981). In humans, it is cortisol (Baxter and Rousseau, 1979). The following section is concerned with the factors that cause the release of this hormone group.

2.3.2 Control of Secretion of Corticosteroids

2.3.2.1 The input side: stressors

The HPA axis starts within the CNS, at the hypothalamus, which is a crucial focus for stress. However, factors beyond the axis impinge upon the hypothalamus and thereby affect activity in the axis. Impulses from various parts of the body are relayed by means of the central, peripheral and autonomic nervous systems to the hypothalamus, which serves as a common path for their influence upon the HPA axis. In this way, the hypothalamus is a transducer between neural impulses and hormonal secretion (Allen et al., 1973). It might be useful to consider a background or 'tonic' influence of the CNS upon this axis (Mason, 1972). Events can then either exert excitation or inhibition relative to this level.

In the paraventricular nuclei of the hypothalamus (PVN), the cell bodies of neurons that synthesize and release *corticotrophin-releasing hormone (CRH)* (often termed *corticotrophin-releasing factor; CRF*) are located (Dallman et al., 1987; see also Figure 2.3). These CRF-containing neurons secrete their contents into small blood vessels, known as hypothalamic–hypophyseal portal vessels. In these vessels, CRF is carried the short distance to the anterior pituitary where it has its effect as part of the HPA axis. Excitatory neurons that impinge upon the CRF-containing neurons cause them to release their contents. Such neurons are activated by stressors.

Although CRF plays the principal role at the level of the HPA axis (Ritchie and Nemeroff, 1991), other hormones (or, as some might prefer to term them, neuromodulators) are also implicated. The PVN contains neurons that synthesize and release, for example, oxytocin, arginine vasopressin (AVP) and vasoactive intestinal peptide (VIP; Plotsky, 1988; Herman et al., 1989; Ritchie and Nemeroff, 1991) (see also Figure 2.4). Some neurons that synthesize CRF also synthesize

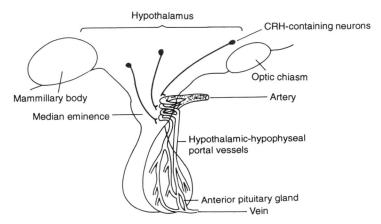

Figure 2.3. The hypothalamus and pituitary showing the vessels that transport corticotrophin-releasing factor from hypothalamus to pituitary. (Source: Guyton, 1991 with permission)

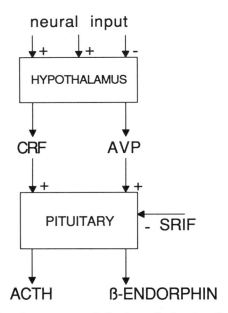

Figure 2.4. The first stages of the hypothalamic–pituitary–adrenocortical axis. The CNS acts as a transducer between external events and neurosecretory cells in the hypothalamus. Neural input excites (+) the release of corticotrophin-releasing factor (CRF) and arginine vasopressin (AVP). Note also inhibitory inputs (−). CRF and AVP then activate the release of adrenocorticotrophic hormone and β-endorphin from the pituitary

and release vasopressin (reviewed by Krishnan *et al.*, 1991). VIP might also play a part. Release of these hormones is influenced by both excitatory (shown in Figure 2.4) and inhibitory neurotransmitters. Also oxytocin secretory cells are found at this level and appear to play a part, albeit somewhat unclear one, in the reaction to a stressor (Sawchenko, 1991; reviewed by Krishnan *et al.*, 1991).

Following their release, the hormones CRF and AVP are then carried by the hypothalamic–hypophyseal portal vessels to the anterior pituitary. In response to such excitatory hormones, the pituitary gland secretes a hormone into the blood, known as *adrenocorticotrophic hormone* often abbreviated as ACTH (sometimes termed adrenocorticotrophin or simply corticotrophin). CRF and AVP have a synergistic effect upon the release of ACTH (Herman *et al.*, 1989; Dunn and Berridge, 1990; Sawchenko, 1991). Figure 2.4 includes the possibility that somatostatin (SRIF) can inhibit the release of ACTH.

The details of biochemical conversions are relevant to the study of stress. ACTH is formed from a precursor substance known as proopiomelanocortin (POMC). The cleavage of POMC yields not only ACTH but such substances as *N*-pro-opiomelanocortin (N-POMC) and β-endorphin (see Charlton and Ferrier, 1989 for a review). These probably also play a significant part in the state of stress. There also appears to be a negative feedback effect of endogenous opioids on the HPA axis. In one study on rats, the opioid blocker naloxone triggered an increase in ACTH and corticosterone levels (see McCubbin, 1993).

ACTH exerts its effect at a distant site, the cortex (outer layer) of the adrenal gland, known as the adrenal cortex. The effect at the adrenal cortex is one of promoting the synthesis and secretion of corticosteroids. The extent to which the adrenal cortex depends upon ACTH in order to secrete corticosteroids varies with species. Mammals depend upon the presence of ACTH more than do birds (Siegel, 1980).

Although the hypothalamus is a principal focus of interest in the study of the neural mechanisms underlying release of hormones of the pituitary–adrenocortical axis, other neural structures are also important in their influence on the hypothalamus. The hippocampus is one such site of prime interest. Removal of the hippocampus is followed by a hypersecretion of corticosteroids, caused by increased secretion of ACTH (Herman *et al.*, 1989). Conversely, stimulation of the hippocampus causes a reduction of corticosteroid levels. Such results led Herman *et al.* (1989) to the hypothesis that '. . . the hippocampus plays a role in tonic neuronal inhibition of the HPA axis'. Though the net effect on the axis of the hippocampus input is generally thought to be inhibitory, under certain conditions it might exert an excitatory role (McEwen *et al.*, 1986).

2.3.2.2   Neural and systemic stressors

A distinction is sometimes drawn between what are termed *neural stressors* and *systemic stressors* (Fortier, 1966; Allen *et al.*, 1973; Palkovits, 1987). The distinction is based upon the presumed route by which activation of the pituitary occurs. An example of a neural stressor would be confrontation with a predator, whose ability to activate the pituitary depends upon processing of information within the nervous system. Such a stressor is sometimes also termed a *cognitive stressor*, indicating the kind of level of presumed CNS processing involved. One mode of action of neural stressors is as follows. Consider, for example, surgery or a broken limb. Information is carried in neural pathways to the hypothalamus and the integrity of these pathways (e.g. spinal cord) is necessary for obtaining a response by ACTH.

By contrast, a systemic stressor is one assumed to act via the systemic circulation, not involving the nervous system. Certain metabolic disturbances seem to fall into this category, as do toxic agents (Allen *et al.*, 1973; Palkovits, 1987; Turnbull *et al.*, 1994). To establish that a particular stressor is systemic rather than neural, some researchers have studied the pituitary surgically isolated from the hypothalamus (Fortier, 1966).

2.3.2.3   Extrapituitary factors

Although the best documented account of the release of corticosteroids is that via the HPA axis, in recent years there has been a recognition that other factors can also be implicated. In some cases, a rise in plasma cortisol level cannot be accounted for by a preceding activity of ACTH (Fehm and Born, 1989). The nature of the process underlying this release is not entirely clear but there is evidence for sympathetic activation of the adrenal cortex and for a cascade involving interleukin-1 (see also Chapter 4) and interleukin-6 exerting direct effects on the adrenals (Turnbull *et al.*, 1994).

2.3.2.4   The circadian rhythm

In humans, under basal conditions, there is not a continuous mode of operation of the HPA system (reviewed by Carroll and Mendels, 1976; Dallman *et al.*, 1987). Rather, it shows a circadian rhythm of activity. Furthermore, its activity comes in bursts or 'episodes'. In the periods between such bursts, the system is quiescent. In humans, cortisol secretion occurs for only some 6 h each day, most of this being concentrated into the period around waking. The long quiescent periods arise because the brain is exerting an inhibitory influence upon the HPA axis. The rhythmic changes in the basal level of activity in the system appear to arise as a result of the influence of an input from the suprachiasmatic nuclei of the hypothalamus to the PVN.

Figure 2.5 shows the circadian rhythm of ACTH and corticosterone in rats (Dallman *et al.*, 1987). Note that the corticosterone rhythm is more pronounced than that of ACTH. At any time throughout the circadian cycle, the effect of stressors is superimposed upon this basal level of activity. As a rough guide, in both dogs and rats, plasma ACTH ranges from about 30 pg/ml in the lowest point in the cycle under basal conditions to about 1000 pg/ml when the animal is maximally stressed.

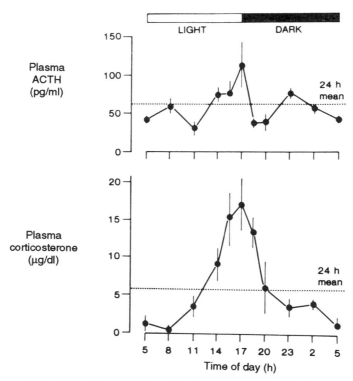

Figure 2.5. Circadian rhythm of adrenocorticotrophic hormone and corticosterone in young male rats. Mean values over 24 h (......). (Reproduced with permission from Dallman *et al.*, 1987, figure 2, p. 130)

In rats maintained on a 12 h light/12 h dark cycle, corticosteroid level normally peaks just before the onset of the rat's active period, the dark (Johnson and Levine, 1973; Krieger, 1974). The phase of this rhythm can be shifted by making food available at specific times in the light–dark cycle (see Section 5.11.1).

2.3.2.5 Receptors for corticosteroids and feedback

At various sites throughout the body, in the CNS and elsewhere, there are receptors for corticosteroids. There is evidence for feedback inhibition on HPA activity exerted by corticosteroid receptors at the pituitary, at the level of the CRF-secreting neurons and other sites in the brain (Keller-Wood and Dallman, 1984; Dallman *et al.*, 1987). At the pituitary, corticosteroids are apparently able to inhibit both the synthesis and release of ACTH (Axelrod and Reisine, 1984). Removal of the negative feedback effect of corticosteroids, by means of adrenalectomy, is associated with activation of CRF and ACTH. Translating the HPA axis into the terms of control theory (Toates, 1975; Cabanac and Russek, 1982), the excitatory input corresponds to some extent to the set-point of the system and plasma corticosteroid level to the regulated (some would say, controlled) variable or output (Yates and Urquhart, 1962). The set-point is not fixed but can be raised, e.g. as a result of stressors.

A large population of corticosteroid receptors has been identified in the hippocampus, and this has led Herman *et al.* (1989) to argue that this is a site for corticosteroid negative feedback upon the HPA axis. Compared with other brain regions, in rats the hippocampus has a particular affinity for corticosterone (McEwen *et al.*, 1986). It shows much less affinity for other corticosteroids (e.g. cortisol and dexamethasone). Depending upon the author in question, there are various conceptual schemes for classifying corticosteroid receptors. According to McEwen and Brinton (1987), there seem to be two populations of receptors which they term corticosterone and glucocorticoid receptors. The corticosterone receptors have a selective affinity for corticosterone whereas the glucocorticoid receptors have a broader affinity, which includes synthetic corticosteroids such as dexamethasone. The corticosterone receptors are particularly dense in the hippocampus whereas the glucocorticoid receptors are distributed more broadly, e.g. hypothalamus, pituitary and kidney.

Rosenfeld *et al.* (1993) describe intracellular receptors for glucocorticoids. Their distribution in the brain defines the target regions for glucocorticoids. They are also assumed to form the basis of the developmental effects of corticosteroids, upon cellular differentiation and other processes. Thus the level of neonatal exposure to corticosteroids affects the subsequent CNS processes underlying the HPA system. In the classification system of Rosenfeld *et al.*, there are two populations of such intracellular receptors: (1) 'type 1', 'mineralocorticoid receptors' (MRs) and (2) 'type 2', 'glucocorticoid receptors' (GRs). The latter type shows the highest concentration in brain regions traditionally most closely associated with the stress response, e.g. hippocampus and locus coeruleus. The evidence suggests that MRs are responsible for regulation of the basal level of activity of the HPA system. There is also some suggestion that they are implicated in circadian rhythms within the HPA system. GRs seem to be primarily involved in the feedback effect accompanying the stress reaction of the organism (see also McEwen *et al.*, 1991; Oitzel and de Kloet, 1992).

Figure 2.6 shows how, involving such receptors, negative feedback loops exist between plasma corticosteroid concentration and the

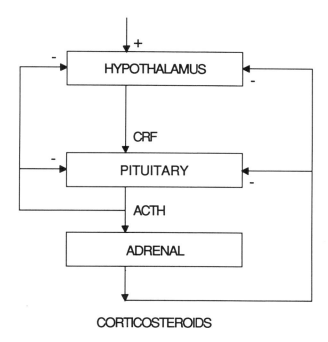

Figure 2.6. Negative feedback effects of corticosteroids at both the hypothalamic and pituitary levels. CRF = corticotrophin-releasing factor; ACTH = adrenocorticotrophic hormone

secretion of ACTH; acting both directly and via CRF, rising levels of corticosteroids tend to inhibit the secretion of ACTH (Yates and Urquhart, 1962; Ritchie and Nemeroff, 1991).

The net output of ACTH depends upon the difference between the excitatory afferent input and the inhibitory feedback effect arising from the detection of plasma corticosteroids, among other possible factors (Motta *et al.*, 1970). There is also evidence for a 'short' negative feedback loop from ACTH level in the blood to its own secretion rate (Motta *et al.*, 1969). However, the efficacy of such feedback in inhibiting the ACTH response to a stressor depends upon the exact nature of the stressor. The site at which the receptors mediating this short feedback are located seems to be mainly at the brain, particularly the hypothalamus, although the pituitary plays some part (Motta *et al.*, 1969). Evidence suggests that some of the negative feedback effect is mediated via inhibition upon CRF secretion.

The characteristics of the HPA feedback system are such that, following corticosterone infusion, there is evidence for two different phases of suppression (de Kloet and Veldhuis, 1985; Ritchie and Nemeroff, 1991). The first (dynamic) phase is evident in the first few minutes. This phase is sensitive to the *rate of change* of corticosterone level and is short-lived. It acts at the level of the pituitary and appears not to involve neural mediation (Ritchie and Nemeroff, 1991). The second phase is more slowly exerted and is relatively long-lasting. It seems to be mediated via the hippocampus and hypothalamus (Ritchie and Nemeroff, 1991). The mechanisms underlying the phases can be distinguished by the agonists that are effective in producing a feedback signal. The only agonists found to be effective for the fast feedback are cortisol and corticosterone. The other natural and synthetic corticosteroids are not effective. However, they are effective in exerting a role in the long-term negative feedback pathway.

The inhibitory effect of the intravenous application of dexamethasone on corticosteroid levels is only seen some 45–90 min after injection (Smelik and Papikonomou, 1973). What accounts for the lag? It is not penetration of receptor cells nor is it conversion of the injected substance into another form. The lag suggests that inhibition is at the level of the synthesis of CRF or ACTH or both. There are reports that, following adrenalectomy, ACTH level in the blood takes a matter of days to rise to its maximum value (Smelik, 1970).

Injection of the synthetic corticosteroid, dexamethasone, exerts a powerful inhibition upon ACTH secretion by the pituitary, both at its resting level and at a stress-induced elevated level (McEwen, 1979). Evidence suggests that the site of this inhibition is at the pituitary itself

(McEwen *et al.*, 1986). Treatment of rats with corticosteroids can prevent the rise in secretion of CRH and AVP which normally follows stressor application (see discussion in Dallman *et al.*, 1987). However, application of dexamethasone is better able to inhibit the corticosterone response to some stressors (e.g. ether, electric shock) than it is to others (e.g. haemorrhage) (Yates, 1967). Inhibition of corticosterone secretion is seen at up to 72 h of fasting but not at 96 h (Mitev *et al.*, 1993). This leads to the concept of stressors exerting their effect upon CRF secretion by either corticosterone-sensitive or corticosterone-insensitive pathways.

The relationship between plasma corticosteroid level and receptor density is a dynamic one. Expressed in control theory terms (Stewart, 1991, p. 79), not only does the regulated variable (corticosteroid level) change over time but also the parameters of the control system change. On the basis of the hippocampus having a role in mediating negative feedback from corticosteroids, Sapolsky *et al.* (1984) postulated that a decreased number of corticosteroid receptors at this site might be associated with activation of the HPA axis. Regarding this negative relationship between hormone level and receptor density, the HPA system is peculiar among hormonal control systems (McEwen *et al.*, 1986). In rats, the elevation of corticosterone associated with the stress of handling and social crowding can lead to a reduced number of steroid receptors in the brain, particularly the hippocampus (McEwen *et al.*, 1986). There is an increase in the receptor number following adrenalectomy. Aged rats show a decreased number of such receptors and do indeed show, relative to younger animals, a continuing HPA response to a stressor that is delayed after stressor offset. Elevated corticosteroids lead to a decreased receptor population, leading to increased corticosteroids, and so the system has the potential of forming a positive feedback loop. Excessive levels of corticosteroids can also exert a destructive effect upon neural tissue (McEwen *et al.*, 1986). To what extent such a situation prevails in certain pathological states, e.g. Alzheimer's disease, is one of urgent investigation (Deshmukh and Deshmukh, 1990).

Sometimes in a chronic stress situation, a decrease in ACTH secretion is seen while the level of corticosteroids is maintained. This might be due to increased efficiency of synthesis and release of corticosteroids for a given level of ACTH secretion (Endröczi, 1972), in control theory language an increase of gain in a component of a negative feedback system (Toates, 1975). Alternatively, or in addition, it might reflect an input to the adrenal outside the HPA axis (see earlier discussion in this chapter).

The notion of negative feedback is important in understanding an abnormality of the HPA axis termed Cushing's syndrome. This is characterized by excessively high levels of corticosteroid release from the adrenals (Liddle, 1967). The initial cause of this might either be due, primarily, to excessive secretion of corticosteroids or the high corticosteroid level might be an effect of elevated ACTH secretion. In the former case, ACTH level will be suppressed.

As briefly noted earlier in this section, there are developmental effects on the brain exerted by corticosteroids and acting upon corticosteroid receptors. Thus, the binding capacity of GRs in the adult brain depends in part upon early experience, e.g. whether the animal has been handled or not. This should alert us to the possibility of effects of early experience on the subsequent development of stress reactions (Rosenfeld *et al.*, 1993). There is evidence that in adult animals the capacity to switch off HPA activation following stressor termination is importantly influenced by early experience, as mediated via the population of hippocampal GRs. Rats handled shortly after birth tend, when adult, to show less fearfulness in a novel environment, a lower activation of glucocorticoids and a faster return to baseline (Meaney *et al.*, 1993). Meany *et al.* suggest that 'these findings represent a biological basis for individual differences in "responsivity" to stress'.

2.3.3 Loss of Corticosteroids

Corticosteroids are removed automatically from the circulation, such that a constant level in the blood implies that secretion rate and loss rate are equal. Cortisol has a plasma half-life of about 60 min (Baxter and Rousseau, 1979). Various tissues metabolize cortisol to the extent that only some 2% of that secreted appears in the urine. An artificial corticosteroid, dexamethasone, which is a useful endocrinological tool discussed at various points in the present study, has a much longer half-life than cortisol (Baxter and Rousseau, 1979).

2.3.4 Effects of Corticosteroids

2.3.4.1 Carbohydrate metabolism

The alternative name 'glucocorticoids' given to corticosteroids provides a clue as to what is their most widely recognized function: it means 'hormones derived from the cortex of the adrenal gland and having to do with the metabolism of glucose'. This distinguishes them from the 'mineralocorticoids', hormones similarly secreted from the adrenal cortex but which regulate mineral balance (e.g. salt loss through the kidney).

The term 'gluconeogenesis' refers to the synthesis of glucose and glycogen from non-carbohydrate precursors (Exton, 1979). A substrate for gluconeogenesis is termed a gluconeogenic substance. One of the effects of corticosteroids is to stimulate gluconeogenesis (see Guyton, 1971; Baxter and Rousseau, 1979). Among other hormonal contributions to gluconeogenesis, two sites need to be considered: (1) directly at the liver and (2) more indirectly at sites peripheral to the liver by controlling the availability of gluconeogenic substances. This occurs at sites such as muscle and fat. Part of the effect of glucocorticoids is to increase the net release of amino acids from peripheral tissues (Exton, 1979), increasing plasma amino acid concentration. Glucocorticoids promote the deposition of glycogen in the liver (Stalmans and Laloux, 1979). Corticosteroids also have the effect of stimulating breakdown of fats (termed lipolysis), which increases plasma free fatty acid concentration to deliver metabolizable fuels (Fain, 1979; Dunn and Kramarcy, 1984). Some tissues (liver, brain, heart and red blood cells) are not subject to the catabolic effects of corticosteroids (de Kloet and Veldhuis, 1985).

Corticosteroids lower glucose transport into cells (e.g. Becker, 1992), specifically at fat, skin, muscle and lymphoid tissue (de Kloet and Veldhuis, 1985). Corticosteroids also inhibit the production of insulin (Weiner, 1992, p. 207). (However, there is also one report of no overall decrease in glucose utilization as a result of corticosteroid action; Ashmore and Morgan, 1967.) Both the increased gluconeogenesis and any decreased uptake of glucose would have the effect of increasing plasma glucose. Adrenalectomy is followed by a fall in blood glucose level (Baxter and Rousseau, 1979). The role of corticosteroids is invariably assumed to be that of providing readily metabolizable fuel. Yet, apparently, utilization of that fuel is inhibited. Similarly, adrenaline both inhibits insulin secretion and antagonizes insulin-dependent uptake of glucose by skeletal muscle (Taborsky and Porte, 1991). For the newcomer to this daunting territory, there is something of a paradox here. Just when the body is preparing for action, hormonal events are triggered that serve to decrease glucose uptake by cells. However, there is, at least in part, a logical resolution. Although the uptake is in general decreased, there are special local processes to ensure that the specific muscles that require large amounts of nutrients obtain them (Sapolsky, 1994, p. 63). Corticosteroids both make glucose available and slow its metabolism, thus keeping significant amounts in reserve in the bloodstream. De Kloet and Veldhuis (1985) report that the effect of an elevation in corticosteroid level is to increase glucose supply to the liver, brain, heart and red blood cells. However, Becker (1992) reports a 20–30% inhibition of glucose uptake of neural tissues as a result of corticosteroid action. Similarly, Sapolsky (1991) describes a decrease in glucose utilization in the hippocampus as a result of the action of glucocorticoids, an effect which might be implicated in the toxic effects of excessive corticosteroid levels (see Chapter 10).

Corticosteroids serve a number of other functions which Arthur (1987) subsumes under the heading of suppressing 'the less important ongoing activity', such as suppressing growth, sleep and reproduction. By these actions, glucose, amino acids and free fatty acids are made available as a source of energy. However, the emergency function should be seen in context; even under resting conditions a basal level of corticosteroid secretion is necessary for normal metabolism.

Perhaps most commonly corticosteroids best serve their physiological role in *preparation* for action, that is in the inactive time prior to action (Arthur, 1987). Thus they promote the availability of glucose to the blood but also tend to conserve it. Arthur concludes that: 'Corticosteroids appear to do their work during anticipation, not during confrontation with stressors'. Arthur reviews evidence showing that in general cortisol levels do not increase during exercise. Further evidence in the same direction is afforded by looking at circadian rhythms. In humans, the highest levels of cortisol are observed in the hours prior to rising and they then decline throughout the day. Arthur argues that if corticosteroids served their primary function during confrontation with stressors one might expect the highest levels during active periods of the day.

There is evidence that high levels of cortisol improve the ability of cells to produce energy anaerobically (Mason, 1972). This could prove crucial at times of maximum exertion.

2.3.4.2 General metabolic effects

Although the effects of corticosteroids on carbohydrate metabolism are the most widely recognized, there is evidence for a wide variety of effects of these hormones, a role that can perhaps best be termed as 'biological amplifiers' of metabolic processes (Granner, 1979). In this capacity, they have very general effects that are evident in most, if not all, bodily organs. For example, sex hormones exert an effect on Leydig cells and catecholamines play a part in cardiovascular function, effects that are amplified by corticosteroids.

2.3.4.3 Inhibition of processes

Traditionally, the various roles of corticosteroids were seen to have in common that they protect the integrity of the organism against the effect of stressors (see Munck *et al.*, 1984 for review). In time, anomalies to this generalization were noted. For example, corticosteroids were found to have an *anti*-inflamatory action and to suppress the immune system (see Chapter 4). These effects were often explained away in terms of a *pharmacological* rather than any natural physiological role. However, in an influential review, Munck *et al.* (1984) attempted a more general and unifying functional account of the role of corticosteroids. They marshalled evidence that, at a variety of sites and involving various processes, the natural physiological role of corticosteroids is one of mediating *negative feedback*. That is to say, they *switch off* several of the body's defence mechanisms. A stressor induces, for example, inflammation, and corticosteroids inhibit this process. Thus, the production or action of a number of substances known to be mediators of inflammation are inhibited by corticosteroids. Munck *et al.* argue that the role of the corticosteroids is to protect the body against overactivity of its natural defences. There is a delay between application of a stressor and maximum corticosteroid response, during which the defence mechanisms can exert their maximum effect. Similarly, in the terms of Munck *et al.*, the antagonism between the effects of insulin and corticosteroids is to be understood as protecting the body against excessive hypoglycaemia.

Corticosteroids also exert effects upon a number of behavioural systems. One of the better known is the hormonal axis representing the so-called sex hormones. For example, cortisol inhibits production of gonadotrophin-releasing hormone (GnRH), leuteinizing hormone (LH), oestradiol and testosterone. In Cushing's disease, characterized by excessive secretion of cortisol, there is a suppression of both reproductive function and a diminution of libido for both men and women (reviewed by Rabin *et al.*, 1988).

2.4 INTERACTIONS BETWEEN THE SYMPATHETIC NERVOUS SYSTEM AND HYPOTHALAMIC–PITUITARY–ADRENOCORTICAL AXES

This section briefly discusses some of the interactions between these axes; more will be discussed later in the context of the behavioural evidence that reveals them. The SAM and pituitary–adrenocortical axes show interactions at all levels (Harvey *et al.*, 1984). At the input side to the system, at the level of the hypothalamus, there are neural pathways that have inputs to both the HPA axis and to the SNS (Sawchenko, 1991). Cooperation between adrenocortical and adrenomedullary hormones is implicated in the maintenance of blood sugar

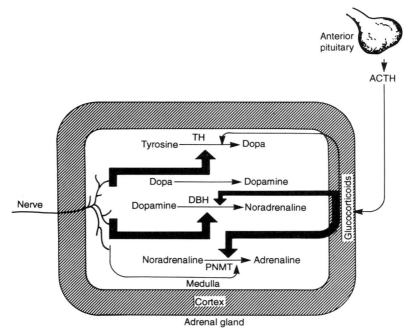

Figure 2.7. Some of the factors involved in the synthesis of catecholamines by the adrenal medulla and the interactions with corticosteroids. Width of lines indicates strength of interaction. By affecting tyrosine hydroxylase (TH) activity, corticosteroids play a small role in the synthesis of dopa from tyrosine, indicated by thin arrow from corticosteroids. Thick arrow to TH indicates the predominant neural determination of this operation. Note thin line from nerve, and thick arrow from corticosteroids, to phenylethanol-amine N-methyltransferase (PNMT), the enzyme that converts noradrenaline to adrenaline. This represents predominant corticosteroid regulation of PNMT. DBH = dopamine β-hydroxylase; ACTH = adrenocorticotrophic hormone. Source: Axelrod, J. and Reisine, T.D. *Science* 224, 452–459

and blood pressure, the latter by means of control exerted over peripheral resistance (Yates and Maran, 1974). The cardiovascular effects of adrenaline and noradrenaline are strengthened by synergistic effects of glucocorticoids exerted at the catecholamine receptor level (Weiner, 1992, p. 208).

Consider the stages in the synthesis of adrenaline: tyrosine to dopa, dopa to dopamine (DA), DA to noradrenaline and, finally, noradrenaline to adrenaline (see Figure 2.7). Note the influence of corticosteroids in these stages. Evidence for the role of corticosteroids in the process of converting noradrenaline to adrenaline was obtained as follows (see

Axelrod and Reisine, 1984). Following hypophysectomy, there is a decrease in activity of phenylethanol-amine *N*-methyltransferase, the enzyme responsible for the formation of adrenaline. Administration of ACTH or corticosteroids reverses this. The width of the arrows in Figure 2.7 indicates the relative weight of the interaction shown. Thus corticosteroids play a rather small part in the conversion of tyrosine to dopa but a large part in the conversion of noradrenaline to adrenaline. The process of synthesis of catecholamines at the adrenal medulla is sensitized by repeated exposure to a stressor, there being a build-up of the enzymes involved in the synthesis (Kvetnansky, 1980). CRF receptors have been located in the adrenal medulla and, acting at this site, CRF is able to increase the secretion of catecholamines (Udelsman *et al.*, 1986). Although the figure shows the influence of corticosteroids on adrenal catecholamines, there also appear to be influences on the synthesis of neurotransmitters within the CNS (Sutton *et al.*, 1994).

Figure 2.8 indicates another aspect of the interaction between the SNS and HPA systems: what Tilders and Berkenbosch (1986) refer to as an adrenomedullary–pituitary axis. Adrenaline of adrenal-medullary origin can stimulate CRF neurons. Also noradrenaline and adrenaline can stimulate the pituitary to release ACTH (Reisine, 1989). Injection of adrenaline to simulate a normal stress response is

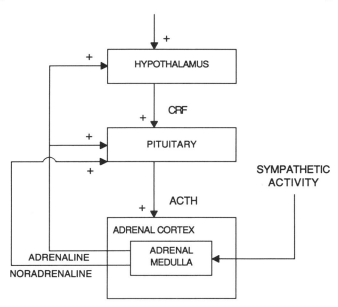

Figure 2.8. Another aspect of the interaction between sympathetic nervous system and adrenocorticotrophic hormone systems

associated with a sharp elevation of ACTH (Smelik *et al.*, 1989). Reciprocally, administration of CRF increases circulating levels of adrenaline and noradrenaline (Tilders and Berkenbosch, 1986).

Henry *et al.* (1976) noted that rats shocked in pairs, as compared with singly, were characterized by a relatively high brain noradrenaline level and low plasma ACTH level (discussed in Section 5.9). However, plasma corticosterone levels did not differ significantly, which is perhaps surprising considering the difference in ACTH levels. Fighting is associated with activation of the SNS. Henry *et al.* suggested that an autonomic innervation of the adrenal cortex might be boosting the levels of plasma corticosterone in the case of the rats engaged in fighting. Henry *et al.* found that, if the nerves supplying the adrenal cortex were cut, the elevation in corticosteroids accompanying fighting was greatly reduced. However, the corticosteroid response accompanying avoidance was not eliminated by this procedure. (There is also evidence for a sympathetic innervation of the adrenal cortex in humans, reviewed by Krishnan *et al.*, 1991.)

Not only are there interactions between the two axes at the level of synthesis and release of hormones, but also in their effects on body tissues (Maickel *et al.*, 1967). The capacity of catecholamines to mobilize free fatty acids depends upon the presence of glucocorticoids (Ganong, 1975; Fain, 1979). Similarly, the effect of catecholamines on the vascular system is influenced by glucocorticoids. According to Williams (1989, p. 81) the interactions between catecholamines and cortisol is of fundamental importance in understanding circulatory disorder. In this context he notes that cortisol acts: (1) to stimulate formation of adrenaline and noradrenaline; (2) to inhibit their breakdown; and (3) to sensitize their receptors.

2.5 OTHER HORMONAL FACTORS IN STRESS

The HPA and SAM axes are the two principal targets of research and theory building in stress. However, other influences are also implicated.

Figure 2.9 shows a wide spectrum of changes that accompany a session of exposure to a stressor in a monkey. In this experiment, the animal was subjected to an avoidance task in which it had to make active responses in order to avoid shocks. Urinary excretion is taken as an index of secretion. Note the rise in urinary adrenaline and 17-OHCS (a metabolite of corticosteroids) excretion during the avoidance period and the return to baseline following its termination. Note also

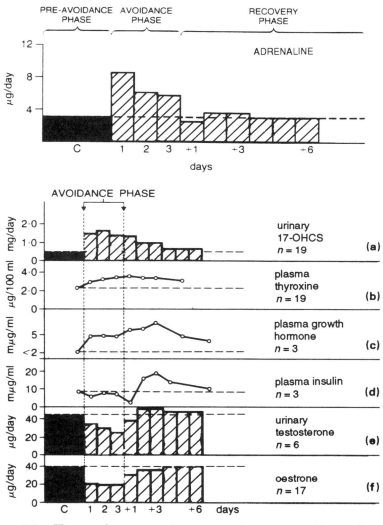

Figure 2.9. Hormonal responses to exposure to a stressor. For explanation, see text. (Reproduced with permission from Archer, J. *Animals under Stress.* Edward Arnold. Copyright Williams & Wilkins 1979)

that plasma thyroxine and growth hormone levels increase during the avoidance period and only slowly return to baseline. By contrast, plasma insulin and urinary testosterone decrease during the stress period followed by an overshoot.

Mason (1968) suggested that the responses of the two major axes discussed in stress, involving the adrenal gland, are only part of a bigger integrated reaction. He noted that those hormones showing an elevation during the period of exposure to the stressor (adrenaline, noradrenaline, glucocorticoids, growth hormone and thyroxine) can be seen as serving an integrated function, their catabolic role in metabolism. Their increased secretion serves to mobilize reserves of energy in anticipation of action. For example, noradrenaline and corticosteroids act to release free fatty acids. Growth hormone decreases the synthesis of triglycerides from glucose and increases the mobilization of free fatty acids from adipose tissue. Thyroxine acts to increase the effectiveness of adrenaline in releasing free fatty acids. (Life is never quite so neat though and there are species differences; whereas in dogs and primates exposure to a stressor stimulates growth hormone secretion, in rodents the effect is inhibitory, mediated by release of somatostatin; reviewed by Smelik, 1984; Tilders and Berkenbosch, 1986; Jurcovicova, Jezova and Vigas, 1989.) Plasma levels of prolactin are also increased by exposure to a stressor (Rivier, 1991b).

The hormones that showed a decrease during the stress session, insulin, testosterone and oestrogen (as indexed by its metabolite oestrone) have an anabolic function (Mason, 1968). The antagonistic action of adrenaline (raising blood sugar) and insulin (decreasing blood sugar) are well known (Mason, 1972). Hormones such as insulin and testosterone tend to show a rebound effect of increased secretion relative to baseline after the period of stressor application is terminated. Their integrated function post-stress can be understood in terms of the breakdown of energy reserves during the stress period. They serve, post-stress, to build up depleted energy reserves and lost body tissue. For example, insulin promotes the storage of glucose and fats and androgens promote protein synthesis.

In conclusion, Mason notes the 'catabolic–anabolic sequence' and suggests a process of reciprocal antagonism between the processes underlying secretion of the two hormone groups. This would be analogous to antagonistic muscles or the antagonistic relationship between sympathetic and parasympathetic divisions of the ANS. Based upon the catabolic–anabolic model and glucagon's capacity to raise blood sugar level, Mason (1972) made the prediction that exposure to a stressor would be associated with an elevation of glucagon secretion. It has subsequently become apparent that, in a variety of species, stressors do indeed induce an almost immediate rise in plasma glucagon concentration (Freeman, 1975). (This might play a part in the mobilization of glycogen stores in the liver.) Mason (1972) raises the interesting question of the nature of the process underlying this co-ordinated array of hormonal actions: 'Are all the hormonal responses initiated as a "package" by a common neural coordinating mechanism?'. The alternative could be that one hormonal change is a consequence of another. Looking at the rapidity with which the hormonal changes occur, leads Mason to suggest a central neural co-ordination process.

Rivier (1989) discusses interactions between the HPA axis and the processes controlling reproductive function. She proposes the model shown in Figure 2.10. Note the three routes by which CRF exerts inhibition upon GnRH, direct and through the mediation of catecholamines and opiates. In turn, this reduces GnRH-stimulated LH release. Such secretion of LH is also inhibited by increased corticosteroid levels during stress. This suggests a functionally coherent suppression of reproductive function.

There is a reduction in urine production during the period of exposure to the stressor. Is it possible to attach any functional significance to this? Mason (1972) suggests that the antidiuretic response, assumed to be mediated via vasopressin release, could be advantageous in anticipation of muscular exertion. Such exertion might elevate body temperature, which would necessitate water use in

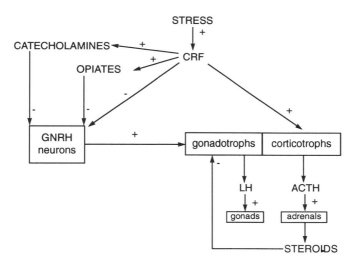

Figure 2.10. Interactions between the hypothalamic–pituitary–adrenocortical axis and reproductive processes as proposed by Rivier (1989, figure 5; Alan R. Liss, Inc., 41 East 11th Street, NY, NY 10003). GnRH = gonadotrophin-releasing hormone; CRF = corticotrophin-releasing factor; LH = luteinizing hormone; ACTH = adrenocorticotrophic hormone

thermoregulation. Also, by-products of increased metabolism would necessitate loss of water through the kidney. Thus the array of hormonal changes that are associated with a stressor should be seen in broader terms simply than those of energy mobilization. As another example, adrenaline increases blood coagulation which can be viewed as serving a function in anticipation of possible injury (Mason, 1972).

As described earlier, concomitantly with the release of ACTH from the pituitary, endorphins are also released (Amir *et al.*, 1980). Stressors exert these effects via the action of CRF and vasopressin. Stressors also release endorphins within the brain itself (described in Chapter 8). Release of both ACTH and endorphins from the pituitary is blocked by the synthetic glucocorticoid dexamethasone. There are some reports that endorphins stimulate synthesis of corticosteroids and opiate receptor binding sites have been located in the adrenal cortex (reviewed by Amir *et al.*, 1980). Endorphins seem to play a part in the release of catecholamines from the adrenal medulla (reviewed by Amir *et al.*, 1980). This might represent an axis in parallel to the SAM axis that is normally associated with release of catecholamines. Enkephalins and enkephalin-like peptides are stored in the adrenal medulla. They are released by sympathetic activation in response to stressors (Lewis *et al.*, 1982). Opioids play a part in the phenomenon of stress-induced analgesia that is discussed in Chapter 8.

2.6 CONCLUDING REMARKS

Activation of both the sympathetic branch of the ANS and the HPA system places the animal in a good physiological state for the exertion of effort, associated with fight or flight. In addition, other hormonal effects in response to a stressor (e.g. suppression of insulin and testosterone secretion) can be understood in terms of the mobilization of resources for activity. A theme that will be developed later is that protracted activation of these systems when behaviour is ineffective constitutes an aspect of stress. Activation of the parasympathetic system generally has opposite effects to that of sympathetic. It will be argued that another form of stress is associated with prolonged and ineffective activation of this system.

The pituitary plays a part in integration. There are inputs that act synergistically at the pituitary level in promoting release of ACTH (e.g. CRF and vasopressin) and also inhibitory effects (e.g. corticosteroid feedback) are exerted at this level.

Chapter 3

Neurochemicals and Stress

3.1 INTRODUCTION

Chapter 3 looks at some of the neurochemicals that underlie the reaction to a stressor. Of course, a large number of different neurochemicals are bound to play a part in any neurophysiological process and associated behaviour, so this section has had to be selective. The criterion for inclusion is where there seems to be the possibility of forming links between the neurochemical evidence and the kind of theoretical modelling that was developed in Chapter 1.

Chapter 2 looked mainly at the sympathetic branch of the autonomic nervous system (ANS) and the hypothalamic–pituitary–adrenocortical (HPA) system, two systems that respond to the application of potential stressors. This chapter considers some of the controls that are exerted over these two systems from within the central nervous system (CNS). A question posed will be—are there neurotransmitters which play an integrating role in co-ordinating the autonomic and behavioural responses to stressors? This section looks at some neurotransmitters implicated in stress with the hope of finding principles of integration.

3.2 NORADRENALINE

One neurotransmitter that has formed a popular target of researchers into stress is noradrenaline (NA). However, the possibility that changes in activity levels of noradrenaline neurons are centrally involved in any motivated behaviour rather than being specifically implicated in aversively motivated behaviours is a caution that needs bearing in mind. A similar logic applies to dopaminergic neurons, discussed in Section 3.4. For example, destruction of catecholamine neurons by 6-hydroxydopamine is associated with deficits in exploratory behaviour as well as behaviour shown in an active avoidance task (Endröczi and Nyakas, 1976).

The cell bodies of noradrenergic neurons are to be found in their highest concentration in the brain regions of the nucleus locus coeruleus (LC) and lateral ventral tegmental area (Glavin, 1985). Studies starting in the early 1960s implicated a role for noradrenaline in attack and defensive behaviours. Exposure to a variety of stressors increased brain noradrenaline activity and turnover whereas when the stressors were of extreme magnitude a depletion of brain noradrenaline was seen (discussed in Chapter 5). Behavioural depression can occur following exposure to uncontrollable stressors and according to some accounts this is associated with depletion of noradrenaline in the LC. Other neurotransmitters, dopamine (DA) and serotonin, and other brain regions were not affected to the same extent (see Glavin, 1985 and Chapter 5).

Both adrenaline and noradrenaline are involved as neurotransmitters in the brain processes that underlie the control of the ANS (De Souza and Appel, 1991).

The role of noradrenaline as a neurotransmitter implicated in stress will be considered further in Section 3.5 where the controls exerted over the HPA system are discussed.

3.3 CORTICOTROPHIN-RELEASING FACTOR

Corticotrophin-releasing factor (CRF), often termed corticotrophin-releasing hormone (CRH), was introduced in Section 2.3.2.1 in its role as part of the HPA axis (further consideration of this topic will be made in Section 3.5). This same substance is also involved, serving in the role as a neurotransmitter (or, possibly, neuromodulator) in the CNS. The substance was first recognized in its capacity as a hormone. However, the effects described in this section are ones that appear not to be attributable to CRF acting in its role as a hormone (Dunn and Berridge, 1990a).

There is some evidence to suggest that CRF might serve an integrating role, which, when stretched to beyond an adaptive range, would implicate it as a 'stress neurotransmitter'. CRF has a role in both the HPA and sympathetic–adrenal–medullary systems as well as in behavioural control. Endogenous opioids that lower reactivity in both axes appear to do so via their action upon CRF (McCubbin, 1993).

The amygdala features prominently in discussions of the neural bases of stress and, as such, CRF-containing neurons are identified as among those that project from the amygdala of the rat (T. S. Gray, 1991). It is of relevance to the present study to note that the amygdala has direct connections with the hypothalamus, cortex and regions of the brainstem involved in autonomic control. Thus this region might serve as an integrator linking, on the one hand, the regions responsible for detection of stressors involving cognitive processing, (e.g. cortex and hippocampus) and, on the other hand, the effectors of the stress response (e.g. hypothalamus and brainstem autonomic controls). Stimulation of the amygdala causes signs of fear. The region is associated with a high density of benzodiazepine receptors, suggesting that it might form a natural target for anxiolytic drugs (T. S. Gray, 1991).

CRF serves as a neurotransmitter in the LC among other regions (Valentino, 1988). Neurons containing CRF are located within regions of the brainstem concerned with the control of the ANS and with affect and emotion, which is compatible with it serving a co-ordinating role that is stretched in stress states (Nemeroff, 1988; Dunn and Berridge, 1990a). CRF is found in brain regions associated with catecholamine (noradrenaline and DA) and indoleamine (serotonin) transmission, thus facilitating a CRF interaction with these systems (Nemeroff, 1988). Following application of a stressor, CRF concentration in various brain regions changes. Activation of the EEG and changes in activity of neurons in various brain regions follows application of small amounts of CRF to the brain. In humans, CRF has been shown to improve attentional processes (Fehm and Born, 1989). In rats, intra-cerebroventricular (i.c.v.) infusion of CRF causes an improvement in learning capacity and an increase in firing of neurons within the LC, a region of importance in selective attention (reviewed by De Souza and Battaglia, 1988; Koob et al., 1988; Valentino, 1988). CRF causes an excitation of neurons in the hippocampus (Cole and Koob, 1991).

A criterion for considering CRF to be a stress neurotransmitter would be the appearance of behavioural autonomic and endocrine changes following application of CRF to the brain. These changes would need to correspond to those normally seen in response to a stressor. Indeed, changes normally part of the 'fight or flight' response are observed following CRF injection. Increased sympathetic outflow and decreased parasympathetic outflow, as indexed by elevated heart rate, blood pressure, cardiac output, glucose utilization, oxygen consumption and increases in blood concentrations of adrenaline and nor-adrenaline, are seen (Koob, 1985; Lenz et al., 1987; Valentino, 1988; Brown, 1991; Wiersma et al., 1993). After administration of CRF, i.c.v., increased sympathetic activation of the heart, accompanied by decreased parasympathetic activation (Brown and Fisher, 1985), is observed. An increase in sympathetic nervous system (SNS) activity is implicated in a decrease in natural killer cell function (Brown, 1991). In rats, CRF increases the magnitude of the acoustic startle response and the amount of shock-induced fighting (Tazi *et al.*, 1987b; Koob, 1991). Furthermore, a CRF antagonist reduces the amount of shock-induced fighting even in rats uninjected with CRF, suggesting a normal role for CRF in the mediation of aggression (Tazi *et al.*, 1987b).

CRF-mediated decreases in parasympathetic tone or increases in sympathetic tone (or both) are also indexed by a decrease in secretion of gastric acid and decreased gastrointestinal motility (Lenz *et al.*, 1987; Dunn and Berridge, 1990a; De Souza *et al.*, 1991). Associated with such decrease is a stimulation of large bowel transit. Such a combination of actions are commonly seen in response to stressors (Lenz, 1990). In dogs but not in rats, pretreatment with naloxone reduces the gastric inhibitory action, suggesting opioid involvement (see Lenz, 1990). The site of action of CRF on gastric secretion under natural conditions would appear strongly to be within the CNS, possibly regions of the hypothalamus (Lenz, 1990). The effects of CRF are not blocked by hypophysectomy or adrenalectomy, leading Koob (1985) to propose a direct activating effect upon the SNS.

Concerning the behavioural effect of i.c.v. injection of CRF in rats, a 'general activation' as measured by increased locomotor activity, sniffing and rearing in a familiar environment is reported (Koob, 1985; Valentino, 1988; Cole and Koob, 1991). There are reports that signs of anxiety are increased by CRF injection (reviewed by De Souza and Battaglia, 1988; Koob, 1985; Koob *et al.*, 1988). The same dose that is associated with activation in a familiar environment causes behavioural inhibition in a novel environment (reviewed by Bond *et al.*, 1989). Thus, on exposure to a novel environment, an 'open-field' piece of apparatus, the CRF-injected rat's behaviour is consistent with increased fear: decreases in locomotion and rearing are seen, accompanied by increased grooming. Also the suppression of appetitive behaviour (e.g. lever-pressing for food) by a cue predictive of shock is increased by CRF (Koob, 1991).

Takahashi and Kalin (1989) observed rats injected with CRF or vehicle when placed in an open arena with the opportunity to hide within a small tunnel. The amount of time spent in the tunnel was taken as an index of emotionality. Injection of CRF, i.c.v. significantly increased the amount of time spent in the small tunnel. This effect was central; it did not occur when the CRF was injected peripherally. The authors concluded that these effects of CRF on behaviour were not mediated via the HPA system and that CRF 'mediates the display of defensive behaviour'. In a further study, injection of a CRF antagonist increased the amount of time spent in the main arena, increased exploration and decreased withdrawal. The tendency of odours from a stressed conspecific to trigger the defensive withdrawal response was attenuated by a CRF antagonist. Time spent in exploration and social interaction tend to be decreased by CRF (Dunn and Berridge, 1990b). These seem to be the result of direct actions on the CNS.

Possibly at least some of the effects of CRF might be described in general terms as an increase in 'arousal', characterized as an increased salience of the environment. Ritchie and Nemeroff (1991) describe a change in firing pattern of neurons in the hippocampus and change in EEG in response to CRF that might be described as increased arousal or activation (Koob, 1991). Cole and Koob (1991) suggest that 'CRF in the central nervous system may be crucially involved in the generation of arousal by aversive (stressful) stimuli'.

Approach to food and feeding are suppressed by CRF injection. Interestingly and perhaps surprisingly, also there is a suppression of the feeding that is normally induced by pinching the tail, so-called stress-induced eating (Cole and Koob, 1991). Release of luteinizing hormone, growth hormone and gonadotrophin-releasing hormone is suppressed, as is sexual behaviour (De Souza and Battaglia, 1988; Rabin et al., 1988; Dunn and Berridge, 1990a). In male rats, testosterone level is lowered by prolonged i.c.v. CRF administration (Dunn and Berridge, 1990a). Such hormone changes are also commonly seen after prolonged application of a stressor. The fact that these effects of a stressor can be either reversed or attenuated by a CRF antagonist suggests that under natural conditions they are mediated by CRF. Similarly, the fact that the responses that occur to CRF injection can be attenuated by a CRF antagonist argues against the interpretation that such injections act merely as a non-specific stressor. The effect of CRF on sexual behaviour appears to be mediated by neurons that have receptors for both luteinizing hormone-releasing hormone and CRF (Nemeroff, 1988). These effects of central administration of CRF do not appear with peripheral administration. At least some of the effect survives removal of the pituitary and adrenal glands, indicating a role of the transmitter in the CNS. However, some of the effect of CRF on the control of reproductive processes appears to be mediated via the HPA axis in that at least part of the suppression effect of CRF on plasma testosterone level can be mimicked by injection of adrenocorticotrophic hormone (ACTH; Rivier, 1989; see also Chapter 2). Adrenalectomy interfered with CRF inhibition. Koob (1985) also reported signs of repetitive behaviour (termed stereotypy) following injection of CRF.

An important focus in the brain for investigators into the stress responses is the LC (Valentino, 1988). Changes in noradrenaline in this region in stressed animals were discussed in Section 3.2 and will be further considered in Chapter 5. Changes in electrical activity in this region correlate with changes in general activity; LC activity is low in sleep and high when the animal is engaging in commerce with the environment. A wide variety of external stimuli cause excitation of neurons in the LC and therefore LC activation under conditions of stress would be predicted, and is indeed found (Valentino, 1988). Stimuli that would be termed stressors (e.g. shock, stimuli that have been paired with noxious events) are particularly effective in increasing firing rate.

Berridge and Dunn (1990b) reported that i.c.v. injections of CRF caused increased turnover of brain catecholamines. Valentino (1988) raised the question whether stressors are able to produce release of CRF from nerve fibres that innervate the LC and thereby activate the LC. Of relevance to this question is the observation that, in anaesthetized rats, i.c.v. injection of CRF causes an increase in firing rate of LC neurons. In terms of the time course and dose–response magnitude, the effects of injected CRF on LC activity correspond to its effect on behaviour and autonomic reactions. Increased LC activity correlates with increased vigilance and orientation towards external stimuli, so any natural CRF-induced excitation of the LC might be seen as part of the adaptive response to a stressor. Valentino admits that the effects she describes might be pharmacological rather than physiological. Although the role of CRF in the LC is still somewhat speculative, these data yield useful pointers to underlying processes.

In summary, much of the effect of CRF within the CNS can be interpreted in terms of activation of defensive behaviours accompanied by increased sympathetic activation and parasympathetic inhibition. However, not all of the effects can be interpreted in this way. For instance, increased freezing in a novel environment and increased latency to emerge are suggestive of an increased parasympathetic activation. Thus, CRF seems to play a part in both active (e.g. fighting, exploration) and passive (e.g. freezing, suppression of appetitive responses) reactions to stressors (Koob, 1991; Wiersma et al., 1993). (A distinction between active and passive strategies is one that will appear at various places in the subsequent chapters of this book.) This would place CRF in a position to be regarded as a neurotransmitter whose activity is a possible measure of stress. In the terms developed in Chapter 1, CRF secretion seems to be sensitive to disparity between Sollwert and Istwert.

3.4 DOPAMINE

A number of experiments indicate that exposure to a stressor (e.g. foot shock, restraint, conditioned foot shock, a passive avoidance situation) increases DA metabolism and release in the brain (Dunn and Berridge, 1990b), possibly in some situations more specifically in the mesolimbic system (Imperato *et al.*, 1992). In rats, an active avoidance task (Chapter 7) is disrupted by systemic injection of DA antagonists (McCullough *et al.*, 1993). In rats, Imperato *et al.* found that stress restraint was associated with increased DA output but so was cessation of restraint. When restraint was imposed on the second and third days, only a slight increase in DA release was seen but the increase on cessation of restraint remained the same. These researchers suggested that DA release in the nucleus accumbens is related to the meaning that the stressor has for the animal. Thus DA release might be the neural correlate of behavioural attempts to cope. Repeated presentation of the stressor and the decline of DA response might then correspond to acquisition of a passive strategy. The DA activation on termination of the stressor could be the correlate of a continuing active attempt at escape from the situation.

Dunn and Berridge (1990b) reported that certain stressful situations (e.g. infection with the influenza virus) that cause the appearance of elevated plasma levels of corticosteroids and the catabolites of noradrenaline are not associated with signs of elevated DA activity. This is suggestive that DA systems are responsive not to stressors in a general sense (as traditionally defined) but to stressors with which goal-directed behaviour is associated.

The fact that stressful situations elevate DA turnover illustrates the argument that we need to be cautious about calling DA a 'stress neurotransmitter' as appetitive situations are also associated with elevated turnover (Blackburn *et al.*, 1989; Salamone, 1994). It could be that DA is reactive in situations where an animal is being required to execute any type of goal-directed behaviour whether appetitively or aversively motivated. In keeping with such an interpretation is the observation that passive avoidance is not disrupted (or is less disrupted than an active task) by DA antagonists (Salamone, 1994). Also escape is less disrupted than avoidance, suggesting a role for DA in the exploitation of conditional cues (Salamone, 1994).

Rats given tone-shock pairings when under the influence of a DA-receptor blocker learn the association, as indexed by a conditioned emotional response (CER) (Beninger, 1989). That is to say, the tone subsequently suppresses appetitive behaviour. However, they fail to learn one-way shock avoidance (Fibiger *et al.*, 1975; reviewed by

McCullough *et al.*, 1993). Beninger (1989) is specific about what it is that DA-depleted rats fail to learn in an avoidance task: 'acquisition by the safety-related environmental stimuli of the ability to elicit reactions that involve instrumental responses that serve to bring the animal closer to them'.

Why do DA-depleted rats fail to learn avoidance? Consider first the case of where physical movement is concerned. Avoidance involves not simply getting away from somewhere but getting to a safe situation (Masterson and Crawford, 1982). Under the influence of a DA block, they seem to fail to attribute positive salience to the safe platform or side of the shuttle-box as cued by the conditional stimulus (Crow and Deakin, 1985). They are unable to organize goal-directed behaviour involving physical locomotion.

The role of nucleus accumbens DA in appetitive motivation is established (Blackburn *et al.*, 1989). Recent evidence has also implicated this brain region in aversively motivated behaviour, lever-pressing to avoid shock (McCullough *et al.*, 1993). DA depletion disrupted this behaviour. McCullough *et al.* suggested that in this situation DA plays a part in attributing motivational significance to temporal cues predictive of shock. By lever-pressing, the rat is not moving anywhere and so, to assimilate this result into Beninger's account (see above), a modification is needed. The rat is achieving a shock-free period by its active behaviour, so if in Beninger's statement 'closer to them' is replaced by 'a situation of safety' the result might be encompassed. That neither freezing (McCullough *et al.*, 1993) nor a CER is disrupted by a DA blockage suggests that the animal is still: (1) sensitive to aversive stimulation and (2) able to effect passive behaviour in response to its expectation, but active goal-directed behaviour is disrupted.

Scheel-Krüger and Willner (1991) note the paradox that not only secondary positive incentive stimuli but also stress activates the mesolimbic system. What have the two in common? They suggest that stimuli predictive of both reward and stress are stimuli to action. Therefore, under either condition, mesolimbic activity could facilitate appropriate goal-directed action. Willner *et al.* (1991) write:

> . . . activation of the system, whether by reward-related incentive or by stress, leads to active behaviour that has reinforcing consequences in both cases: the delivery of a reward following the successful execution of a sequence of appetitive behaviour, or stress reduction following the successful execution of an avoidance or escape response.

Glavin (1993) investigated the role of DA in the susceptibility of rats to the so-called stress ulcer (see Chapter 10). Injection of the DA agonist SKF 75670C provided considerable protection against the development of gastric ulcers in response to the stress of immobilization. This was particularly marked in rats showing high anxiety and a correspondingly greater susceptibility to gastric ulcers. Gastric damage was also induced by intragastric loading of ethanol and the DA agonist afforded protection here too. Evidence was obtained showing that highly anxious rats have a higher DA turnover in the amygdala and striatum than do rats with low anxiety. Three hours of restraint in a cold environment led to a loss of 70–80% of the DA from the amygdala. Rats with high anxiety show a more rapid decline of DA.

3.5 SEROTONIN

Serotonin has effects both at the level of the brain and directly at the pituitary in affecting the secretion of pituitary hormones (De Souza and Appel, 1991). There is some evidence for its direct effects upon ACTH and prolactin secretion.

3.6 OPIOIDS

Opioid receptors are located in various brain regions (e.g. LC, amygdala). Opioids have a central part in the discussion of stress (De Souza and Appel, 1991). Opioids both play a part in the release of such hormones as ACTH and, as will be discussed in more detail in the chapters that follow, influence the nervous system processes underlying the animal's reaction to a stressor. Opioid receptors have been classified into such subtypes as mu, delta and kappa, which might well play different parts in the processes underlying the stress response (De Souza and Appel, 1991). For example, kappa and mu opioid receptors at the hypothalamus seem to play a part in ACTH secretion.

In conscious animals, opioids injected into the brain tend to affect such autonomic functions as heart rate and blood pressure, mediated via hypothalamic and other sites (De Souza and Appel, 1991). There is a suggestion that the subtypes of receptors (kappa and mu) might mediate opposite effects concerning the sympathetic–parasympathetic balance.

A caution is in order regarding species differences in the effects of opioids on the HPA axis; in rats their effect is primarily one of stimulation whereas in humans it is inhibitory (De Souza and Appel, 1991).

3.7   GAMMA-AMINOBUTYRIC ACID AND BENZODIAZEPINES

Benzodiazepines potentiate the effect of gamma-aminobutyric acid (GABA) at its receptor (De Souza and Appel, 1991). The benzodiazepine receptor is of interest in the present study in that agonists to the receptor (e.g. diazepam) both have an anxiolytic effect and inhibit the HPA axis. GABA receptors have been identified at the hypothalamic and pituitary levels and seem to play a part in inhibition of the HPA axis (De Souza and Appel, 1991).

3.8   NEUROTRANSMITTERS AND THE HYPOTHALAMIC–PITUITARY– ADRENOCORTICAL AXIS

The following account presents the main features of the system determining the release of CRF, β-endorphin and ACTH within the HPA system. (Other factors are also implicated and the reader is referred to Brush and Shain, 1989, for a discussion of these.) Thus in this section CRF is being described in its role as a hormone, albeit a somewhat peculiar one, rather than as a neurotransmitter.

A number of reports indicate that there is a pathway employing acetylcholine that exerts an excitatory effect upon the release of CRF (Bradbury *et al.*, 1974; Hillhouse *et al.*, 1975; Buckingham and Hodges, 1979; Laborit, 1986, p. 139; De Souza and Appel, 1991). The normal response of elevated ACTH to several different stimuli, e.g. ether and surgical stress, is blocked by atropine implants in the anterior hypothalamus, suggesting cholinergic mediation of HPA activation (Hedge and Smelik, 1968). Serotonergic neurons also exert an excitatory effect (Plotsky, 1991). There is evidence for a catecholaminergic effect upon the pituitary–adrenal axis. However, both inhibitory and excitatory (Feldman, 1989) effects have been reported. Both effects might indeed occur in parallel (Plotsky, 1988). Possibly, species differences are implicated.

Evidence for an inhibitory role (represented in Figure 2.4 by the minus sign) was obtained by Buckingham and Hodges (1979), Hillhouse *et al.* (1975) and Roth *et al.* (1981). Axelrod and Reisine (1984) show adrenaline-containing neurons to exert an inhibition upon CRF secretion and note that depletion of brain adrenaline can be induced by stressors. Drugs that inhibit phenylethanol-amine *N*-methyltransferase, the enzyme in the pathway leading to adrenaline synthesis, were found to lead to a dose-related increase in plasma corticosterone in rats. There is evidence to show that noradrenergic neurons in the hypothalamus and preoptic area exert a tonic inhibition on CRF secretion and ACTH release (Ganong *et al.*, 1976; reviewed by Anisman, 1978; Depue and Kleiman, 1979). Thus, large-scale depletion of noradrenaline with the drug reserpine is followed by increases in CRH and ACTH secretion. This effect can be countered by drugs that boost noradrenaline, such as the monoamine oxidase inhibitors. GABA and opioid peptides exert an inhibitory role (Grossman, 1991; Plotsky, 1991).

Evidence for an excitatory effect on ACTH by injections of noradrenaline and adrenaline was obtained by Krieger and Krieger (1970) and Szafarczyk *et al.* (1987). There appear to be both CNS (involving synapses upon CRF-producing neurons) and pituitary (involving synergistic activity with CRF) sites of excitatory action of catecholamine (discussed also by Plotsky, 1987, 1991; Plotsky, *et al.*, 1989). Szafarczyk *et al.* (1987) postulated an adrenergic innervation of CRF-producing neurons in the paraventricular nuclei (PVN) by neurons originating in the brainstem.

3.9 CONCLUSIONS

A certain amount of insight into the organization of the processes that underlie what are generally termed stress responses can be gained by looking at the role of specific neurotransmitters such as noradrenaline, DA and CRF in the organization of behaviour. We shall have cause to return to the roles of these neurotransmitters when behaviour is more closely examined in subsequent chapters.

Chapter 4

The Nervous, Endocrine and Immune Systems

4.1 INTRODUCTION

The goal set at the start of the present study was to construct a theoretical model of stress that could integrate diverse aspects of the phenomenon. One aspect of stress that has come into particular prominence in recent years is its influence on the immune system; there has been a growing awareness of interactions between the nervous, endocrine and immune systems. These interactions are such that for some purposes the systems, traditionally described one-by-one, are perhaps best thought of as one large system serving an integrated function, rather than three distinct systems. The immune system is immensely complex and this section can do no more than introduce some of it in the context of looking at how the immune, nervous and endocrine systems interact in states described as stress.

In the present context concerned with general principles of organization and function, understanding of the immune system and its interactions might be helped by noting certain similarities between the nervous system and the immune system (Ballieux and Heijnen, 1987). Both maintain the integrity of the body in what is often a hostile world. The nervous system recognizes external threats and organizes specifically targeted action by the body. The immune system has the function of recognizing foreign materials (termed *antigens*), targeting and eliminating them from the body. Both nervous and immune systems involve communication over distance and preserve a 'memory' of past events. Both employ chemical messengers. Of course, some of these features are shared with the endocrine system.

4.2　THE BASICS OF THE IMMUNE SYSTEM

The human immune system is composed of some 10^9 million or more white cells, also termed leucocytes. These cells circulate throughout the body, within the lymphoid system and also in the blood and other body fluids; their influence penetrates throughout. A high concentration of such cells is found in particular locations of the body, e.g. the lymph nodes and spleen. The class of leucocytes that we know most about in terms of interactions with neuroendocrine systems are the *lymphocytes* and *monocytes* (Sapolsky, 1992). There are two major classes of lymphocytes, both of which start their lives in the bone marrow. B lymphocytes (also termed B cells) develop to maturity in the bone marrow. The other type of cell, the T lymphocytes (T cells), leave the bone marrow while still in an immature stage. They complete their development in the thymus.

One type of T cell that we shall discuss is termed a *T helper*. Another class of cell is known as *natural killer cells* (NK cells). An example of a monocyte that we will need to consider is a *macrophage*.

T cells play a part in what is termed *cell-mediated immunity*. A macrophage recognizes a pathogen and forms a bond. The bond between the pathogen and the macrophage has the effect of releasing *interleukin-1* (IL-1) from the macrophage. IL-1 is an example of a chemical messenger of a class termed cytokines. The other line of defence, this time mediated by B cells, is termed *antibody-mediated immunity*. It is also sometimes termed 'humoral-mediated immunity'.

4.3　OVERVIEW OF THE INTERACTIONS BETWEEN NERVOUS, ENDOCRINE AND IMMUNE SYSTEMS

Table 4.1 shows a summary of the kind of evidence on which the existence of interactions between nervous, endocrine and immune systems is based. Note the reciprocal nature of the interactions. Items 1–3 are suggestive of causation from the nervous system to immune system, whereas 4 is evidence for interaction from the immune to the nervous system. Table 4.2 shows a summary of the suggested processes linking the nervous and immune systems that are responsible for the phenomena of Table 4.1. There are two main routes of interaction. There is the route (items 1, 3, 4 and the adrenal medulla part of 2) that involves the mediation of hormones, the so-called *soluble connection*. In this domain, corticosteroids are the most commonly discussed means for the central nervous system (CNS) to influence the immune

Table 4.1.   Evidence for nervous and immune system interactions

1   Immune responses can be conditioned
2   Electrical stimulation or lesions of specific brain sites can alter immune function
3   Stressed experimental animals have altered immune responses
4   Activation of the immune system is correlated with altered neuro-physiological, neurochemical and neuroendocrine activities of brain cells

Reprinted from Dunn 1989. Copyright 1989, with kind permission from Elsevier Science Ltd, The Boulevard, Langford Lane, Kidlington OX5 1GB, UK

Table 4.2.   Potential links between the nervous and immune systems

Mechanisms by which the nervous system might affect the immune system (in most cases with hormonal mediation):

1   Glucocorticoids secreted from the adrenal cortex
2   Catecholamines secreted from terminals of the sympathetic nervous system and by the adrenal medulla
3   Endorphins secreted by the pituitary, the adrenal medulla and sympathetic terminals
4   Other hormones secreted by the pituitary and the gonads

Mechanisms by which the immune system might affect the nervous system:

5   Cytokines secreted by activated immune cells

Reprinted from Dunn 1989. Copyright 1989, with kind permission from Elsevier Science Ltd, The Boulevard, Langford Lane, Kidlington OX5 1GB, UK

system. There is also the direct link (item 2; terminals of sympathetic nervous system, or SNS) from nervous system to lymphoid tissues, what Ballieux and Heijnen (1989) term the *wiring system* link. A sympathetic innervation of the thymus and spleen, important components of the immune system, exists (Ballieux and Heijnen, 1987; Dunn, 1989). Item 5 represents a blood-borne means by which the immune system could influence the nervous system.

The next two sections will look in more detail at these interactions.

4.4   EFFECTS OF THE NERVOUS AND ENDOCRINE SYSTEMS ON IMMUNE FUNCTION

4.4.1   Causal Processes

The importance of the stress response and its associated hormones in mediating the relationship between the nervous and immune systems is suggested by a number of things. For example, adrenalectomy generally enhances the functioning of the immune system and applying adrenocortical steroids generally suppresses it (Ader, 1987).

There are a variety of ways in which corticosteroids can depress immune system function and, as Sapolsky (1992) notes, 'some of the means are subtle, some extraordinarily crude'. As an example of a more subtle interaction, corticosteroids influence the role of cytokines. They do this by: (1) inhibiting the release of cytokines and (2) decreasing the sensitivity of their target cells. For example, corticosteroids decrease the number of IL-2 (another cytokine) receptors. They inhibit the release of IL-1. As an example of a more crude means, Sapolsky gives the blocking of the maturation of developing lymphocytes by corticosteroids. Such a process is seen at a gross level in the shrinkage of the thymus gland at times of hypothalamic–pituitary–adrenocortical (HPA) activation. In some species, corticosteroids are able to remove lymphocytes from the circulation, and finally there exists a process by which they are able literally to destroy lymphocytes.

A rich density of steroid-receptor sites has been located on lymphocytes (Craddock, 1978), and these are one route that mediates the immunosuppressive effects of corticosteroids. Craddock notes that circadian changes in immune system activity are a function of the normal circadian rhythm of corticosteroids. This led him to propose that the interaction between the pituitary–adrenocortical axis and the immune system should be seen as an aspect of normal homeostasis rather than simply something that represents pathology. In such terms, the corticosteroids would be seen as playing a vital negative feedback role (see also Chapter 2). Their absence would risk over-activity on the part of the immune system. This view is discussed later.

A concentration of corticotrophic-releasing factor (CRF)-binding sites in the mouse spleen in regions of high macrophage concentration suggests that CRF might play a part in regulation of the immune system, which (in line with the message of Chapter 3) might give it an integrating role in nervous, hormonal and immune responses to stressors (De Souza et al., 1991).

Although most attention has been directed to the HPA axis in consideration of effects upon immune function, the autonomic nervous system (ANS) also needs consideration. Axon branches of the ANS terminate throughout the lymphoid organs at the surface of lymphocytes. Thus there are SNS pathways running to the spleen, thymus and bone marrow, all sites of crucial importance in the synthesis and storage of lymphocytes. The evidence suggests that sympathetic activation exerts an inhibitory effect upon the immune system (Sapolsky, 1992).

A further factor that mediates immunosuppression appears to be release of natural opioids at a time of stress (Shavit and Martin, 1987). Opioid receptors are found on various cells of the immune system (Sapolsky, 1992). Immunological deficits have been observed in opiate addicts. Shavit and Martin investigated the pathways involved in opioid-based immunosuppression, suggesting three possibilities as to how opioids might act: (a) directly upon receptors on individual cells of the immune system; (b) via modulation of the ANS; or (c) via an effect upon the HPA axis as this axis has a suppressing effect upon immune function.

Evidence suggestive of factor b and/or c was that injections of morphine made into the lateral ventricle of the brain caused a suppression of NK cell activity that was equivalent to the effect of a 3000-fold larger systemic injection. The effect was blocked by naltrexone. NK cell activity was unaffected by a systemic injection of a morphine analogue that could not cross the blood–brain barrier. Adrenalectomy prevented the suppressive effect of morphine from appearing, pointing to a role for the adrenal gland in mediating the effect. Further evidence pointed specifically to the adrenal cortex as being responsible.

In summary, there seems to be a rich collection of fire-power with which a state of stress is able to inhibit the immune system. Why should things have evolved this way?

4.4.2   Considerations of Function

The fact that HPA activation tends to suppress immune function might come initially as something of a surprise; surely a time of stress is one that might be associated with infection (e.g. as a result of tissue damage inflicted by a predator) and one during which the immune system should be activated. Again, it is necessary to reiterate the caution made in Chapter 1, the processes underlying stress and the immune system evolved under rather different conditions from those seen today. Domestication of animals and our own life in urban cultures might be revealing a pathological mode of interaction that was rarely seen in an earlier evolutionary history.

One possible, although highly speculative, way of making some sense of the suppression is to consider that immune activation is costly as an anabolic process, an idea which Sapolsky (1992) discusses. It might be a small price to pay to suspend such activity for a while, as tumours and infectious agents can be fought later. Sapolsky applies a similar logic to inflammation which is also inhibited by HPA activation. Suppose, for example, that a zebra injures a knee in a confrontation with a lion. An inflammatory response would consist of an accumulation of fluid in the local extracellular space, with a migration of leucocytes into the area. As a result the knee is difficult to use and a source of pain. These are conditions favouring rest and recuperation which could be maladaptive if the external environment is still sufficiently threatening to maintain elevated corticosteroid activation. Thus there might be a certain evolutionary logic to be seen in a temporary inhibition of inflammation by activity in the HPA system. This view requires: (1) a natural anti-inflammatory effect of HPA activation under natural conditions and (2) a time course of the events, such that when HPA activation occurs, inflammation is thereby delayed. Accompanying HPA activation is an analgesic process (Chapter 8), which will tend to favour activity in the face of injury. As Sapolsky (1992) notes, perhaps evolution simply could not achieve a suppression of inflammation without a parallel suppression of immune function. In this context, he observes that most of the cytokines exert a positive effect upon inflammation.

By a similar logic, it is possible to make evolutionary sense of a sympathetic inhibition upon the immune system. Sympathetic activation would normally correspond to bodily exertion in fight or flight and might well be followed by a parasympathetic rebound on the termination of immediate danger (see Section 6.9.3). Any possible parasympathetic innervation of the immune system (its involvement seems less certain at the time of writing than the sympathetic involvement; Sapolsky, 1992) might then boost the immune system.

However, attractive as the idea of a temporary suspension of immune activity in the interests of conservation of resources might seem, there is a serious objection to it as being the whole answer. As Sapolsky (1992) argues, all that would appear to be needed to prevent costly anabolic processes would be a process of inhibition upon the immune system. This would suspend both production of new lymphocytes and proliferation of those already in the system. It would hardly seem necessary to destroy lymphocytes. By analogy, the costs of reproduction at a time of stress seem to be avoided by nothing more drastic than various levels of inhibition, e.g. upon testosterone secretion (Section 2.5).

Perhaps a short-term suppression might serve a functional end, but long-term suppression must surely be maladaptive. By analogy, in primates following parental loss, processes of behavioural protest and later apathy might be adaptive in the short-term but maladaptive if the situation remains unresolved and something like full-blown depression results (Section 10.5.2). In a similar vein, Sapolsky (1992) notes:

The answer lies in the sort of disclaimers that one gets with the instruc-
tions for a new appliance: The stress-response, just like a new microwave
oven, must be used properly. It is an ideal system for allowing an organism to deal with short-term physical stress, and that is exactly the sort of
stressor that most organisms face most of the time.

Presumably the costs associated with long-term stress (pathology for
which immunosuppression is responsible) have not proven sufficient to
offset the benefits (whatever they might be) derived from short-term
inhibition of immune function. Of course, in general, we do not know
the extent to which such long-term costs have in reality been encountered during the course of evolution or whether they are the product of
such things as domestication; though some studies suggest that
chronic stress is endemic in baboon colonies (see Section 6.6). Stress-
related disorders tend to occur when the stress response has been
activated: (1) for too long to be of adaptive value and (2) when there is
no physiological justification (e.g. activation by psychological processes
associated with being submissive; Sapolsky, 1992). One might speculate that those animals being in such a state sufficient to compromise
the immune system will not generally be those of high fitness in the
ethological sense. But such discussion should not detract from the
truth: that, at the time of writing, we do not know the function *if any*
(to commit an ethological heresy) served by immune suppression.

4.5   EFFECTS OF THE IMMUNE SYSTEM UPON THE NERVOUS SYSTEM ENDOCRINE STATE

So much for the effects of the nervous system, acting directly or via
hormones, on the immune system, this section will now look at the
effects of the immune system on endocrine state and on the nervous
system. Some of the effects on endocrine state are direct ones and
others are mediated via the nervous system.

In both humans and laboratory animals, infection is followed by
increased levels of plasma corticosteroids (Rivier, 1991; Sapolsky,
1992). As Figure 4.1 shows, part of this causal link is effected via the
production of interleukins by activated macrophages. There would
seem to be a role for interleukins in effecting an integrated pattern of
metabolic and behavioural changes on the part of the infected host, e.g.
fever (the pyrogenic effect of interleukins, discussed in Section 9.3,
seems to be distinct from their endocrinological role), sleep and increased availability of nutrients, as well as activation of the HPA system (Rivier, 1991). In rodents, it has been shown that IL-1 can activate

the HPA axis by promoting the secretion of CRF from hypothalamic neurons (Dunn *et al.*, 1991; Rivier, 1991), possibly through mediation of an aversive state (Tazi *et al.*, 1988). In some respects, it might provide a missing link as the 'stress agent' (or at least a hint leading us to one), as in addition to activation of the HPA axis, its effects include loss of appetite and activation of noradrenergic systems in the brain and the sympathetic–adrenal system.

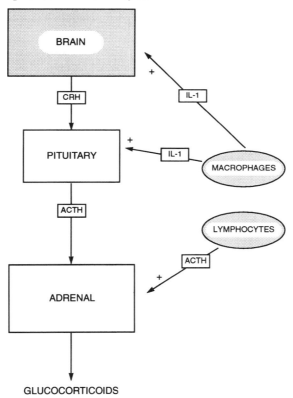

Figure 4.1. Possible effects of the immune system upon the hypothalamic–pituitary–adrenocortical (HPA) axis. To the left is the classical HPA axis as described in Chapter 2. To the right are the suggested influences of the immune system upon this axis. Note the release of interleukin-1 from activated macrophages and its excitatory effects upon both the brain and (perhaps more tentatively) the pituitary gland. Again somewhat tentatively, there is a suggestion of the secretion of adrenocorticotrophic hormone from lymphocytes. Whether this is sufficient on its own to cause corticosteroid secretion from the adrenal is not certain. (From Sapolsky, 1992 in *Behavioural Endocrinology* (eds Becker, Breedlove and Crews). Reproduced by permission of the MIT Press)

It was normally assumed that any influence the immune system was able to exert upon corticosteroids was mediated via the HPA system. However, a route 'short-circuiting' this has also been described. Smith *et al*. (1982) found that a virus could induce a rise in plasma corticosterone levels even in hypophysectomized mice. They suggested that lymphocytes are a source of an 'adrenocorticotrophic hormone (ACTH)-like' substance that promotes corticosterone release (see Figure 4.1). These authors argue: 'In contrast to the pituitary–adrenal axis, the putative lymphoid–adrenal axis would be stimulated by non-cognitive factors recognized not by the central nervous system but by lymphocytes'. In this way, the immune system could be seen to be serving a sensory function; although see also Dunn *et al*. (1987) and Blalock (1987) for a further consideration of this claim. Such release of ACTH seems to be accompanied by β-endorphin release, based upon the precursor pro-opiomelanocortin molecule (see also Chapter 3; Ballieux and Heijnen, 1989).

As a further possible process, Blalock (1988) describes a new axis parallel to the HPA axis and similarly involving the sequence CRF → ACTH → corticosteroids (see Figure 4.2). This axis is mediated via leucocytes, where CRF is able to synthesize and release ACTH and β-endorphins. Blalock speculated that, in response to stressors, leucocytes might produce ACTH as a result of their passage through the portal circulation between the hypothalamus and the pituitary. It is

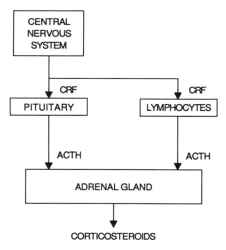

Figure 4.2. Parallel pathways between CNS and corticosteroid release. The pathway via the pituitary release of adrenocorticotrophic hormone (ACTH) and that involving the mediation of lymphocytes. CRF = corticotrophin-releasing factor

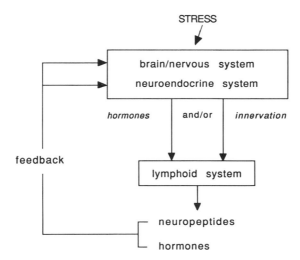

Figure 4.3. Summary of relationship between nervous, endocrine and immune systems. Typically, a stressor will evoke activity first in the nervous system. This will then, either directly or via the endocrine system, influence the lymphoid system. Activity there will feed back to influence the nervous and endocrine systems. (Source: Ballieux and Heijnen, 1987, figure 2, p. 75)

here presumably that their chances of an encounter with CRF would be greatest. Figure 4.3 shows some of the relationships between CNS, endocrine and immune systems that Blalock proposes.

A response on the part of the immune system is followed by an increase in the activity of neurons located in the ventromedial hypothalamus and an increase in plasma corticosteroid levels (Dunn, 1989). Accompanying the immune response, Besedovsky *et al*. (1983) found a decreased turnover of noradrenaline in neurons that project into the hypothalamus. Besedovsky *et al*. (1983) suggested that removal of an inhibitory noradrenaline influence might be associated with increased activity in the medial hypothalamus.

Besedovsky and collaborators (see Dunn, 1987) were able to find a factor produced by *in-vitro*-stimulated lymphoid cells which had the effect of increasing hypothalamic activity. This stimulated the search for a 'lymphoid cell-derived neurohormone' (Ballieux and Heijnen, 1987), or as Dunn (1987) describes it, an *immunoneurotransmitter*. As Figure 4.3 shows, we are dealing with another feedback system. It appears strongly that IL-1 might be such an immunoneurotransmitter, acting via the hypothalamus to cause CRF secretion. Infection could be described as 'stressful' according to standard criteria: (1) decreases in

paraventricular nuclei noradrenaline and increases in the noradrenaline catabolite, 3-methoxy, 4-hydroxyphenylethyleneglycol, in
the hypothalamus and (2) increased activity by the pituitary–
adrenocortical system (Dunn, 1988, 1989). Figure 4.4 summarizes the
proposed interactions. Following the appearance of an antigen, macrophages produce IL-1. IL-1 then activates brainstem noradrenergic
neurons that innervate the hypothalamus. This results in CRF secretion, exciting the HPA axis and increasing plasma glucocorticoid levels. The loop is closed by the inhibitory effect of glucocorticoids upon
the immune system.

One interesting interaction between the immune system and the
nervous system is seen on examining body temperature (discussed in
Section 9.3). Exposure of rats, rabbits and humans to a stressor is
rapidly followed by a rise in body temperature (Singer *et al.*, 1986). It
has been suggested that prostaglandins are the primary mediator of
such stress-induced hyperthermia. In an experiment with rats exposed

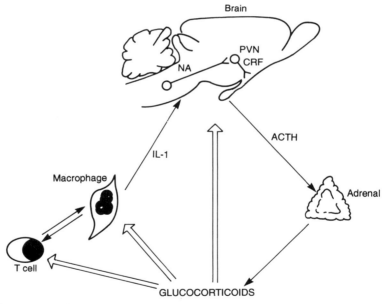

Figure 4.4. Interactions between interleukin-1 (IL-1) and the hypothalamic–
pituitary–adrenocortical axis. For explanation, see text. NA = noradrenaline;
ACTH = adrenocorticotrophic hormone; PVN = paraventricular nuclei; CRF =
corticotrophin-releasing factor. (Reprinted from Dunn, 1989. Copyright 1989,
with kind permission from Elsevier Science Ltd, The Boulevard, Langford
Lane, Kidlington OX5 1GB, UK)

to the stress of being placed in an open field, Singer *et al.* found that 69% of the rise in body temperature could be blocked by application of a drug that inhibits the synthesis of prostaglandins. Singer *et al.* compare stress-induced hyperthermia with fever induced by IL-1 following infection. IL-1 is thought to elevate the set-point of the temperature regulation system by means of stimulating the production of prostaglandins. Singer *et al.* speculate that exposure to a stressor might cause the release of IL-1, which in turn stimulates the release of prostaglandins. However, if this is the means by which stress-induced hyperthermia is mediated it implies something interesting about the source of IL-1. Stress-induced hyperthermia occurs more rapidly than the hyperthermia seen following intravenous IL-1 injection. Thus, IL-1 would be centrally produced, and Singer *et al.* speculate that it could be produced in the hypothalamus.

4.6   CONCLUDING REMARK

Even this cursory glance is sufficient to reveal something of the complex reciprocal interactions that occur between nervous, endocrine and immune systems. The existence of these interactions and their effects raise profound questions for understanding their functional significance and for developing a theoretical model of stress. At various points in the subsequent chapters the discussion will return to the immune system in the context of its reaction to particular stressors. For instance, the implications of effects upon the immune system will be discussed in later chapters in the context of depression and tumour growth, among other things. It is difficult to exaggerate the degree of care needed in discussing stress and the immune system and in considering the kind of interactions discussed in Chapter 4. We need to be careful about unitary concepts of stress and to avoid a simple blanket assumption that stress inhibits immune function. Rather, we need to investigate more cautious claims of the kind that '*some* stressors under *certain* conditions can depress *some* parts of the immune system'. Also we must not forget that stressors can have an effect on disease through means other than immune suppression (Maier, Watkins and Fleshner, 1994). For example, stressors change a variety of physiological parameters such as blood flow to various body regions. As will be discussed later, stressors such as divorce or bereavement can change many behaviours, e.g. decrease sleep and exercise, whilst increasing alcohol and cigarette consumption. Any of these obvious factors (or less obvious ones) might crucially increase susceptibility to disease.

Neurons in the hypothalamus secrete CRF in response to activation of the immune system, a criterion by which immune activation could be termed a stressor. This connection between immune and nervous systems is mediated by cytokines, especially IL-1, normally released by cells engaged in an immune response. The involvement of IL-1 is evidenced by the observation that its injection produces the effect on CRF even in the absence of infection or an immune response (Maier, Watkins and Fleshner, 1994). In addition to this effect upon stress hormones, IL-1 affects behaviour. A time of immune activation requires co-ordination of activities throughout the body and in interaction with the environment. Only the CNS can do this and so it is possible to make some sense of the existence of interactions between the immune system and the nervous system. Thus rats injected with IL-1 exhibit a reduction in exploratory, feeding and sexual behaviour. The animal is motivated to sleep, and especially slow wave sleep is shown, which reduces the brain's metabolic demands.

It is a challenging task to view the interactions between nervous and immune systems from the perspective of function. For instance what is the adaptive value in corticosteroids suppressing the immune system? Is this just of pathological interest or is it a useful adaptive physiological reaction? There are both costs and benefits attached to either immune activation or inhibition. The question concerns therefore when the *net* benefit of a reaction is greater than the *net* cost. Depending upon the circumstances, it might be more appropriate sometimes to restrain the immune system. So when is an immune response adaptive and when is it adaptive to put a brake on it? To attempt to answer this, it might be useful to distinguish two types of stressful situation.

First, there is a primarily local infection as a result of injury and invasion of pathogens, e.g. an unfortunate individual being bitten on a finger by an infected wild dog that then proceeds to harass for an hour or so as the individual takes avoidance action. Stress hormones would be activated by the traumatic encounter. Secondly, there is the kind of infection that is perhaps more 'whole body' as with AIDS or influenza and for this the process of infection was not accompanied by a stress reaction.

To make sense of the interactions between stress and immune systems, it could be useful to distinguish two phases of corticosteroid activation. The wild dog encounter would involve both of these but the influenza infection only one. For each of these we might be able to see adaptive reasons why corticosteroids might usefully inhibit the immune response.

Consider first the corticosteroid activation that comes from confrontation with an external stressor, e.g. an angry wild dog. In our evolutionary history, there might have been frequent encounters with jstressors that involved fight and flight. In the course of such encounters, tissue damage might well have resulted. Placing a distance between the victim and the source of the stress would have required a supply of nutrients to the skeletal muscles and a temporary suspension of inflammation and attending to wounds. When the danger has passed, corticosteroid levels would return to normal and this might be a better time for inflammation to proceed and wounds to be licked. The second phase of corticosteroid activation is not in response to the external stressor but to cytokines secreted by cells of the immune system. This phase would be common to both the wild dog bite situation and a non-traumatic source such as an infection with influenza. In both the wild dog and influenza situations, corticosteroids might serve to stop the immune response from getting too large.

Attempts to make sense of the link from nervous system to immune system via hormones commonly focus upon the role that corticosteroids serve in terminating inflammation. One possible line of logic is as follows. Inflammation is a crucial local response to local infection, a vital first line of defence. If successful, it serves to limit the damage to the local site. Cells of the immune system are brought in large numbers to the local site, which is richly supplied with blood. Components of the immune system enter what is termed positive feedback loops as a result of these events. For example, IL-1 stimulates further IL-1 release (Maier, Watkins and Fleshner, 1994). However, there is a danger that things can get out of control and the immune response can damage even uninfected intact tissue. Hence a restraint mechanism is needed and this is provided by corticosteroids. The commonly made assumption is that inflammation is rather rapid but the corticosteroid response to cytokines will be delayed following the onset of infection, so corticosteroids would offer their braking action after inflammation has had time to proceed (Maier, Watkins and Fleshner, 1994).

Chapter 5

Types of Stressor and their Effects

5.1 INTRODUCTION

This chapter looks at a range of different stressors and their effects upon the body. First, in the traditional mode, we look at separation distress, novelty and various kinds of aversive stimulation. A later section considers challenges to the physiological homeostasis of the body and what the body's response tells us about the nature of stressors. Then we look at how appetitive situations (e.g. gaining food) can reveal something about the processes responsible for stress reactions. The appropriateness of the model of stress proposed in Chapter 1, involving failed attempts at control, will be considered in the context of the animal's reaction to various stressors.

5.2 SEPARATION DISTRESS

In the terms of Chapter 1, separation might be understood in terms of disparity being created between a situation of social contact and one of loss, the animal being motivated to restore the previous state. Some observations on the hormonal and behavioural responses of infant squirrel monkeys to separation were made by Levine and Coe (1985). The condition of: (1) total separation from the mother was compared with (2) partial separation in which the infant could maintain auditory and olfactory, but not visual, contact. In condition 1, plasma cortisol concentration increased steadily over the 24 h of separation, reaching a value of 10 times basal level. In condition 2, the level peaked at 6 h. Infants in condition 2 showed significantly more distress vocalization than in condition 1. The disparity between the two possible stress indices, vocalization and corticosteroid response, points to the need to see such indices in context. One needs also to take strategy into account. As Levine and Coe argue: '. . . the calling frequency is a very poor index of the degree of emotional disturbance, but instead reflects the infant's attempts to reestablish contact with its mother and thereby cope with the stressful situation'. The animal in condition 1 might be described as having no active coping strategy, whereas that in condition 2 would seem to be making active, albeit unsuccessful, attempts to restore the *status quo*. There is some evidence that the cognitive processes that detect attachment and separation are closely connected with an endogenous opioid system, as is now discussed.

Herman and Panksepp (1978) observed infant guinea-pigs separated from their caregivers. Distress vocalizations were decreased by a morphine injection and increased by the opioid antagonist naloxone. This result led to the suggestion that the basis of separation distress is 'an endogenous endorphin withdrawal process'. Distress might then share some neural circuitry with pain. In such terms, social attachment would reflect a process analogous to addiction; the infant depends upon social contact to maintain endorphin levels.

Herman and Panksepp (1978) also observed the degree of proximity that infants showed to their mother when she was restrained in a small cage within the test arena. The amount of time spent in proximity was decreased by morphine and increased by naloxone. Both of these experiments suggest that the opioid agonist morphine can serve as a partial substitute for the caregiver. A somewhat analogous effect was observed by Keverne *et al.* (1989). They found that cerebrospinal β-endorphin levels increased during grooming in Talpoin monkeys. Grooming invitations and time spent grooming increased following administration of the opioid blocker naltrexone. Conversely, morphine administration reduced the number of invitations and time spent grooming.

The notion that an animal tracks its levels of endogenous opioids as indexed by a central affective state and that behaviour is motivated towards the end of maintaining this state seems a reasonable one. Opioids seem to meet the criteria of being rewards (Eikelboom and Stewart, 1982; Bozarth, 1987) and rats will adjust their levels of operant responding to maintain levels of exogenous opioids. That distress vocalizations might be reflections of a lowered central affect level is suggested by the observation that cocaine injections dramatically lower such vocalizations (Kehoe, 1989).

Hennessy *et al.* (1991) note that, in squirrel monkeys and guinea-pigs, separation is associated with both a high rate of vocalization and rising levels of cortisol. After a period of separation (60–90 min in guinea-pigs), vocalization falls to a low level in spite of an elevated level of activity in the hypothalamic–pituitary–adrenocortical (HPA) axis. They speculated that HPA hormones inhibit vocalization. Hennessy *et al.* found that that peripherally applied corticotrophin-releasing factor (CRF) caused a dramatic drop in the vocalization of guinea-pig pups separated from their mothers. The effect appeared not to be mediated via either adrenocorticotrophic hormone (ACTH)/ glucocorticoids or β-endorphin. It would appear then that one function of CRF is to shut down vocalization. Hennessy *et al.* speculate that peripherally administered CRF is able to cross the blood–brain barrier of guinea-pig pups and that the effect observed was a central one.

In neonatal rats, Kehoe (1989) observed ultrasonic vocalization (30–50 Hz) as a response to separation from the parent. Such a response can serve as a cue for retrieval by the parent. A role of opioids was implicated in this response (see Figure 5.1). The results cited earlier in this section indicated that social contact maintained endogenous opioid levels. However, Kehoe's results suggest that this is not true under all conditions. Isolation was associated with analgesia (see Chapters 1 and 8) which was reversible with the opioid antagonist naltrexone. Relative to saline-injected controls, morphine decreased the number of distress calls and increased the latency to lift the paw from a hot object. Naltrexone had quite the opposite effect of increasing the number of calls and decreasing the paw-lifting latency. This suggests that, under natural conditions, calling is inhibited by endogenous opioids. When their action is blocked by an antagonist, the bias is shifted towards calling.

A logical interpretation is that either the cognitive appraisal of separation or loss of some basic sensory input (or both) causes: (1) increased distress vocalization and (2) increased opioid levels. The latter then causes increased analgesia. However, it would appear that the effect of the increased opioid level is to decrease distress vocalizations from the level at which they would otherwise be.

As indexed by paw-lifting latency, it seems that proximity to an adult female, even to an anaesthetized virgin, decreased opioid levels. Similarly, distress vocalizations were sharply reduced by such proximity.

Naltrexone administered to pups in the nest did not induce vocalizaton but resulted in very high levels of vocalization when the pup was isolated. This suggests that vocalization is not a response to a blocking of the opioid system *per se* but rather a combination of the detection of separation and a blocking of opioids can act to induce vocalization.

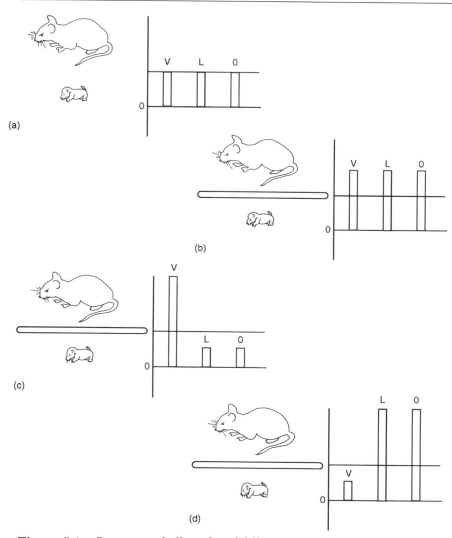

Figure 5.1. Summary of effects found following separation of neonatal mice based upon results of Kehoe (1989). (a) Normal condition of proximity to female with associated levels of opioids (in this case purely endogenous), distress vocalization and latency of paw-lifting; (b) the results following separation (saline injected), all three variables have increased; (c) separation combined with naltrexone injection indicating, in effect, decreased opioid levels, de-creased analgesia and increased distress vocalization; and (d) separation com-bined with morphine injection, indicating increased opiod levels, decreased vocalization, increased analgesia. O = effective opioid activity; L = latency of paw-lifting; V = distress vocalizations

The result raises the question of whether the action of endogenous opioids is to be understood in a broader context of giving a bias towards passivity as opposed to activity, in this case activity being represented by calling. Such an interpretation would fit with the evidence just given that activity on the part of the HPA axis seems to exert inhibition on the vocalization accompanying separation. In functional terms, it might be that with protracted separation the benefits of calling (presumably, in a natural situation, being found by the mother) are outweighed by the costs and an increased opioid-mediated bias towards passivity is exerted.

Clearly, theorists need to direct attention to the issue of when opioid levels are maintained or reduced by social contact. It is possible that different opioid sub-types are involved under the different conditions.

5.3 NOVELTY

The model (Chapter 1) suggested that animals are sensitive to disparity between the actual state of the world and some kind of reference value for that state. If this is so, then novelty might be expected to be a trigger for a stress reaction. For instance, placing an animal in a new environment would involve sensory inputs for which it has no pre-existing representation.

A change in stimulus input within an animal's environment can sometimes trigger activity in the HPA system. For rats and mice, increasing the degree of novelty of the animal's environment by increments was reflected in correspondingly incremented increases in corticosteroid levels (Hennessy and Levine, 1978; Natelson *et al.*, 1981). Electric shock causes a response that is only some 50% higher than that of simply being placed in the test box (Natelson *et al.*, 1981). By contrast, catecholamines show little response to novelty but respond in proportion to the intensity of sudden electric shock.

5.4 LOUD NOISE

Figure 5.2 shows the result of applying a loud noise to a group of rats three times in rapid succession. Note the immediate rise in plasma concentration of adrenaline and noradrenaline, and the delayed rise and fall of plasma corticosterone level. The delay in the rise of corticosterone can be attributed to the fact that it is the end-product of a series of hormonal events (De Boer *et al.* (1988); see Chapter 2). Note also the decline in response to the stressor over the three presentations. Whether a decline, no change or an augmentation in response as a result of repeated presentation is seen depends upon a number of parameters such as intensity, modality and any consequences, as well as individual differences between animals (Natelson *et al.*, 1988). One might reasonably assume that in this case the noise comes to be interpreted as relatively benign. Presumably, the noise was not intrinsically aversive and when the animal learned that it heralded nothing aversive, it was assimilated into its model of the world. By contrast, repeated exposure of rats to foot shock was found to be associated with no habituation of the response of either corticosterone or prolactin (Ratner *et al.*, 1989).

That there can be a diminution in response to the repeated presentation of a stressor that heralds no adverse consequences is used by Mikulaj and Mitro (1973) as an index of successful adaptation.

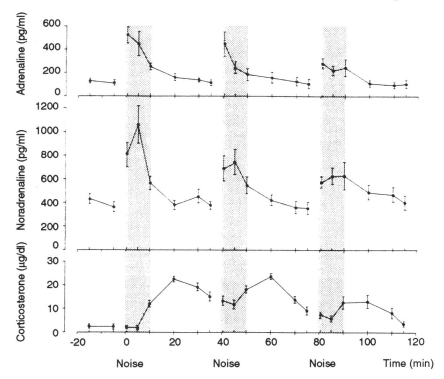

Figure 5.2. Responses of adrenaline, noradrenaline and corticosterone to repeated application of a 100 dB white noise stimulus in rats. (Reprinted from De Boer *et al.*, 1988. Copyright 1988, with kind permission from Elsevier Science Ltd, The Boulevard, Langford Lane, Kidlington OX5 1GB, UK)

Mikulaj and Mitro's way of considering adaptation is opposite to the assumption commonly found that '. . . the more intensive the adrenocortical reaction, the better the adaptation of an organism to stress'. As Mikulaj and Mitro note, this assumption would only be valid if the increasing reaction could be metabolically justified in terms of the energy needs of, say, fight or flight.

5.5 SOCIAL CONFRONTATION

Schuurman (1980) noted a rise in plasma corticosterone level following conflict in both winner and loser rats. The rise was higher and of longer duration in the losers than the winners. Following defeat, and after plasma corticosterone level had returned to normal, Schuurman looked at the effect of confronting the defeated animal with a non-aggressive conspecific. An elevation of corticosterone was seen. Controls not having a history of defeat showed only a minor elevation. This suggests the possibility of a learning process involving prediction of an aversive consequence of a social encounter. In the terms developed in Chapter 1, it suggests an estimation of future action required. This subject is looked at more closely in the next section.

Researchers have also investigated adrenomedullary events that accompany a history of victory or defeat in mice (Brain, 1980; Hucklebridge *et al.*, 1981), looking at adrenaline, noradrenaline and the enzyme that converts noradrenaline to adrenaline, phenylethanolamine *N*-methyltransferase (PNMT) (see Chapter 2). Victors but not losers showed an increase in the adrenal noradrenaline content. Compared with controls, the adrenaline content of the adrenal gland was increased little if at all in victors. However, a significant increase was measured in losers. Defeat increases PNMT activity. Victory was associated with some elevation of PNMT compared with the controls but to a much less extent than was seen in the losers. Brain (1980) suggests that the elevated PNMT activity of losers might be the consequence of elevated activation of the pituitary–adrenocortical axis accompanying defeat, an example of interaction between the two principal stress axes (see Section 2.4). Brain reports an accumulation of noradrenaline in the adrenals of victors but little increase in conversion of noradrenaline to adrenaline. There is a time lag between the experience of defeat and the conversion of noradrenaline to adrenaline and this is presumably accounted for by the time taken for corticosteroids to stimulate PNMT activity. This activity is at a maximum 12 h after defeat.

In interpreting these results, Hucklebridge *et al.* (1981) note that the rate of synthesis of noradrenaline from tyrosine is controlled by enzymes tyrosine hydroxylase and dopamine (DA) β-oxidase. In turn, they are stimulated mainly by neural activity in the sympathetic outflow to the adrenal. PNMT activity, the process responsible for conversion of noradrenaline to adrenaline, depends upon activity in the HPA axis. The authors also note that the anatomy of the mammalian adrenal is important here. Thus, chromaffin cells, which produce adrenaline are situated in proximity to blood coming from the adrenal cortex, which would be rich in corticosteroids. Hucklebridge *et al.* suggest that adrenocortical activity might play a part in the release of adrenaline. By contrast, noradrenaline cells are situated in proximity to medullary arteries, which would have a much lower level of corticosteroid activity. Such an organization, facilitating chromaffin cell stimulation by corticosteroids, is not seen in other vertebrate classes.

To place these results in context, Hucklebridge *et al.* (1981) note some findings showing that aggressive mice have been found to have higher adrenal noradrenaline contents than more docile animals. Also a number of researchers into human stress reactions have found an elevation of noradrenaline secretion to occur in situations of outwardly directed aggression. The more inwardly directed states described as fear and anxiety are associated with elevated levels of adrenaline.

5.6   AVERSIVE EVENTS THAT ARE PREDICTED

Central to understanding stress is the observation that the consequences of applying aversive stimulation can vary according to context. Section 5.6 looks at some of the contextual determinants starting with that of the role of prediction of aversive events. In terms of learning theory, learning that a stressor is predictable is expressed as learning a (stimulus$_1$) → (stimulus$_2$) cognition (Bolles, 1970; Dickinson, 1980; Ursin, 1988; Toates and Slack, 1990). The animal learns that a cue (stimulus$_1$) predicts the stressor (stimulus$_2$). If an animal is subjected to repeated presentation of a stressor, the effect can depend upon whether the stressor is predictable. For example, if a warning signal is sounded a few seconds before shock onset then the effect of the shock, as indexed by stomach ulceration, is less severe than for unsignalled shock (Weiss, 1971; Guile and McCutcheon, 1984). One possible explanation for this effect that is commonly offered is as follows. When shock is signalled by a tone, the tone acquires a fear-eliciting capacity. In the absence of the tone, the animal can relax. However, if the shock is unpredictable, then the whole apparatus acquires a fear-eliciting capacity and the animal can never escape from the stress-inducing cues. The elevation in corticosterone level is greater following unpredictable than following predictable shock (Weiss, 1970).

If a stressor is applied repeatedly then, in terms of its hormonal response, there can be signs of anticipation. For example, rats were exposed to the stressor of a cold environment for 10 min per day (Burchfield, 1979; Burchfield *et al.*, 1980). After 3 months of such daily exposure, a clear anticipatory response was observed in that as much corticosteroid was secreted before exposure to the stressor as during it. Burchfield *et al.* assume the conditional stimulus to be something such as noise made by the experimenter. This result might be interpreted in terms of activation of corticosteroids as a result of the anticipation of future demands to be made upon the body; the significance of the cue is assessed.

Arthur (1987) argues that the 'stress response', as indexed by corticosteroid changes serves an essentially *anticipatory* function regarding noxious, or at least challenging, stimulation. This would accord with the theoretical model proposed in Chapter 1, a trigger for corticosteroids being the anticipation of future demands. Arthur virtually equates stress with high levels of corticosteroids. He cites evidence to show high levels before combat in the Vietnam war and prior to a visit to the dentist. Anticipation of engaging in sport also evokes release, whereas muscular exertion tends not to do so unless the psychological element of competition is present (reviewed by Michael and Gibbons, 1963). In animal research, adrenocortical hormones are elevated in anticipation of a session of shock avoidance, sometimes even more so than during the session. They are elevated when the animal is uncertain as to which of several experiments it is destined, suggesting that a failure to be able to anticipate can trigger the HPA system (in accordance with the definition proposed in Section 1.4). Resolution of the uncertainty, even in the case of being allocated to a shock avoidance experiment (where presumably, if accomplished at the task, the animal can predict that coping is possible), can result in a lowering of level. Even for an animal having been exposed to sessions of inescapable shock, sometimes the corticosterone level is higher before the session than following the onset of shock.

Arthur (1987) notes a number of cases where corticosteroids are not elevated at times of actual confrontation with a potential stressor but during its anticipation. Whereas hospitalization was associated with high cortisol levels, the time immediately before surgery was not (certainty of future?). Yet he acknowledges that the latter time is distressing by the criterion of subjective feelings. Similarly, anticipation was associated with higher levels of cortisol than was confrontation in the case of phobics undergoing exposure therapy. Such indices of distress as screaming, weeping and labile heartbeat were exhibited during confrontation. Arthur notes that several studies have shown that parents experience elevated corticosterone levels during the time of their children's hospitalization but these levels dropped with the death of the child. He concluded that '. . . neither human beings nor animals show high levels of corticosteroids during exposure to repeated and expected stressors'.

It is not difficult to imagine that corticosteroid activation as a learned response to certain cues could be adaptive. For example, a cue predictive of a rival, a predator or cold exposure could help prepare the body for the physical/metabolic exertion that might shortly follow. Considering exposure to aversive stimuli, evidence suggests that evolution has programmed a simple rule into the system: activate the HPA system in situations in which aversive events are expected. For this effect to be shown, it is not a necessary condition that the animal should have learned to react in an active way (involving metabolic cost) to the aversive event that is predicted. For example, in rats, a cue predictive of shock in an enclosed environment for which the only obvious reaction is an inhibition of ongoing appetitive behaviour accompanied by cardiac deceleration, is associated with HPA activation (Auerbach and Carlton, 1971). It is perhaps not surprising that HPA activation does not depend upon the rat having an active response available to perform to the predicted event; animals can learn about events in the outside world for which no response was performed at the time of learning (Dickinson, 1980). Also the context might change and, in the case of a cue predictive of shock, the animal might be able in the future to perform an active response to the cue (with associated metabolic cost). Thirsty rats confronting a solution that in the past had predicted gastrointestinal discomfort also show HPA activation (Smotherman et al., 1976a).

Anticipation is, however, broader than simply to anticipate aversive events. As will be shown later, anticipation of food is also associated with a rise in corticosteroid levels. In a more metaphorical sense, it might be said that, in rats, corticosteroids are also activated towards the end of the light period of the 24 h light/dark cycle (see Sections 2.3.2.2 and 5.11.1) in 'anticipation' of the active period to follow. A broader formulation for which some evidence has already been brought is that anticipation of the *possible future need to take action* triggers corticosteroid release. If the demands of such action are uncertain or if the anticipated event is aversive, then the response is relatively large. The anticipatory response will also be high even if the anticipated event is unavoidable shock for which no response has, in the past, been helpful. The notion of anticipation of 'possible action' also might be appropriate here.

Arthur (1987) interprets the role of the pituitary–adrenocortical system in permitting:

> . . . organisms to anticipate dangerous events and to take action to avoid them, to escape them, or to modify their impact before they occur, not at the time they occur. Organisms who are able to anticipate dangers and able to take appropriate coping action before the dangers occur, can survive better than organisms who do not have this ability.

The physiological function of corticosteroids was described in Chapter 2. An additional function attributed to them by Arthur is that of arousal and vigilance in the face of oncoming threat (see Chapter 7). In these terms, if we equate stress with corticosteroid levels, as Arthur notes: 'Physiological stress seems to be more closely related to the intention of the organism to be vigilant and to be ready to take corrective action than to distress and suffering'.

Given a choice between exposure to an environment associated with predictable or unpredictable shocks, animals mostly, but not always, tend to favour the predictable (Abbott et al., 1984). Logically from this, as Abbott et al. note, one would tend to argue that predictable shock is less stressful than unpredictable shock. By the indices of ulceration, weight loss and plasma corticosterone levels, this sometimes is the case but it is not always so. Regarding the animals for which this does not apply, Abbott et al. argue: '. . . it seems intuitively unreasonable that subjects would prefer those conditions that were sometimes found to be more physiologically debilitating'. Intuitively unreasonable it may be but there is evidence of animals opting for that which physiologically seems least desirable. For example, on some schedules animals actually act so as to deliver shock (McKearney, 1968), rats sometimes show a preference for non-nutritive saccharine solution over nutritious foods (Valenstein, 1968) and will risk hypothermia for a highly palatable meal even in the presence of free food (Cabanac and Johnson, 1983). It is perhaps not altogether surprising that, in the predictable versus unpredictable choice, animals occasionally opt for that which can be shown to be physiologically harmful. Nature's wisdom is severely constrained. Evolution has equipped animals with highly effective survival mechanisms but these might not be manifest in obvious ways under the contrived situation of a laboratory experiment. Damage due to exposure to a stressor (e.g. weight loss, ulceration) is of a relatively long-term nature. Animals can form associations over long intervals, such as (taste) → (gastric illness) but these tend to be particular adaptations in situations that might well have been encountered in the species' evolutionary history. It is difficult to see how long-term future effects of stressors could be expected to influence present choice, and there is some evidence that the preference for predicted shock is more evident under conditions of short-term exposure (Abbott *et al.*, 1984).

An animal might be able to predict a stressor but it might instead, or in addition, be able to exert control over it. The next section looks at the role of control.

5.7 THE ROLE OF CONTROL

Having control over the environment can involve learning; in terms of contemporary learning theory (Bolles, 1970; Ursin, 1988; Toates and Slack, 1990), animals that are able to exert control might do so by learning a (response) → (outcome) cognition. They learn that the consequence of their action is termination of aversive stimulation. In terms of the model proposed in Chapter 1, learning a (response) → (outcome) cognition and successfully acting upon it in the face of aversive stimulation is a way of completing the feedback loop; behaviour closes a loop that would otherwise be open. Having control over a stressor can affect its impact in terms of the corticosteroid and catecholamine response as well as the ulcerogenic effect.

A study on the effects of control over high-intensity noise in rhesus monkeys was reported by Hanson *et al.* (1976). Animals having control showed normal levels of plasma cortisol whereas those *exposed to the same noise* but lacking control had elevated levels. It is important to emphasize that the difference between groups was not in the amount of exposure to external noise as animals in the two groups were exposed to identical load noises. The group with control were able to terminate the loud noise by responding whereas those 'yoked' to them were passive in the face of the stimulation. In monkeys, there is some evidence that, on first exposure to aversive stimulation, corticosteroid activity is high but, if with time action can be taken to avoid the stimulation, so the corticosteroid activation diminishes (Mason, 1968). What seems to be particularly stress evoking is to have control over a situation and then to lose that control, i.e. a closed-loop situation goes on open-loop and an established expectation is disconfirmed.

This appears to be more stressful than never having experienced control at all (Overmier *et al.*, 1980).

In an experiment by Weiss (1968, 1971), rats were subjected to electric shocks applied to the tail. Animals were shocked in pairs both receiving identical shocks. One rat of each pair, the active rat, could terminate the shock by turning a wheel at the front of the cage. The other rat, although having a wheel available, was not able to influence the shocks by its behaviour. It was yoked to the behaviour of the first rat. Active rats gained weight faster and had fewer stomach lesions than the yoked passive rats. By these measures, an aversive situation over which the subject can exert some control is less stressful than one over which no control can be exerted. Weiss argues that making the response yields *relevant feedback*. Behaviour that provides such relevant feedback is sometimes termed a *coping strategy*. The information is gained that a shock-free period will follow the response. Any such responses on the part of the yoked rat will not yield useful information.

However, by other physiological measures there might not always be a differentiation of impact between controllable and uncontrollable stressors. Maier *et al.* (1986) looked at the plasma ACTH and corticosterone levels following exposure of rats to either controllable or uncontrollable shock. The elevation and subsequent decline in plasma levels were not significantly different between the two conditions. Similarly, in a study on mice, Prince and Anisman (1990) found that controllable and uncontrollable stressors were both associated with elevations in corticosteroid level. Prince and Anisman suggested that, where a *prepared response* can be utilized in exerting control, there will be a discrimination in hormonal response between controllable (relatively low HPA activation) and uncontrollable (relatively high HPA activation) conditions. A prepared response is one that in such a situation the animal is most likely to perform, a species-typical response in the context considered, e.g. attack in response to an intrusion or shock.

Under some conditions, there seems to be a correlation between the degree of ulceration and the levels of corticosterone reached during exposure to a stressor (Weiss, 1971). It is tempting to suggest in the spirit of Selye (see Chapter 1) that different levels of corticosterone might cause the different levels of ulceration. However, there is reason for caution here. In fact, the high levels of corticosterone and ulceration appear to represent a correlation rather than a causal link. Ratner *et al.* (1989) tried independently manipulating corticosterone levels in rats exposed to stressors and found ulceration to be independent of corticosterone level. (Interestingly, Weiss, 1970, found unpredictable shock to be associated with both more ulceration and higher corticosterone levels than the same shock delivered predictably.) Other evidence also points to there being no causal link between cortico-steroid levels and ulceration, as discussed next.

Not only are the effects of exposure to a stressor different, depending upon whether control can be exerted, but also subsequent effects of stressor exposure can depend upon whether there has been a history of exposure to controllable shock. By the criterion of gastric ulceration, exposure to a controllable shock has a protective effect upon the animal when it is subsequently exposed to restraint stress (Overmier et al., 1985). By contrast, exposure to an uncontrollable shock tends to have a harmful after-effect. Overmier et al. investigated the nature of the process underlying the protective effect of controllable shock. They reasoned that the response constituted a predictive signal, a signal that a shock-free period will now occur. So could a similar protective effect be obtained if an instrumental contingency was not in operation but an auditory signal was given at the end of shock? This would convert a state of control to one of prediction. Overmier et al. found that exposure to such a shock-signal combination did offer significant protection against the subsequent stressor of restraint. Interestingly, such rats, although protected against gastric ulceration, had elevated levels of plasma corticosterone relative to restrained controls not hav-ing prior shock exposure. By contrast, rats able to exert control show decreased levels of plasma corticosterone. This result also argues against there being a simple causal link between high corticosterone levels and gastric ulceration.

Swenson and Vogel (1983) looked at yoked rats subjected to electric shocks where one rat, termed the 'coper', could terminate the shock by manipulating a pole and the other, the 'non-coper', could not. The lev-els of peripheral and central catecholamines and plasma corticosterone were investigated before and after a 1 h exposure to the stressor. Both copers and non-copers showed an increase in plasma corticosterone levels. The increase was longer lasting in the non-copers. The effect of the coping variable was shown also for plasma adrenaline levels. For coping rats, plasma adrenaline was elevated relative to baseline be-tween 1 and 30 min. For rats without control, plasma adrenaline was elevated relative to baseline and to the coping rats between 5 and 90 min. For both groups, plasma noradrenaline rose within 1 min of shock onset. In the coping rats, plasma noradrenaline was significantly ele-vated for the first 30 min. Non-coping rats had plasma noradrenaline levels elevated relative to coping rats at 5 and 15 min.

Concentrations of noradrenaline and adrenaline and DA in the hypo-thalamus were measured. For noradrenaline, coping rats were not different to unshocked controls at any time. Non-coping rats were depleted of noradrenaline in the hypothalamus relative to both copers and unshocked controls, this achieving statistical significance at 60 and 90 min. This difference had disappeared by 3 h after shock termination. There were no significant differences between the three groups in adrenaline levels in the hypothalamus at any time. Thus, in this particular study, having control over a stressor was, relative to lack of control, associated with: (1) a lower adrenal catecholamine response; (2) lower corticosteroid response; and (3) maintenance of hypothalamic catecholamine levels.

This section has considered active coping but another technique is to study so-called passive avoidance, where an aversive stimulus can be avoided by not responding. Goesling *et al.* (1974) claim that not only active but also passive strategies that succeed in avoiding shock also provide an ameliorating effect on bodily measures of stress. Thus rats placed in a passive avoidance situation showed less severe gastric ulceration than yoked controls whose behaviour was not instrumental in ameliorating shock stimulation. However, there is a problem in interpreting this study; the rats were food deprived and placed in running wheels. The yoked controls showed more running by a factor of about 100–200 than their partners. As running in a hungry rat is ulcerogenic (Chapter 6), one cannot be sure that controllability *per se* was implicated or whether the results reflect a difference in running. In other words, would the same result have been obtained in an avoidance task in which the master rat simply had to stay on a platform and not stepdown?

The effect of shock on brain catecholamines, briefly introduced in this section, is explored further in the next section.

5.8   EFFECTS OF UNCONTROLLABLE AVERSIVE STIMULATION

Suppose that a group of rats has been exposed first to a series of uncontrollable shocks. Subsequently, they are tested in a situation where control can now be exerted: for instance, they can avoid shocks by shuttling from one side of a box to another when a warning signal is sounded. Typically, the experience with uncontrollable shock causes a deficit in behaviour to be revealed in the second phase of the experiment where the opportunity for control is provided (Weiss *et al.*, 1979). Similarly, if the second phase of the experiment requires the rat to swim rather than shuttle, then prior experience with uncontrollable shock is followed by less active swimming and struggling and more passive behaviour, such as floating (Weiss *et al.*, 1981). (Subsequently, less grooming in the home cage is also shown.)

This phenomenon is termed *learned helplessness* by some authors (Seligman, 1975). Some recognizable biochemical changes occur in the brain following exposure to uncontrollable aversive stimulation and some authors focus upon learning as the explanation and some upon the biochemical events. Controversy surrounds which is the most appropriate formulation, with authors noting a similar failure to learn following exposure to uncontrollable positive events (e.g. food reward) (Overmier *et al.*, 1980). However, there is no reason why both learning of cognitions about the world and the biochemical changes are not jointly implicated.

Weiss *et al.* (1981) argue that the behavioural deficit can be explained in terms of depletion of brain noradrenaline levels (particularly in the locus coeruleus; LC) arising from exposure to uncontrollable shock. Part of their argument is that, in an experiment in which a behavioural deficit was manifest 24 but not 48 h after exposure to uncontrollable shock, levels of noradrenaline had returned to normal by 48 but not by 24 h. On exposure to a stressor, both utilization and synthesis of noradrenaline and DA are increased (Anisman and Zacharko, 1986). Depletion will occur if synthesis is unable to keep pace with utilization. According to this model, depletion of noradrenaline removes a source of *inhibition* that the noradrenaline neurons normally exert within the LC. Thereby, another set of neurons are activated. These now abnormally activated neurons project beyond the LC (Weiss and Simson, 1988).

Correlation does not of course prove causation; the neurochemical changes might simply parallel the behavioural changes without mediating them, a point acknowledged by Weiss *et al.* (1981). However, they favour the idea that the noradrenaline changes mediate the behavioural changes. Their grounds, among others, are that pharmacological disruption, reducing noradrenaline concentrations or increasing acetylcholine concentrations, can have very similar effects to uncontrollable shock (reviewed by Anisman and Zacharko, 1986). On exposure to uncontrollable shock, pharmacological protection of noradrenaline levels prevents the appearance of the behavioural deficit.

Anisman and Zacharko (1982) suggest that initial amine release might be the basis for coping attempts and so long as such heightened amine activity occurs the animal will make coping attempts. However, such elevated release might set the scene for subsequent reduced amine levels and failure to make coping attempts. In the extreme, under these conditions and with exposure to subsequent aversive stimulation, the setting might be the one that, in humans, we associate with depression (see Chapter 10).

Weiss *et al.* (1981) argue that noradrenaline depletion produces a 'motor activation deficit', meaning a deficiency in performing *active* behaviour in response to the stressor. Exposure to an uncontrollable stressor can sometimes cause what might be termed 'neurochemical sensitization'. Relatively little depletion of noradrenaline is seen and yet, on the next day, what would be considered a mild stressor is associated with a sharp reduction in noradrenaline levels (Anisman and Zacharko, 1986). It was argued that conditioning might well play an important part in this. Weiss *et al.* (1981) also consider this factor. They suggest that behavioural deficits seen on occasion 48 h after the session of uncontrollable stress cannot be explained in terms of an intrinsically low noradrenaline level at that stage, as recovery has occurred by then. Rather, the level of noradrenaline might be classi-cally conditioned. Simply removing an animal from the home cage and placing it in an experimental context might, by Pavlovian conditioning, cause a lowering of brain noradrenaline levels.

Conversely and somewhat paradoxically, under some conditions, re-peated exposure to an uncontrollable stressor is associated with nei-ther noradrenaline depletion nor a behavioural deficit, but a process that Weiss *et al.* term 'neurochemical habituation'. It is believed that this is due to an increase in activity of the enzymes that are involved in amine synthesis, thus enabling noradrenaline synthesis to keep pace with its depletion (Anisman and Zacharko, 1982, 1986).

Anisman *et al.* (1980) also observed a depletion of brain nor-adrenaline as a result of exposure to uncontrollable stress. By contrast, a controllable stressor did not cause a reduction in brain noradrenaline but rather 'immunized' against the effects of a subsequent uncontroll-able stressor. The depletion of brain noradrenaline that normally fol-lowed application of an uncontrollable stressor was prevented by a prior 'toughening-up' session of exposure to a controllable stressor. For severe stress, depletion of noradrenaline is accompanied by an in-crease in brain acetylcholine. Controllable stressors appear not to cause the increase in acetylcholine. It is possible that the rise in acetyl-choline is a consequence of the fall of noradrenaline (Anisman, 1978).

In the light of later developments, a rather specific hypothesis was advanced by Weiss and Simson (1985). The behavioural depression caused by exposure to uncontrollable shock was found to correlate most closely with depletion of noradrenaline at a specific brain region, the LC (Chapter 3). This is, in turn, associated with decreased noradrenaline release. In support of this interpretation, it was found that 'immunization' against the effect of uncontrollable shock could be obtained by infusing into the LC a drug that prevents the breakdown of noradrenaline. Emphasis on the importance of abnormalities in noradrenaline at the base of behavioural depression does not preclude a role also for other transmitters, such as DA, acetylcholine and serotonin. Indeed, as Weiss and Simson note, the LC is influenced by, and influences, neurons employing such transmitters.

Kvetnansky et al. (1976) subjected rats to 150 min of immobilization stress. During this period, hypothalamic catecholamines fell by about 50%. A dramatic rise in plasma ACTH and corticosterone levels was observed. Of course, correlation does not prove causation, but Kvetnansky et al. suggested that this result lends support to the notion that central catecholamines serve to inhibit ACTH release (see Discussion in Chapter 3). Another possible causal explanation which is not mutually exclusive with this one is that elevated levels of ACTH depleted brain catecholamines. It is known that injected ACTH can deplete brain noradrenaline (Endröczi and Nyakas, 1976).

Recently, a new interpretation of immobility and helplessness has been presented by Minor et al. (1994a,b). They address the issue of the unconditional mediation of the effect and suggest that the metabolic homeostasis of the CNS (see Chapter 1) is disrupted by uncontrollable shock. In their argument adenosine plays a crucial part. Recovery corresponds to a restoration of the metabolic disturbance of the CNS. They argue against an interpretation in terms of the fundamental cause being disruption of a classical neurotransmitter.

5.9   AVERSIVE STIMULATION AND AGGRESSION

Considering hormonal reactions, one effective coping strategy in the face of noxious stimulation seems to be to perform aggressive behaviour. Rats housed in pairs and subjected to electric shocks normally fight each other immediately after the onset of shock. This is termed 'shock-elicited aggression'. Conner et al. (1971) and Levine et al. (1979) measured plasma ACTH and adrenocortical levels in rats following electric shock. They compared the condition when animals were housed individually with when they were housed in pairs (facilitating shock-induced aggression). For both groups, plasma ACTH was higher following shock than that of control animals. However, animals able to fight were significantly lower in ACTH than those shocked alone. Henry (1976) discusses what common-sense logic, rather than an

understanding of coping, might have predicted: 'Since paired animals
fight at the onset of shock, it might have been expected that the combination of shock with fighting would have elicited a greater pituitary
adrenal response than either stimulus alone'. However, in terms of
coping: 'It would appear that pairing changed the animals' perceptions.
Instead of experiencing helplessness and depression, the fighting was
associated with arousal of the classic Cannon sympathetic adrenal–
medullary response'.

As will be discussed later, an animal having some perception of
being able to control a stressor by an active strategy is one whose
sympathetic nervous system (SNS), rather than HPA, system is predominantly activated. However, quite how a result of Williams and
Eichelman (1971) should be interpreted in these terms is unclear. They
looked at blood pressure in the tail of rats subjected to shock, which
showed an elevation. Rats subjected to the same shock but paired,
hence showing shock-induced aggression, showed a *fall* in tail blood
pressure. Williams and Eichelman suggest that the result might be
due to differential release of adrenaline and noradrenaline under the
two different conditions, associated with escape and attack, respectively (see Sections 5.11.2 and 6.7). A similar effect to this was reported
by Laborit's group (see Laborit, 1986, p. 244). They tested rats under
one of three different conditions: (1) with the possibility of escape from
a shock-associated compartment; (2) with no possibility of escape; or
(3) with no possibility of escape but shocked in pairs, hence providing
the possibility of fighting. Only group 2 were found to show signs of
hypertension and Laborit refers to the protective effect of motor activity. Laborit associates this with different levels of peripheral noradrenaline secretion between, on the one hand, groups 1 and 3 (low)
and, on the other, group 2 (high) but it might be that different levels of
HPA activation underlie the difference. Either way, as Laborit argues,
this result does not fit with the common assumption that a defence
reaction lies at the origin of the development of hypertension.

Levine *et al*. (1979) argue that '. . . the reason shock-induced fighting
reduces arousal is that, like eating or drinking, fighting may also be a
consummatory response . . .'. In a similar vein, Weinberg *et al*. (1979)
suggest that there is an 'element of self-reinforcement' to fighting,
analogous to the act of feeding (in this context, feeding is discussed in
Section 5.11). They go on:

> We suggest that the reinforcement provided by engaging in this be-
> haviour serves to reduce arousal, thus enabling animals to cope with
> shock more effectively, and to exhibit altered pituitary–adrenal

responsiveness that more closely resembles that of controls rather than that of singly shocked animals . . .

Based upon experiments of the kind described here, homeostatic models of stress and coping are found in the literature. The explicit or implicit assumption is that by behaving in a way termed coping the animal can correct an abnormal and potentially harmful neurotransmitter or hormonal level. For example, Dantzer and Mormede (1983) discussed the fact that rats, exposed to shock and having the opportunity to fight, exhibited smaller rises in ACTH than animals housed singly. They argued: 'Fighting behaviour might therefore be seen as a very effective way for the animals to cope with the shock situation, because it enables them to reduce hormonal activation that would otherwise result from exposure to the physical stressor'. Similarly, Conner *et al*. (1971) argued that: 'This mechanism can serve an adaptive function by dampening the internal response which may be excessive and have damaging consequences'.

As this quotation illustrates, coping tends to be defined by the efficacy of a strategy in reducing activity of the HPA system. However, we have no unambiguous evidence that the actual level of ACTH or corticosteroids is monitored somewhere and a reduction in level serves to feed back and strengthen successful strategies that lead to it. This is what might have been expected from a control systems perspective on these claims. The claims also raise an interesting issue on the adaptive function served by HPA activation. Presumably there *is* an adaptive function and so is it necessarily adaptive to suppress secretion? It would seem to be an easier solution for evolution to have made the axis less sensitive rather than to produce processes that encourage the animal to inhibit it. Clearly, behavioural systems that serve to terminate a stressor are adaptive in their own right and there is evidence that stress-related pathology is less when species-typical behaviours can be recruited (see later in this section), quite apart from any associated effects upon the HPA axis.

Weiss *et al*. (1976) compared three conditions of receiving shock insofar as the gastric ulceration was concerned: (1) shocked alone; (2) shocked in the presence of a companion allowing aggression; and (3) shocked in the presence of a companion but with a glass partition dividing the two rats. The latter condition allowed the rat to perform aggressive-type behaviour but with no consequence as far as the opponent was concerned. Rats in condition 1 had much more severe gastric ulceration than in conditions 2 or 3. That 2 and 3 had a similar degree of ulceration indicates that performance of the aggressive response was instrumental. Weiss *et al.* consider aggressive behaviour in this situation to be a *coping response*. They add that for a non-circular definition of a response constituting a coping response, the response must provide 'relevant feedback'. They list three possible ways in which fighting might give such feedback: (1) the animal would have been fighting at the time of shock termination and therefore might have formed an association between its behaviour and shock termination; (2) fighting might in some way distract the animal; and (3) 'Certain highly prepotent responses in danger situations, such as fighting, might inherently produce their own relevant feedback'. Such feedback would not depend upon the outcome of the fight.

That the *performance* of certain defensive actions plays a part in ameliorating the effect of stressors, even though the response does not yield useful effects on the external world, was suggested by experiments of Guile and McCutcheon (1980). They argued that such responses are ones the animal is *prepared* to perform in an aversive situation. One such is struggling in response to shock. Preventing such struggling by restraint increased ulceration. Conversely, allowing a block of wood for the animal to chew reduced ulceration. It was suggested that chewing is a natural defence reaction for a restrained animal in an aversive situation and would, under natural conditions, serve the function of forming an escape route. (An anecdotal report by Marx (1972) described chewing of the walls of the cage in response to a shift of incentive (sucrose solution) to one that is less favoured.) In a similar vein, Anisman (1978) referred to fighting as a *species-specific defence reaction* (Bolles, 1970), performance of which might be expected to have comparable physiological effects to fleeing.

A notion of 'prepared response', albeit in a slightly different sense to that discussed so far, is central to Phillips' (1989) analysis of stress, which dovetails with some of the assumptions made here. He writes:

> Behavioural certainty is present when an organism is able to emit a behavioural response that *in the past* has led to a successful outcome. That response may then be described as 'a prepared response'; it exists as a behavioural unit that may be emitted at known energetic cost to an appropriate discriminative cue.

The expression 'in the past' is used by Phillips implicitly with reference to the life history of a given animal. An equally valid and not mutually exclusive interpretation would be in the life history of the species. Phillips did not intend the expression 'known energetic cost' to imply knowing in the cognitive sense and in this vein, looking at the species history, one might interpret 'known' to mean selected by evolutionary fitness. Thus, prepared responses would be those that not only have proven effective in terms of eliminating disparity but also can be associated with appropriate metabolic activation.

Parenthetically, it is worth noting that the research discussed here is relevant to broader issues of motivation and reinforcement in ethology and psychology. Under certain conditions, i.e. when an animal is in what might be termed an 'aversive state' as a result of pain or frustration (Cohen *et al.*, 1985), performance of aggression constitutes positive reinforcement. However, from this it is necessary to be cautious before claiming that animals have some intrinsic need, a spontaneous internal drive, to behave aggressively (Cherek *et al.*, 1973; Toates and Jensen, 1991) even though under some conditions aggression does seem to share certain features with appetitive motivations (Hogan and Roper, 1978; Potegal, 1979). There is some evidence of an effect that could be described as positive reinforcement or positive feedback underlying the control of aggression (see Section 9.5.3.7), as evidenced by such things as a priming and warm-up effect of aggressive behaviour upon further aggression (Potegal, 1979). Potegal postulates various positive and negative feedback processes between aggressive behaviour and an underlying motivational state. It is interesting to speculate in terms of such processes as to what might be responsible for mediating the effects of aggressive behaviour on gastric physiology.

A model of the relationship between noxious stimulation, behaviour and brain biochemistry was proposed by Stolk *et al.* (1974). It is similar to the model of Weiss and associates designed to account for the behaviour of isolated rats having access to a wheel. The model is based upon what happens when rats are subjected to foot shock under one of two conditions, alone or together. In the latter condition, rats engage in fighting, which can be viewed as a coping response. In the 'shock with partner' condition, aggressive behaviour is associated with an increased turnover of noradrenaline which, in turn, facilitates further shock-elicited aggression. By contrast, placing rats in the 'shock without partner' condition is followed by a decrease in turnover of noradrenaline, which in turn biases future behaviour away from displaying shock-elicited aggression. (Considering having control over shock by lever-pressing to have some similarities with performing aggression, as coping strategies, the model is congruent with the results of Swenson and Vogel (1983), discussed in Section 5.7.) The effects of two drugs are considered in terms of the model. Lithium carbonate treatment has effects on the brain which are similar to those observed postshock in the 'shock without partner' condition and decreases shock-elicited aggression. By contrast, rubidium chloride treatment causes changes similar to those observed after fighting and promotes shock-elicited fighting.

Sections 5.1–5.9 have considered various situations, e.g. exposure to novelty, infant separation and electric shock that might intuitively be felt to be more or less stressful. Section 5.10 discusses physiological regulation. This is in the face of such things as exposure to cold, which might be described as another example of aversive stimulation. However, Sections 5.10 and 5.11 show that the stress hormones can also react in the context of physiological regulation and appetitive situations. This will suggest a modification of the concept of what actually triggers these hormones from being in terms of events necessarily having aversive connotations to a broader concept of activation by events that call for action.

5.10   HOMEOSTASIS: REGULATION AND CONTROL

5.10.1   The Hypothalamic–Pituitary–Adrenocortical System

A number of challenges to the physiological homeostasis of the body stimulate an increase in ACTH secretion. The larger the magnitude of the disturbance, the larger the response (Dallman *et al.*, 1987). For example, insulin-induced hypoglycaemia in fasted rats, hypoxia and haemorrhage are potent stimuli. Stretch receptors at various points in the circulatory system are responsible for the ACTH response to haemorrhage.

Sometimes, after first responding, the pituitary–adrenal system returns to a pre-stress level in spite of continued chronic application of a stressor, such as cold (Sakellaris and Vernikos-Danellis, 1975). Decreased responding to repeated acute cold exposure can also be seen (Burchfield *et al.*, 1980). Without further examination, a number of possible explanations might be offered, such as depletion of hormones. However, in some such cases, application of a second stressor is associated with an *enhanced* response as a result of the exposure to the chronic stress. Clearly, depletion is not the answer in such cases. The system exhibits a form of memory and is changed by its exposure in spite of a return to pre-stress levels of hormones. Burchfield *et al.* (1980) refer to *adaptation* of the stress response on repeated exposure to a stressor that does not place undue demands upon the organism. A similar explanation presumably applies to the decreasing response to what is initially a novel environment (File and Peet, 1980).

An interesting question at the centre of discussions on what constitutes a stressor concerns the effect of a physiological challenge such as food or water deprivation, on the HPA system. Does a challenge to physiological homeostasis *per se* act as a trigger? Although some physiological challenges to homeostasis can be potent stimuli to ACTH secretion, it is not always the actual systemic physiological shift *per se* that is responsible. The challenge to homeostasis is sometimes inextricably associated with cognitive processing, emotional connotations and plans for behavioural action. Mason (1971) argued that, in many cases in the past study of stress, physiological challenges really owed their potency as stimuli for a stress response to their psychological impact. For example, there is evidence that muscular exertion is accompanied by HPA activation and it might be supposed that metabolic factors trigger it. However, Mason (1972) reports that 'when emotional reactions can be minimized, muscular activity *per se* may not elicit substantial changes in corticosteroid levels'. For another example, consider the case of food deprivation and the associated physiological challenge to homeostasis. Food-deprived animals often show elevated corticosteroid levels, suggesting that deprivation serves as a stressor. However, on closer examination it seems that deprivation is a state that *sensitizes* the system to potential stressors, such as the presentation of food to other animals in neighbouring cages. Such external stimuli would become actual stressors during food deprivation.

A similar logic applies to temperature 'stress' imposed by either hot or cold environments. Mason argued:

> Perhaps the only bodily response which might conceivably be equally appropriate, in a homeostatic sense, under conditions of both heat and cold would be a *behavioural* response of emotional arousal or hyperalerting preparatory to flight, struggle or other strenuous exertion which might serve to eliminate the source of heat or cold or to remove the subject from its presence.

and he continues '. . . if this interpretation is correct, then the "stress" *concept should not be regarded primarily as a physiological concept but rather as a behavioural concept*'.

Mason (1975) noted that, in the laboratory situations designed to study the role of so-called 'purely physiological' stressors, such as heat and exercise, it is extremely difficult to eliminate the psychological component of, for example, disturbance. Further he argues that when the psychological component is eliminated, activation of the pituitary–adrenal system is not seen. For example, giving fasting monkeys so-called 'placebo food', fruit-flavoured, non-nutritive cellulose fibre, prevents the rise in plasma corticosteroid level that would otherwise be associated with food deprivation. According to Mason, the stressor is not the energy state *per se*. From such a result, one might assume that the stressor is seeing another animal being fed or the presence of familiar cues to feeding but no food appearing, while being in an energy-deficient state. For another example, Mason argues that heat *per se*, if anything, depresses corticosteroid activity. Any activation on exposure to heat would be from the psychological discomfort rather than a rise in body temperature.

Ursin (1988) makes a similar claim to that of Mason, in terms of his activation model (Chapter 1). Ursin notes that activation does not increase as a linear function of hours of deprivation of, say, food or water, unless cues indicate that 'the actual value of that particular variable may be corrected'. For example, when an animal is housed in a cage where it has ascertained that no food or water is present, the optimal strategy is to sit still, thereby conserving resources. When a cue indicating that the deprivation period might be over is presented, then: (1) the animal is active and (2) activation as measured by hormones also increases.

Research subsequent to Mason's claim is not always easy to interpret in a way that would allow support or refutation. However, some evidence supports both Mason's claim and Ursin's related model. In humans, Santiago *et al.* (1980) found that plasma cortisol was relatively insensitive to falls in blood glucose level (as compared with the responsiveness of adrenaline and noradrenaline). Rovensky *et al.* (1981) found a diminution rather than an increase of plasma cortisol level in humans exposed to a hot water bath. In pigs, plasma catecholamine responses were found to be similar in both hot and cold environments (Ingram *et al.*, 1980).

In chickens, although some researchers have reported a rise in corticosteroid level as a function of food deprivation in immature birds (Scanes *et al.*, 1980), others have found that it does not occur in mature birds. In 16-week-old chickens, Freeman *et al.* (1983) found no consistent rise in corticosterone level as a function of food-, water- or combined food/water-deprivation. In a further experiment, using 3-week-old chicks, Freeman *et al.* (1984) obtained a result entirely congruent with Mason's theory. Water deprivation *per se* (removal of the water source) did not cause a rise in plasma corticosterone. However, if the birds were denied access to water by the source being covered with a nylon mesh such that it could still be seen, a rise was observed. In sheep, Parrott and Matthews (1991) reported that water deprivation *per se* did not cause elevated cortisol levels, although it could enhance the effects of restraint on activating cortisol.

In rats, Smotherman *et al*. (1976a) found that a single experience of quite severe combined food/water deprivation did not elevate corticosteroid level. Similarly, Mitev *et al*. (1993) found that a single experience of food deprivation had to be extended to somewhere between 48 and 72 h before an elevation of corticosterone level was seen. This was in spite of the fact that 48 h of deprivation was associated with a 40% fall in serum glucose concentration. This lack of response is perhaps surprising given the widely held assumption that corticosteroids are a powerful defence against a fall in blood glucose level.

Also using rats, Levine and Coover (1976) found that 24 h food and water deprivation was associated with a large increase in plasma corticosterone concentration. However, this does not necessarily argue against Mason's interpretation. Levine and Coover measured corticosterone concentration at the time when the rats would normally have received food. It is known that, by the index of their locomotor activity, rats are able to anticipate the time of feeding even in the absence of extrinsic cues (Bolles and Moot, 1973). It seems that what Levine and Coover and others in similar studies were observing was a corticosteroid response to *anticipated* feeding, sensitized by the state of deprivation (Coover *et al*., 1984). In rats, Lucke *et al*. (1980) observed a large (presumably ACTH-mediated) increase in plasma corticosterone concentration as a function of water deprivation. It would appear that this was in the absence of cues signalling the return of water availability, but we cannot be certain.

Mason's challenge to Selye's non-specificity theory complicates an already complex area. However, as Mason (1975) points out, the notion that a whole variety of different physiological conditions, heat, cold, fasting and so on, can all communicate at a common locus of hormonal release, is itself a profound challenge. Maybe invoking the CNS as the site of mediation makes it easier to grasp. As he notes: 'Of all the known responses of higher organisms, *emotional arousal is certainly one of the most ubiquitous or relatively "nonspecific" reactions common to a great diversity of situations'*.

Certainly, Mason's argument suggests that the applicability of simple stimulus–response or input–output models to understand stress will be very limited. Complex neural processing intervenes between the potential stressor and the reaction. Mason argues that such a perspective shifts the focus of the search: rather than asking how a hormonal response can be evoked by a variety of physiological stimuli (possibly implying a reflex arc), one needs to ask how emotional arousal is generated by a variety of stimuli (involving more complex information processing) and how this one factor then comes to effect endocrine release.

Mason (1975) also notes that, in terms of the principles of homeostasis, need generally determines response. But, he asks, how could a given physiological response be adaptive in serving the needs arising from, for example, both heat and cold? The specific physiological adjustments evoked by the temperature regulation system are indeed appropriate for loss and conservation of heat, respectively, and it is not clear as to how a unidirectional, non-specific adaptation would aid these physiological processes. The pituitary–adrenal response to heat might be maladaptive in terms purely of physiological homeostasis. He argues that the only general response that might be appropriate to any temperature stress is one of moving to a new environment and it is in this psychological/behavioural context that the stress response has evolved. Resources are mobilized for coping with the demand of finding a new environment.

Mason (1975) did not go so far as to argue that the pituitary–adrenal system responded only to psychological stimuli. There is some evidence to suggest that cold, hypoxia and haemorrhage are effective stimuli even in the absence of psychological concomitants. Furthermore, as Selye (1975) notes, lower animals that lack a nervous system and even plants show something like a stress response. He notes use of the terms 'psychogenic' and 'neurogenic' for the particular class of stressors whose role is mediated via the nervous system. However, it seems that in the context of homeostasis much of the input to the HPA system derives from the motivation and activation of behaviour in the context of appropriate cues. Normally behaviour so motivated would serve to restore equilibrium.

5.10.2   The Autonomic Nervous System

In pigs, Ingram *et al.* (1980) found no increase in plasma catecholamines as a function of food deprivation. The return of food was associated with an increase in plasma noradrenaline.

An effect of deprivation and incentive object availability on physiological responses, somewhat analogous to that of the HPA response discussed in the last section, can be seen in the autonomic nervous system (ANS), as indexed by heart rate (reviewed by Fowles, 1982). In rats, heart rate increases as a function of the length of water deprivation, provided that it is measured at, for example, the time of bar-pressing for water, but not in the absence of cues predictive of water. Food deprivation has a similar effect. The effect is seen in the presence of conditional stimuli predictive of food even in the absence of instrumental responding and therefore seems essentially anticipatory, rather than responsive to effort exerted. Along with active avoidance of shock, the effect of appetitive cues was interpreted by Fowles (1982) in terms of 'a preparation for the activation of behaviour', a topic addressed again in the next chapter.

Thus evidence from both the HPA system and from the ANS shows that under some conditions activation is associated with external stimuli acting in association with physiological states. The external stimuli are ones that signal the need for activity on the part of the animal.

5.11 APPETITIVE SITUATIONS

Section 5.10 discussed homeostasis and, in order to understand the role of physiological states, it was necessary to consider incentive objects. Section 5.11 looks more closely at incentive presentation and what it tells us about the control of stress hormones.

5.11.1 Effects of Returning Food and Water after Deprivation

In rats maintained on a 12 h light/12 h dark cycle and *ad libitum* food and water, the circadian rhythm of corticosterone level shows a peak just before the rat's active period of 12 h lights off. If, however, food or water is made available for only a (regular) period of time during the 24 h cycle, corticosteroid will come to peak just before the missing commodity is made available, in other words there is a powerful shift of the phase of the circadian rhythm (Endröczi, 1972; Johnson and Levine, 1973; Krieger, 1974). On a water deprivation schedule, the rise in corticosterone just before restoration of water shows some adaptation over days of repeated deprivation–restoration (Endröczi, 1972), which one might theorize reflects a learning effect: the situation becomes more predictable. As noted in Section 5.10.1, Levine and Coover (1976) maintained rats on a schedule of 23 h deprivation and 1 h access to food and water. At the end of the 23 h period, plasma corticosterone was elevated six-fold compared with *ad lib* fed and watered controls.

If at the time of the expected return of water, the water fails to materialize there is a further elevation in secretion of corticosterone (Endröczi, 1972). Replacing the missing food and/or water leads to a very rapid drop in plasma ACTH and corticosterone level (Levine and Coover, 1976; Heybach and Vernikos-Danellis, 1979a,b). So rapid is the drop that it cannot be accounted for by metabolic changes from assimilation of food or water.

Merely replacing an empty drinking bottle causes a fall in corticosterone level similar to returning water. Presumably, the rat discovers rather soon that it has been duped by the empty spout. Thus the rapid decline in plasma corticosteroid is, not surprisingly, followed by an elevation, in fact to a level above that at the end of the 23 h deprivation period.

In a similar vein to discussions of aggressive behaviour (Section 5.9), Gray *et al*. (1978) suggest the possibility: '. . . that adrenocortical suppression represents a neuroendocrine correlate of the process of reinforcement'. Interestingly, electrical self-stimulation of the brain, which seems to have features in common with the reinforcement associated with performance of species-typical behaviour (Glickman and Schiff, 1967), causes inhibition to be exerted on the HPA system (Endröczi, 1963, p. 63).

Looking more closely at the situation where a missing commodity is returned, what is it exactly that has the effect of suppressing the HPA axis? Levine *et al*. (1979) discuss two processes. They argue that '. . . performance of the consummatory response *per se*, rather than thirst reduction, satiation or some peripheral effect of water intake . . .' is implicated (a similar argument to that applied to aggression; see Section 5.9). They suggest that conditioning is also implicated, as do Coover *et al*. (1977), who noted that stimuli associated with daily feeding, e.g. entry of the experimenter, caused a drop in corticosterone. Such conditioning would presumably be strongly implicated in the situation where merely returning an empty spout was associated with HPA suppression. Endröczi (1972, p. 80) suggests that, in rats, the increased activity that occurs at about the time of the light to dark transition in 24 h light/dark cycle plays a part in the lowering of plasma corticosterone seen at this time.

Logically, one would suppose that the fall in plasma corticosterone level on return of a missing commodity is due to a fall in plasma ACTH level. Heybach and Vernikos-Danellis (1979a,b) concluded that it was due to an active CNS inhibition of ACTH secretion. However, observations by Wilkinson *et al*. (1982) showed that the decrease in corticosterone level is too rapid to be accounted for by the fall in ACTH level alone, suggesting active inhibition at the adrenal (this possibility was also discussed by Gray *et al*., 1978). Various mechanisms that might be implicated were considered (Section 2.4 discussed a neural input to the adrenal cortex).

One possible interpretation of these results is that activation of the HPA system is triggered by the information processing underlying the search for a strategy of goal-directed (often termed 'appetitive') behaviour, usually involving locomotion. The goal in this case would be to obtain food. Thus both the situation of no cues to incentive availability (deprivation of food/water in the absence of any cue to food/water res-toration) and the situation of availability of food/water following de-privation is associated with low HPA activation. Logically, it might be argued that neither situation would be associated with the information processing involved in finding a goal-directed strategy. The intermedi-ate situation of cues being present predictive of availability (e.g. on a regular feeding schedule, the lapse of time corresponding to when food is normally given), but with some uncertainty (e.g. food has not yet appeared), is one of activation of the HPA system. Such an interpreta-tion is similar to that of Ursin (1988) who argued that both: (1) no food and no cues to food present and (2) food present are situations of certainty, associated with low activation. The situation of some uncer-tainty as to whether food might arrive is associated with high HPA activation.

Interestingly, in pigs, Ingram *et al.* (1980) found that the level of plasma noradrenaline increased following onset of a meal. This point will be taken up again, where it will be suggested that an elevation might be associated with control, certainty and the performance of consummatory behaviour.

5.11.2 Instrumental Tasks

Experiments have studied the hormonal profile of rats performing in-strumental tasks for food in Skinner boxes. Suppose a rat has learned to lever-press for food. The size of reward is then reduced. There is an increase in pituitary–adrenal activity, a so-called 'frustration effect' (Goldman *et al.*, 1973). Conversely, if the actual reward is larger than what the rat has come to expect, an 'elation effect' is obtained, a de-crease in pituitary–adrenal activity to below its basal level. This is strongly suggestive of a process of monitoring the state of the world, a comparison with expectation and an excitatory or inhibitory input to the HPA system based upon the outcome.

In an experiment in which rats were reinforced with food pellets for pressing a lever, Davis *et al.* (1976) obtained results that supported the general assumptions of Weiss' model (described earlier in this chapter) in terms of relevant feedback. After training, a group of rats was put on to extinction, meaning that pellets are no longer delivered for a lever-press. Extinction, i.e. responding but without the normal consequences of food arriving, was associated with an elevation of plasma cor-ticosterone. However, for another group, omitting the lever from the apparatus did not lead to an elevation. Hence, the rise in corticosterone levels of the extinction group could not be attributed to being placed in the Skinner box in the absence of food. Rather it was the performance of lever-pressing but without the feedback of food arriving. In terms of learning theory (Bolles, 1972), the rats had learned a (response) → (outcome) cognition which, in the extinction phase, was not confirmed. Coe *et al.* (1983) observed rats that received food pellets without having to perform a response. When the pellets no longer arrived, corticosterone level increased. Presumably, such rats would simply have learned to expect food in the experimental context and without making any response, an expectation that was subsequently disconfirmed.

Coe *et al.* (1983) found that for both operantly rewarded rats and their passive yoked controls, reinforcement lowered corticosterone level and extinction increased it. The patterns were very similar for active and passive subjects. They suggested that:

> ... when an instrumental response is learned in acquisition, performance of this response may be necessary to evoke corticoid elevations during extinction. However, when an instrumental response has not been learned in acquisition, adrenal responses to extinction can readily occur in the absence of instrumental responding.

In terms of learning theory, these results suggest disconfirmation of response → outcome and stimulus → stimulus expectancies, respectively, as the factor.

The elevated level of corticosteroids that accompany extinction is not seen in rats with lesions to the hippocampus (Coover *et al.*, 1971). In a comprehensive theory of hippocampal function, O'Keefe and Nadel (1978) see this result as evidence for: (1) the role of the hippocampus in the detection of disparity between expectation and reality and (2) an input of information concerning disparity from the hippocampus to the HPA system.

Hennessy and Levine (1979) propose that: 'When animals press levers for rewards, feedback from two sources may be important: (1) response-produced proprioceptive feedback from the appetitive behaviour itself, and (2) stimulus feedback provided by the reinforcing event'. These are, to some extent, separable. Davis *et al.* (1976) trained rats to earn food pellets on a VI schedule (where rewards are spaced apart by varying amounts according to a schedule set by the experimenter), and then various 'extinction-type' terms were imposed on different groups: (1) rats were put on standard extinction terms; (2) the contingency between bar-pressing and reward was removed, but free pellets were delivered on a VI schedule (R-FF); (3) rats were placed in the apparatus with the lever removed; and (4) rats were placed in the apparatus with the lever removed but given free pellets on a VI schedule. Only in condition 1 was there an elevation in corticosteroid level above the normal VI baseline level. However, rats extinguished bar-pressing in conditions 1 and 2. Condition 2 demonstrates that breaking the close contingency bar-pressing → reward, which is necessary for maintaining responding, does not necessarily excite the pituitary–adrenal system. Davis *et al.* state: 'These data are not consistent with a simple model of expectancy. This hypothesis would have predicted an elevation in corticosteroids for the R-FF group insofar as the lever-press response no longer leads to the same consequence'. Of course, this depends upon how simple the simple model in question is. It might be that, given the nature of a VI schedule, the rats did not distinguish between the conditions prevailing during training and those in condition 2. The result for condition 3 shows the importance of the response component in a situation where the expectancy is response dependent.

De Boer *et al.* (1990) examined both catecholamine and corticosterone levels in the plasma of rats during food-rewarded operant behaviour and extinction. The Skinner box had the facility to change between lever retracted and lever available conditions. Figure 5.3 shows the result. A slight anticipatory rise in noradrenaline level was shown in the 30 min period after being placed in the test apparatus and prior to the lever being made available. When the lever was made available in the operant chamber and food available contingent upon lever pressing (condition A), a sharp rise in plasma noradrenaline level was noted relative to the prior lever retracted condition. Plasma adrenaline changed little if at all. For plasma corticosterone, the period in the Skinner box prior to the lever being made available was characterized by a rise in level. Access to the lever in the food available condition (A) was associated with a fall to baseline level.

Under extinction conditions (C), after the lever was made available a very different hormonal response was observed. Noradrenaline level changed little relative to baseline. The elevated level of corticosterone remained elevated. Plasma adrenaline showed a sharp increase. In other words, reinforcement was associated with a high noradrenaline/adrenaline ratio and extinction was associated with a low noradrenaline/adrenaline ratio. When extinction conditions were imposed after 10 min of reinforced responding (condition B), the rise in noradrenaline level was reversed. De Boer *et al.* associate the high noradrenaline/C ratio of reinforced responding with the state of having *control* whereas the low noradrenaline/C ratio of extinction characterizes the state of *loss of control*. By a similar logic, a high noradrenaline/adrenaline ratio characterizes control and a low noradrenaline/

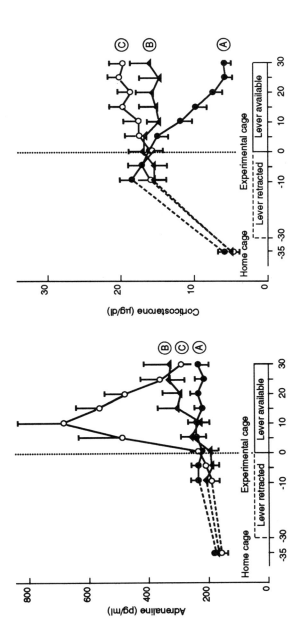

Figure 5.3. Changes in plasma adrenaline, noradrenaline and corticosteroid of rats. In the training phase, all rats were first trained on continuous reinforcement and then switched to a VI schedule. In the testing phase, the results of which are shown, rats were divided into three groups: condition A were on reinforcement available conditions throughout the 30 min lever available period, condition B received 10 min on reinforcement available conditions followed by 20 min of extinction and condition C was on extinction conditions throughout the 30 min period. (Reprinted from De Boer *et al.*, 1990. Copyright 1990, with kind permission from Elsevier Science Ltd, The Boulevard, Langford Lane, Kidlington OX5 1GB, UK)

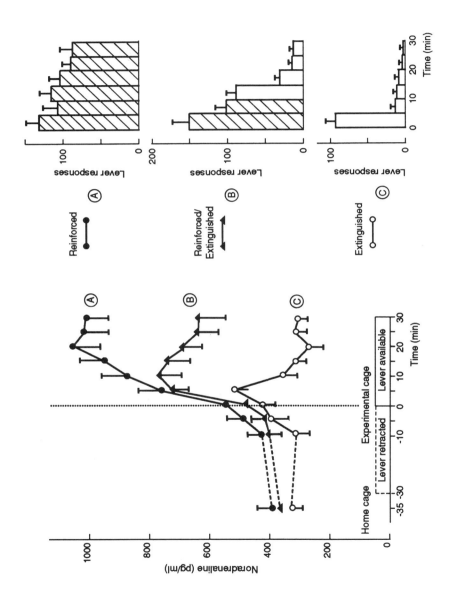

adrenaline ratio loss of control (for a somewhat different interpretation of noradrenaline/adrenaline ratios, see Laborit, 1986, pp. 78 and 190). Similarly, in rats, Steffens *et al.* (1986) found that plasma noradrenaline was elevated during a meal whereas adrenaline was elevated in only the first minute.

The dissociation between noradrenaline and adrenaline here appears to have parallels in studies on human subjects, Frankenhaeuser (1976) reports that gaining control over an aversive situation is associated with decreasing adrenaline secretion but noradrenaline secretion changed little. However, the issue of just how much psychological interest we can attach to the noradrenaline response in the appetitive situations needs further investigation. It should be noted that food intake *per se* appears to influence catecholamines (Steffens *et al.*, 1986) so elevated noradrenaline cannot necessarily be explained in such terms as control. It would be interesting to see whether the result of de Boer *et al.* would be obtained using thirsty rats and water as reinforcement. The elevation in noradrenaline in the rewarded group showed a clear positive correlation with their lever-pressing activity. Extinction was associated with relatively low lever-pressing rates and low levels of plasma noradrenaline. Whether all of the variation in plasma noradrenaline could be explained in terms of activity remains to be seen.

5.12   GENERAL CONCLUSIONS

A number of conclusions can be drawn from the evidence reviewed in this chapter, as follows:

1. Separation is a powerful stressor that seems to affect a natural opioid system.
2. As indexed by corticosterone levels and gastric damage, a potential stressor appears to be less stressful if the animal is able to exert some control over it. For example, control might consist of pressing a lever to terminate the shock. In some cases, performing an appropriate species-typical behaviour (e.g. attack) seems to reduce the stress level even though it might not effect any change on the external environment. However, if the shock is of a brief duration, it might appear to the animal's nervous system processing that behaviour is having an effect in terminating aversive stimulation. (Coping strategies for effecting change on the external world will be discussed in more detail in Chapter 6.)

3. A number of experiments have found that exposure to uncontrollable shock leads to depletion of brain catecholamine levels.
4. Although such generic terms as 'sympathetic activation' and 'catecholamine response' are often made, under some conditions there is a certain amount of independence between adrenaline and noradrenaline responses. Figure 5.3 shows this, with noradrenaline responding more strongly in a situation of control and adrenaline in a situation of loss of control.

From the review, some clear pointers to the determinants of activation of the HPA axis can be given. However, it is difficult to produce a neat summary model or statement that encapsulates the process underlying such activation. Activation is clearly associated with aversive stimulation but it is also triggered by novelty. In many cases, the reaction depends critically upon the psychological context. Although certain disturbances to homeostasis (e.g. haemorrhage) seem to be potent stimuli for activating the axis, other disturbed physiological states (e.g. low energy level) may serve more to sensitize the system so that potential stressors and cues to activity in the outside environment become triggers. The review accords with Grossman's (1991) conclusion that both HPA and SNS activation are triggered when there arises a 'frustrated expectation with no obvious solution, especially when assessed by the organism as being highly significant to its integrity'.

Mason (1972) found evidence that activation of the HPA system accompanies: '. . . a rather undifferentiated state of arousal, alerting or involvement — perhaps in anticipation of activity or coping'. He was led to conclude his review:

> While the system appears to respond to a wide variety of events and psychological stimuli, there do appear to be some conditions which tend to elicit responses of unusual intensity. The element of novelty, uncertainty, or unpredictability appears especially striking in this regard, as was demonstrated in the various 'first experience' effects observed by many workers.

In a variety of situations, both aversive and appetitive, *anticipation of a significant event* leads to activation of the HPA axis. In appetitive situations, access to the commodity (e.g. food or water) is associated with a lowering of HPA activity. Thus activation of the HPA system tends to be associated with *uncertainty* (e.g. when food might appear but has not yet appeared; a rat being in a situation where it does not know in which of several experiments it will be participating) and lack of control (e.g. uncontrollable aversive stimulation). Where the world seems certain and predictable and the animal has an appropriate strategy of action available to switch in, there seems to be a low level of activation or an inhibition of activity in the HPA system. Examples include food becoming available after prior deprivation, either freely or as a result of lever-pressing, and the animal acquiring a strategy for avoiding shock. In an operant situation, when reward is less than expected the axis is activated, which might, by some stretch of the imagination, be described as a loss of some control. When reward is better than expected the axis is inhibited. Thus results in an operant situation are congruent with the results seen at the end of a period of deprivation; obtaining food ('reinforcement') seems to inhibit the HPA axis.

Perhaps the most general statement that can be offered comes from applying a slightly circuitous logic, in terms of a double negative—to consider the situation when the HPA axis is *not* activated. Activation then corresponds to one or more of these conditions not being present. Activation does not occur when the animal is in a familiar situation, having a tried and tested coping strategy available for dealing with any anticipated change in that situation and where action taken delivers results that are as good as expectations. On such a basis, activation corresponds to the situation where the animal might be called upon to find a course of goal-directed behaviour or revise one. For example, in a novel situation the animal might be called upon to perform behaviour that is still unpredictable. In a situation of food deprivation, where cues suggestive of food are presented but no food present, the animal needs to find a course of food-directed behaviour. In a situation of exposure to a cue immediately predictive of food but where it fails to materialize, a new course of action might be called for. In an operant situation, where food of value less than that expected is earned, the animal might need to revise its strategy, e.g. to forage elsewhere. If food better than expected is obtained there is no need to revise the strategy; rather it should be strengthened.

Further theorizing in this direction is needed in order to relate the conditions that trigger the HPA axis with brain states characterized as 'arousal'. In this context it could prove useful to note that the theta rhythm of hippocampal activity is associated with: (1) exploration; (2) organization of goal-directed behaviour; and (3) aversively motivated behaviour. It is absent during consummatory activity (Endröczi, 1972, p. 116). It would thus seem to correlate rather well with the neural situations known to excite the HPA axis.

This chapter has looked primarily at active attempts to ameliorate the impact of potential stressors. The next chapter looks at both passive and active strategies and compares various species in their reactions.

Chapter 6

Strategies of Action

6.1 INTRODUCTION

The last chapter looked at reactions to potential stressors and considered such active strategies as fighting and pressing a lever to terminate a shock. It also looked briefly at the passive strategy of not doing something and thereby escaping or avoiding some aversive stimulus. Chapter 6 looks more closely at such strategies. In response to potential stressors, there is often more than one strategy that can be adopted. In some cases, an animal can switch from one strategy to another if the effect of the first is unsuccessful. One might also expect differences between individual animals as to the strategy that they follow. This chapter looks at the evidence bearing on differences in strategies, considering various species. In interpreting the evidence, the dichotomy active versus passive will be related to the dichotomies sympathetic nervous system (SNS) versus hypothalamic–pituitary–adrenocortical (HPA) system and SNS versus parasympathetic nervous system (PNS).

Chapter 6 looks mainly at the behavioural side of strategies; although to develop an integrated approach, behaviour will be briefly related to associated events in the HPA and autonomic systems. Section 6.9 will more closely examine autonomic reactions that accompany the behavioural strategies.

6.2 RATS

6.2.1 Differences in Avoidance Behaviour

Confronted with an active avoidance task, there are strain differences in learning ability. For example, the Maudsley Reactive (MR) strain are poorer at learning an active shuttle-box avoidance task than are the Maudsley Non-reactive (MNR) strain (J. Gray, 1991). Gray explains this in terms of excessive activity on the part of a response inhibition mechanism in the case of MR rats. This mechanism would promote passivity and act to inhibit active response production. Similarly, Paré and Redei (1993) found that the Wistar Kyoto (WKY) strain of rat showed a long response latency when put in a shuttle-box avoidance task after first being exposed to unavoidable shock. They described this as a tendency to learned helplessness.

On being confronted with a prod that produced an electric shock a number of strains of rat will then attempt to bury the prod. However, WKY rats do not exhibit this behaviour but show immobility (Paré and Redei, 1993). Similarly, WKY rats more readily show passive avoidance than do other strains.

6.2.2 Social Behaviour

Fokkema *et al.* (1988) looked at individual differences in social behaviour and in activity of the SNS. Behaviour, arterial blood pressure, plasma adrenaline, noradrenaline and corticosterone were recorded simultaneously. Those rats that displayed aggression towards an intruder had: (1) higher baseline levels of plasma noradrenaline and (2) a greater percentage increase in plasma catecholamines associated with the encounter. The magnitude of aggression displayed correlated positively with blood pressure reactivity and the response of plasma adrenaline and noradrenaline. The authors suggested that: '. . . the more competitive, socially active male rats are physiologically characterized by a high sympathetic tone'. The level of baseline plasma noradrenaline measured *before* any experience with aggressive behaviour was found to be predictive of future tendency to show aggression.

From studies of this kind, Bohus *et al.* (1987a) divided rats between those whose predominant tendency is towards either *active* or *passive coping strategies*. In a challenging social encounter, active rats display more aggression and less immobility. They are characterized by a relatively high SNS activity. There is a sharp corticosterone response to an aggressive encounter. Passive rats show either no aggressive behaviour or relatively little, more immobility and are characterized by less sympathetic, and more parasympathetic, autonomic activity. Their reactivity to an encounter measured in terms of the sharpness of change in catecholamines or corticosterone, cardiac response or blood pressure is relatively low (Bohus *et al.*, 1987a). This leads the authors to argue that, as with humans, *personality* is a meaningful concept in stress research in the context of rats. In terms of genetic selection, they argue: '. . . that selection for a certain behaviour is in effect selection for general behavioural characteristics (active or passive strategy) in diverse environments and for physiological reactivity that corresponds to these behavioural properties'. According to this interpretation, two behavioural processes are incorporated into the neuroendocrine system of each rat, that underlying active control, heavily involving catecholamines, and that underlying passive control, heavily involving corticosteroids. Genetics and early experience will then exert a bias towards the expression of one of these modes of control, although the less favoured mode of control is still available for expression if circumstances become more appropriate. The sharp increase in corticosteroid secretion associated with an active strategy needs to be distinguished from the chronic elevation of corticosteroids that typically characterize the passive strategy. The increase in corticosteroid level in the active strategy is usually associated with a rapid fall if the strategy is successful.

A colony of rats was observed over a 3 month period by Fokkema (cited by Bohus *et al.*, 1987a). Subdominant males, defined as active on the basis of earlier observations of territorial defence, were in a position of regularly challenging the dominant rat. They were in receipt of the most offence from the dominant. Those defined as submissives showed predominantly a freezing strategy in such social interactions and thereby avoided offensive attention for the most part. Over the 3 months, the mean blood pressure of the subdominants became higher than that of either the dominant or the submissives.

6.2.3 Ulcer Proneness

Paré (1989a) compared rat strains for: (1) their ulcer proneness when on an activity stress test in a running-wheel activity cage and (2) their behaviour when placed in water. The WKY strain of rat showed in situation (1) a large incidence of stomach ulcers and in (2) a strong tendency to float (considered an index of 'behavioural despair') and little struggling. Conversely, Wistars showed a low incidence of stomach ulcers arising from the activity cage and a low tendency to float and much struggling. Rats of a strain that show active coping, specifically struggling behaviour in this case, are ones that show a low incidence of ulceration. The experiment was not designed to demonstrate a causal relationship, rather a genetic bias towards both despair and ulceration was revealed. Paré suggested that such behavioural despair might be a model of human depression.

Interestingly, the rat strain showing least floating and the most struggling as well as the least ulceration (the Wistars) also showed the *least* running activity. Could this strain then be described as predominantly exhibiting active coping strategies? One possible way of viewing this is to see running not as an active strategy of confrontation but as an abortive attempt to get out of the situation (Mather, 1981), a giving up (there is a report by Tazi *et al.*, 1985, of an elevation in corticosteroid levels in rats with access to a running wheel).

In a further study, Paré (1989b) showed that WKY rats were more emotional than the other strains, as defined by their longer latency scores for initiating movement in an open-field test and their lower ambulation in the apparatus. He found that WKY were more ulcer prone than other strains when tested in a water-restraint test, comparable with a higher proneness to ulceration that appears in the activity wheel. Paré found that WKY rats were also more prone to learned helplessness than were other strains, as defined by their latency to initiate an escape response following a session of exposure to unavoidable shock. The WKY characteristics of: (1) greater ulcer proneness; (2) long response latencies; (3) low ambulation in the open field; (4) high tendency to exhibit freezing; and (5) greater tendency to float when given a forced swimming task, suggested to Paré (1989b) that '. . . behavioural depression is a characteristic of the WKY rat'.

6.3   MICE

6.3.1   Experimental Studies

Ely and Henry (1978) studied the behaviour patterns and endocrinological profiles of group-housed dominant and subordinate mice in a complex environment. The dominant mice were more vigilant than the subordinates in that they tended to launch frequent patrols of the territory. After 42 days of group living, the colony was said to have become socially stabilized according to the criterion that aggressive displays gave way to more peaceful gestures of rank. Initially, both types of animal responded to social interaction with a 'general non-specific arousal' involving activation of both sympathetic–adrenal–medullary (SAM) and pituitary–adrenocortical axes. Ely and Henry characterized this phase as being one of ambiguity and uncertainty, during which the animal tests out the new environment.

Over time, a differentiation appeared. The response of dominant males to the social interaction became predominantly one of activation of the SAM system, sometimes termed a 'defence response', involving threat to the subordinate mice. The subordinates' response became predominantly one of pituitary–adrenocortical activation, variously termed an 'alarm response', 'behavioural withdrawal' or 'conservation of energy pattern'.

Ely and Henry studied the effects of role reversal, by: (1) removing a dominant mouse from its familiar environment and giving it the intruder role by placing it in a new colony, and (2) increasing the status of subordinates by replacing the dominant with a subordinate. The former dominants were now subject to attack from members of the established colony. The former dominant males responded to their new status with, as Ely and Henry term it, a 'subordinate-type neuroendocrine profile', consisting of an increase in corticosterone levels and a decrease in catecholamine enzymes. Subordinates responded to the new status with a 'dominant-type response', enhanced levels of catecholamine enzymes and decreased levels of corticosteroids.

Researchers at the University of Groningen have pursued the subject of differences in aggressiveness between individual mice *Mus musculus domesticus*, finding both aggressive and non-aggressive individuals (Benus, 1988). The Dutch researchers dichotomized their aggressive and non-aggressive mice according to their attack latency score when confronted with an intruder. Aggressive mice show a short latency of attack (abbreviated as SAL), whereas non-aggressive show either a long latency or no attack at all (abbreviated LAL). This distinction implies neither that LAL mice would never display attack nor that SAL mice invariably do. It means merely that, under a standard test condition, animals can be dichotomized into these two populations. As Benus observes:

> . . . passive copers cannot simply be characterized as never exerting attempts to actively manipulate events. It is more accurate to state that they have a low tendency to actively control events and a high tendency to switch to passivity when active control is not easily perceived or cannot easily be executed.

Male mice of each class were then introduced into the territory of a highly-aggressive resident and their reaction towards the resident's inevitable aggression observed. SAL mice displayed more flight behaviour than LAL and also a greater percentage of time spent fighting. LAL mice displayed more immobility than SAL mice. Benus (1988) also observed what happened if, subsequent to defeat, the intruder was allowed the opportunity to escape from the resident's territory through a tunnel. Both SAL and LAL males utilized this opportunity, although at first some SAL males failed to notice the escape opportunity. No LAL males failed to do so. Benus associates the behaviour of the SAL mice with the broader concept of fight–flight or active response and the LAL males with the conservation–withdrawal or passive response. Benus suggested that non-aggressive mice predominantly: '. . . adopt a passive behavioural strategy, unless effective instrumental control (i.e. an effective mastering of the external situation) is easily perceived'.

Do the results of social interaction apply also in a non-social context? Does the fundamental difference between two strategies appear here? Benus (1988; see also Benus et al., 1989) observed the behaviour of SAL and LAL mice in an active shock-avoidance task. One might have predicted that the more active flight pattern characteristic of the SAL mice in a social encounter would generalize and thereby better lend itself to this task than the passive strategy of the LAL mice. Indeed, there was a tendency for SAL mice to solve the problem better than LAL mice. However, looking at the population of LAL mice one could dichotomize this into two subgroups. One of these displayed much immobility and the other behaved rather like SAL mice, showing a relatively large number of avoidance responses. Thus SAL mice very strongly go for an active strategy, whereas LAL mice tend towards a passive strategy but if control is perceived will sometimes go for it. (Interestingly, Zhuikov, 1993, found a somewhat analogous result for guppies (*Poecilia reticulata*): fish that were aggressive tended also to be good at solving an active avoidance task.)

In a further study (Benus et al., 1990), the reactions of SAL and LAL mice to inescapable shock were observed. These fitted the pattern seen earlier. LAL mice spent much more of the time between shocks immobile whereas the SAL mice tended to be active. This was an amplification of a difference in behaviour observed simply in response to being placed in a novel environment: SAL mice tended to explore more and LAL mice tended more to remain immobile.

Further experiments looked at the effects of exposure to uncontrollable shock upon subsequent avoidance and escape learning. The result of Benus et al. pointed to an important qualification to the claim, discussed in Section 5.8, that exposure to uncontrollable shock impairs avoidance and escape tasks. They found such an impairment for LAL mice but there was a *facilitation* for SAL mice. For LAL mice, the strategy of freezing adopted in the uncontrollable phase had a carry-over into the controllable phase. Regarding the slight facilitation in the SAL mice, Benus et al. suggested that, provided it does not instigate freezing, fear acquired in the unavoidable shock phase can have a facilitatory effect on subsequent avoidance/escape.

Looking at a population in terms of their tendency to attack, the attackers appear to have intrinsically a predominant sympathetic–adrenal activity, whereas the non-attackers appear to have an elevated adrenocortical activity (Schwartz *et al.*, 1976). Such a hormonal difference and difference in preferred strategy would appear to be genetically determined.

6.3.2 Adaptive Value of Active and Passive Strategies

Benus argues that both: (1) the active strategy of removal of either the challenge or themselves from the situation and (2) the passive strategy, 'to adjust themselves to the situation and accept it as it is', are effective ways of coping and have adaptive value. Under stable conditions, the active strategy is more successful whereas the passive strategy is better under changing conditions. In the natural environment, a number of individuals live together in what are termed 'demes'. Juvenile males and some females will emigrate from the deme to form new colonies elsewhere. Aggression serves to establish and maintain territory as well as dominance within a territory.

Benus argues that we need to qualify the often-made claims that: (1) exposure to uncontrollable events leads to behavioural passivity and (2) that behavioural passivity is, by definition, 'non-coping'. Benus' own results on mice showed that individual differences are large; whereas exposure to uncontrollable shock tended to strengthen the tendency to passivity in LAL mice, this was not so in SAL mice. Benus identifies an instrumental effect of passivity: immobile intruder mice are less often attacked by the resident than are active intruders. As Benus notes, an intruding male is a threat to stability, and: '. . . another means to restore stability is to adjust to and accept the situation as it is. This is another way of diminishing the threatening input. Therefore aggressiveness and non-aggressiveness are two alternative solutions to encounter the threat of an intruding opponent'.

Anisman (1975) makes a similar point in the context of passive shock-avoidance studied in the laboratory; a response–shock contingency exists. One might argue that the animal has two cognitions: (1) (response) → (shock) and (2) (passivity) → (no shock) that are formed and confirmed in such an experiment. As Barry and Buckley (1966) note, under natural conditions, crouching serves to conserve energy. The animal is in a good position to show active escape when this becomes possible. In the meantime, freezing makes the animal less likely to be spotted by a predator.

From the results observed in both rats and mice, as well as the theories discussed in these sections, we would therefore need to qualify the argument presented by Thierry *et al.* (1984): 'The conservation-withdrawal system is a second biological defense organization which comes into play if and when the energy expenditures of the first reaction (flight–fight) threaten the organism with exhaustion before supplies are secured'. The statement is not false, but it would seem that conservation-withdrawal is sometimes the first line of defence for some animals.

Though both active and passive strategies can be viewed in terms of coping, clearly either strategy can also fail in the longer run, described as 'loss of control', as Benus notes. (Failure of the passive strategy might be a suitable model of at least some aspects of human depression, discussed in Chapter 10.) This corresponds to a state of stress as defined in Chapter 1. When population density is very high, immobility might fail to deflect attack. Gastric ulceration and immunosuppression can then occur. Conversely, a dominant male experiencing difficulty in maintaining its dominance by aggression can experience hypertension. Benus argues that the SAL mice will be at an advantage on home territory whereas: '. . . under migratory conditions there will be a selection in favour of the non-aggressive mice. They are the ones that are able to establish a new deme'.

In a study of meadow mice, migration was found to play a crucial part in survival and population dynamics. Certain genotypes were associated with dispersal. There was a suggestion that aggressiveness was a particularly important trait for those animals tolerant of high population density and therefore not migrating (Myers and Krebs, 1974), although migrating animals also displayed aggression (Krebs *et al.*, 1973).

6.4   TREE SHREWS

6.4.1   Experimental evidence

Von Holst (1986) studied tree shrews (*Tupaia belangeri*) following their being placed in an enclosed space with a conspecific. He found that a fight resulted, the outcome of which determined a victor (termed the dominant) and a vanquished.

According to the behaviour exhibited following the confrontation, vanquished animals could be dichotomized into two classes: subdominants and submissives. Subdominant animals showed a strategy of active avoidance. They monitored the moves of the dominant animal and took active steps to pre-empt conflict. By contrast, the submissive animals sat in a corner of the cage and were unresponsive to external stimuli. For example, they neither attempted to defend themselves nor to flee in response to threats and attacks from the dominant animal. They died within 14 days of the encounter. The cause of death was not as a result of such physical consequences of an encounter as wounds or exertion. Rather it was perceiving the presence of the dominant animal. Death still occurred if a wire mesh barrier separated the two. The submissives stopped grooming themselves, their coats becoming rough and dirty. Von Holst described their appearance as 'apathetic or depressive'. Figure 6.1 shows the weight loss of dominant, subdominant and submissive animals.

There was no difference in hormone concentrations between dominants, subdominants and submissives at the start of the experiment. Testosterone concentration fell in both subdominants (by 30%) and submissives (by 60%) after 10 days. For the dominants, serum testosterone had doubled by 20 days after the start of the experiment.

For the first 1–3 days of encounter, serum corticosteroid levels were elevated in all animals, although more so in submissives than in the other two classes. However, once the dominance relationship had been established, in both dominants and subdominants, corticosteroid levels

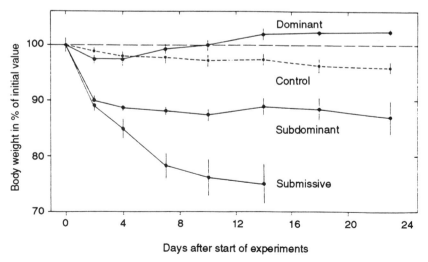

Figure 6.1. Body weight of tree shrews following encounter. Controls are animals undisturbed, kept in their home cages. (Reproduced from Von Holst, 1968 with permission)

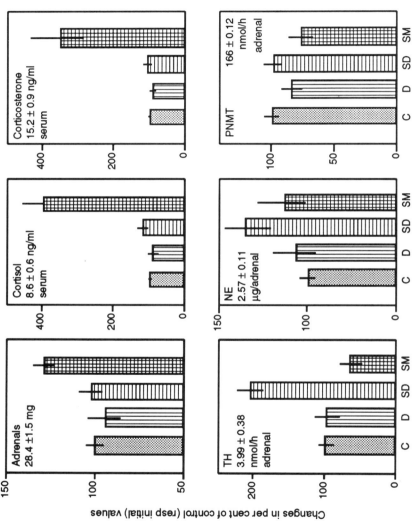

Figure 6.2. Results of Von Holst for tree shrews following social confrontation. C = controls; D = dominants; SD = subdominants; SM = submissives; TH = tyrosine hydroxylase; NE = noradrenaline; PNMT = phenylethanol-amine N-methyltransferase. (Reproduced with permission from Von Holst, 1986)

returned to initial values (see Figure 6.2). These levels were maintained even where fighting occurred daily. After 10 days of confrontation, the mean adrenal weights were no different from controls. By contrast, for submissives, dramatic increases in serum corticosteroid (cortisol and corticosterone) levels (300% up on pre-confrontation) were seen up until death. By day 10, adrenal weight was 30% higher than control. Evidence of an effect on the immune system (Chapters 4 and 10) was present: the numbers of basophil and eosinophil leucocytes and lymphocytes were reduced by 30% of control (unchanged in the other two groups).

Comparing the adrenal tyrosine hydroxylase activity to its control level, this was not different in dominants, decreased by about 30% in submissives and increased by over 100% in subdominants. Tyrosine hydroxylase is involved in the synthesis of catecholamines (see Section 2.4). In subdominants, mean adrenal noradrenaline content was increased by about 30%. Von Holst suggests that the results indicate increased SAM activity in subdominants but reduced activity in submissives. A general increase in heart rate of subdominants supports this (Figure 6.3). Note the increase in heart rate on first confrontation. For the dominants this soon returns to baseline. For the subdominants, heart rate remains elevated. The normal circadian rhythm is

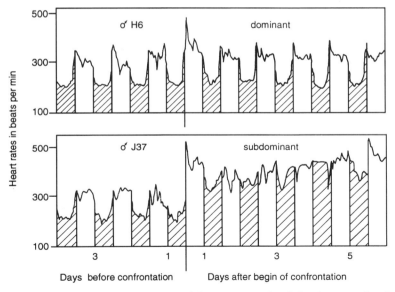

Figure 6.3. Results for heart rate of dominant and subdominant animals following social confrontation. (Reproduced with permission from Von Holst, 1986)

abolished. Measurement of the heart rate of submissives was not poss-ible, but Von Holst's impression was that it was reduced.

6.4.2 Interpretation of Results

Von Holst related his findings to the notion of a general stress reaction of the Selyean kind:

> . . . an adaptation to a stressful situation—respectively a reaction to a stressor—demands interplay among a great variety of central and peripheral nervous and hormonal processes; the activation of the adrenal cortex is only one of these, and can hardly be taken as a 'primary monitor' of the response of the entire organism.

For the dominant tree shrew, there are apparently no negative effects of social confrontation. This is in spite of the need to assert dominance by the occasional fight. Reproductive capacity and body weight show an increase. By contrast, vanquished tree shrews, in both classes, show lowered body weight and lowered gonadal activity. By the criterion of weight loss, a common measure of negative welfare, both subdominant and submissive tree shrews would be described as stressed. By the index of corticosteroid activity, the submissive tree shrews would be described as stressed. Excessive corticosteroid levels, which from adaptive considerations are the preparation for activity, are inappropriate to the lethargic behaviour of the submissive. Using heart rate as an index, the subdominant animals would be described as stressed. It is reasonable to assume that the elevated heart rate, by night if not also by day, is inappropriate to the activity level.

On a more positive note, in established and harmonic pair-bonds, tree shrews showed decreased heart rate and adrenocortical activity.

6.5 MONKEYS

A study by Corley *et al.* (1975) carried out on avoidance learning in squirrel monkeys is relevant to the theme of this section. These au-thors compared animals that could actively avoid shock by lever-pressing with controls (passive subjects) who were yoked to the active subjects and thereby subjected to the same shocks but who were un-able to influence the shocks. In five of six passive subjects (but only one of six active subjects), severe bradycardia with ventricular arrest was observed. The mechanism of this effect is assumed to be parasym-pathetic activation, corresponding, in the terms used here, to a failed passive strategy. Active subjects, by contrast, are more likely to suffer damage arising from excessive sympathetic activity.

6.6 BABOONS

Sapolsky (1990) made a study of dominance and hormonal state in olive baboons (*Papio anubis*) living in the wild in Kenya. Sapolsky reasoned that stress in such baboons might have important similarities to human stress, it being primarily of psychological rather than physical origin. In their natural habitat, there is an abundance of food, and predators are few. As Sapolsky expresses it: 'With the luxury of plentiful resources and free time, the animals can devote themselves to distressing one another'.

Dominant males, i.e. the harassers rather than the harassed, have greater access to such resources as females, food and shelter. Subordinate males are likely to have their food taken from them by dominant animals and can also form the target for displaced aggression by a more dominant animal that has lost a contest. Coalitions can be formed and then betrayed with resultant conflict and power struggles. With the development of sophisticated socially aware brains in such species, a dominant might help to maximize its reproductive success by stressing the opposition. As Sapolsky (1990) so aptly expresses it, 'olive baboons occupy a social landscape of Machiavellian dimension'. Dominance is not necessarily static; over months or years, roles can change with dominants and subordinates exchanging places.

Following exposure to a stressor, anaesthesia, a fall in testosterone levels was observed in both dominant and subordinate males. In part, this fall is mediated by the secretion of β-endorphin, which suppresses the secretion of luteinizing hormone-releasing hormone by the hypothalamus.

Dominant males were characterized by a lower resting level of cortisol than subordinate males and yet their levels rose faster in response to a stressor. Sapolsky (1990) investigated the cause of the difference in basal cortisol levels between dominant and subordinate males. Cortisol was found to be cleared from the blood at the same rate in both classes of animal and so different clearance rates could not be the explanation; therefore, secretion rate must be higher in subordinates. The adrenal glands of subordinates were no more sensitive to adrenocorticotrophic hormone (ACTH) than were those of dominants. Logically, they must be exposed to more ACTH. In turn, elevated production of ACTH could be attributed to a relatively high sensitivity of the pituitary to corticotrophic-releasing factor (CRF) and associated substances, a high secretion rate, or both. In fact, the sensitivity of the pituitary was found to be relatively low in subordinates, from which one can conclude that there is probably a hypersecretion of CRF. (As Sapolsky notes, researchers have similarly attributed the abnormally high basal levels of cortisol in depressed humans to a high CRF secretion rate, as discussed in Chapter 10.) In engineering terms, the subordinate's relatively high basal level of corticosteroids combined with a relatively low response to a stressor constitutes a low signal-to-noise ratio, an inefficient system (Sapolsky, 1988).

How do we explain the high resting level of CRF, and thereby cortisol, in subordinate animals? Some of it can probably be explained by a higher frequency of stressful encounters, whose effects spill over to the 'resting state'. In addition to such a factor, there is a basic difference in the feedback pathway of subordinate animals. It has been suggested that exposure of corticosteroid receptors in the hippocampus leads to what is termed 'down-regulation', a reduction in sensitivity of the structure to glucocorticoids (Sapolsky, 1988; and Section 2.3.2).

Abnormality in the feedback system is revealed by administering dexamethasone, a synthetic version of cortisol. In response to this, as a negative feedback effect, the secretion of CRF, and thereby ACTH and cortisol, is suppressed in both dominant male baboons and healthy people. However, subordinate male baboons are like depressed people in that they are 'dexamethasone-resistant': the secretion of CRF is unchecked by the dexamethasone load.

Sapolsky (1990) asked whether subordinate males are being harmed by the high basal levels of cortisol. There is some evidence to suggest that subordinates are placed at a higher risk of atherosclerosis and thereby heart disease (discussed in Chapter 10). Subordinates have less circulating high-density lipoprotein (HDL) cholesterol than do dominants, this being the kind of cholesterol that can play a part in preventing atherosclerosis. Sapolsky found an inverse relationship between basal levels of cortisol and levels of HDL cholesterol.

Sapolsky (1990) speculated that the healthier hormonal profile exhibited by dominants, lower basal cortisol secretion and a faster response to onset of a stressor, 'derived in part from the sense of control and predictability that comes with sitting atop a stable hierarchy'.

During the formation of a new social group, dominant males have relatively high basal cortisol levels. Once the hierarchy has stabilized, the dominant shows lower basal levels. On the basis of results with captive animals, Sapolsky (1990) argued that the direction of causality ran from dominance to hormonal state. On the formation of a new social group, one could not predict future status on the basis of prior hormonal profile. Prior hormonal status of dominants and subordinates did not differ significantly. Presumably, dominance emerges from a superior ability to predict and effect changes upon events. Optimal physiology, as indexed by a low basal cortisol secretion rate, was found only in males that showed at least one of the following characteristics: (1) a reliable differentiation (as measured by different behaviours) between neutral and threatening behaviour on the part of a rival; (2) initiation of a fight in response to a threat from a rival; (3) different behaviour following the winning or losing of a fight; or (4) displacement of aggression towards a third party on losing a fight.

6.7 HUMANS

Some experimental results on humans lead to the notion of a healthy cortisol profile. McEwen *et al.* (1986) argue that: 'The key to normal functioning of the pituitary–adrenal axis appears to be prompt and efficient turning on and shutting off of the adrenocortical stress response'. They refer to studies of air traffic controllers (Rose *et al.*, 1982), which show that the best-adjusted (characterized by lowest illness rate and highest involvement in work) exhibited a rapid cortisol response with an increase in work-load. They concluded that elevated corticosteroids were compatible with a good adjustment provided an effective corticosteroid switch-off process was also present. Air traffic controllers characterized by relatively poor job adjustment and having psychiatric disorders were associated with above average cortisol levels. They also showed less dramatic rises in cortisol in response to an increased work-load. In some cases, repeated exposure to what most would term a 'stressor' (e.g. parachute jumping) but where an effective strategy has been implemented, leads to adaptation of the cortisol response. Unpredicted events in the same context evoked the cortisol reaction (discussed by Rose *et al.*, 1982).

Lundberg and Frankenhaeuser (1980) examined pituitary–adrenal and sympathetic adrenal responses of healthy humans performing tasks designed to evoke either distressing or positive affective states. Subjective reports of boredom, impatience, tiredness and irritation were subsumed under the label 'distress', were positively associated with cortisol excretion and negatively associated with noradrenaline excretion. The label 'effort' described such psychological states as tenseness and concentration, and was highly associated positively with adrenaline excretion. A controllable task, not perceived as distressing but requiring effort, was associated with an increase of adrenaline excretion but a decrease of cortisol excretion. This implied an active inhibition of cortisol secretion in a situation characterized by a high degree of controllability. Lundberg and Frankenhaeuser summarize their results as: '. . . pituitary–adrenal activation was shown to be associated with negative feelings of distress, and sympathetic–adrenal activation with feelings of alertness and action proneness'.

In general the evidence from human studies suggests that, when confronted by a challenging, ambiguous task for which no obvious strategy is available, the response involves: (1) high SNS arousal, with increased cardiac output, vasodilation in skeletal muscles, increased blood pressure and heart rate, elevated secretion of adrenaline and noradrenaline by the adrenal medulla and (2) activation of the adrenal cortex with increased secretion of corticosteroids. Acquisition of active control over the situation is normally associated with some diminution of the high adrenaline and cortisol reactions (reviewed by Schneiderman and McCabe, 1985). Depending upon the exact circumstances of control acquisition, the noradrenaline response can remain high (reviewed by Schneiderman and McCabe, 1985) or show a diminution (Phillips, 1989).

Phillips (1989) reviews evidence showing that, on confrontation with a task, the sympathetically mediated increase in heart rate and systolic pressure can be greater for a difficult (but, in principle, solvable) problem as compared with either an easily solvable or an impossible task. Phillips' argument is supported by evidence from Bandura *et al.* (1985) who looked at the plasma catecholamine response of phobics as they confronted the object of their phobia. The biggest response was from subjects who rated their self-efficacy as medium, as compared with either those classified as strong or who declined the task on the grounds that it would prove impossible. The response pattern of plasma adrenaline was very similar to that of noradrenaline in this study, suggesting no differentiation in terms of differences in self-efficacy.

Thus, the evidence from rats, mice, tree shrews, monkeys, baboons and humans has something in common: the notion of a distinction between active control, involving predominantly the SAM system (though with some HPA activation) and passivity, involving predominantly the HPA axis. Uncertainty is characterized by a relatively high HPA activity. Within the SNS system there is some evidence to associate high noradrenaline/adrenaline ratios with control and high adrenaline/noradrenaline ratios with loss of control. The following section looks at theoretical models that attempt to integrate such data.

6.8 ACTIVE AND PASSIVE BEHAVIOURAL STRATEGIES: THEORETICAL MODELS

The hypothesis of J. Henry proposes two types of stress, with a distinction between the hormonal axes involved in the processes underlying the two classes of associated behaviour (Henry, 1982). The SAM axis is concerned with fight and flight, and its study was pioneered by Walter Cannon. According to Henry, activity in this axis is evoked: '. . . when the power to control access to desiderata, such as food, water, shelter, mate, and dependants, is challenged and the subject perceives that an adequate response is feasible'. The positive pole of this axis is labelled 'coping' and the negative pole 'relaxation'. There are two subdivisions of activity in the positive pole of this axis: fight/anger associated with noradrenaline and flight/anxiety associated with adrenaline. The opposite (i.e. negative end) of the pole of activity on this axis is associated with relaxation and grooming.

Henry (1982) describes activation of the second axis, the HPA, by: '. . . adverse conditions, such as immobilization, in which the animal is helpless'. The positive pole, i.e. high hormonal level, is labelled as 'dejection' and the negative pole as 'elation'. In this account, '. . . helplessness and loss of control are associated with dejection. The classic behaviour of the depressed animal is to act submissively, its body immobile, and avoid the company of others'.

Henry (1980) argues that, in a complex social environment, there is a clear evolutionary advantage in an animal having the facility to show inhibition of the fight–flight decision-making process. In effect, this involves submission to the dominant animal, neither to fight with it nor flight away from the common territory. In this way, the submissive animal would normally be able to remain within the group and derive the benefits of group membership. Another evolutionary advantage that being on this pole brings, is according to Henry, the influence of ACTH on learning (see Chapter 7): 'The losing animal is freed by ACTH to learn new patterns of behaviour more rapidly which is demanded by those to whom he is subordinated and to whom he has lost control'.

The third axis that Henry describes is the hypothalamic–pituitary sex-steroid axis (discussed briefly in Section 2.5). Henry argues: 'Testosterone appears to support the behavioural effects of high catecholamines and low corticoids, and high levels are associated with vigorous effort and social success'. Some evidence congruent with the latter point was obtained by Bernardi et al. (1989) in a so-called 'behaviour despair test'. They found that, in response to placing mice in water, castration increased the tendency to show immobility, passive floating. Restoration of testosterone had an effect in the same direction as an antidepressant, desipramine: to decrease the tendency to immobility.

Von Holst (1986) sees the difference between subdominant and submissive tree shrews regarding the relative changes in adrenocortical and SAM activity as lending support to the hypothesis of Henry (1980). However, there are some complications to the neat simplicity of the model. A study by Candland and Leshner (1974) in squirrel monkeys found a hormonal profile the opposite of what appears in other species. Subordinate animals showed lower levels of adrenocortical activity than dominants, as measured before and after the establishment of the dominance hierarchy.

Over a number of years both Gray (1987) and Laborit (1986) have developed comprehensive theoretical models of behavioural control which depend upon a dichotomy and antagonism between behavioural activation (active flight or fighting) and behavioural inhibition. Laborit (1986, pp. 60 and 140) argues that a cholinergic process of behavioural inhibition (in distinction to the catecholaminergic system of activation) is switched in corresponding to the animal learning that active behaviour is ineffective in achieving anything (*l'inefficacité de l'action*). In looking at Laborit's analysis, caution is in order: it is undoubtedly the case that learning of the ineffectiveness of behaviour can trigger an inhibition system but it might be wrong to see this simply as a default process only to be activated when all else fails. Evidence reviewed earlier in this section suggested that passive behaviour was as much a strategy in its own right as active behaviour. For instance, in the natural environment freezing by rats is surely not a consequence of their learning that they cannot avoid predators any other way. In the laboratory freezing can be seen as a first line of defence (Bolles, 1970). Whether voles freeze or run on perceiving a predator depends upon information processing connected with the probability of their having been perceived by the predator (Fentress, 1976). Conversely, under some conditions passivity might result wholly, or at least in part, not so much as a result of learning a strategy but as the inevitable (unconditional) consequence of aversive stimulation on the metabolic homeostasis of the CNS (Minor *et al.*, 1994a,b).

Laborit (1986, p. 143) closely associates the behavioural inhibition system with activation of the HPA axis. (There is an activation of the septohippocampal cholinergic system, presumably an input to the HPA system, in response to stressors; Gilad *et al.*, 1985). Situations that trigger behavioural inhibition also trigger the HPA axis but that does not mean that the axis can only be triggered by the perception of inefficacy of active solutions. As Laborit argues that corticosteroids exert a bias towards behavioural inhibition, this amounts to a positive feedback loop and indeed there is some suggestion for the existence of such an effect in the case of, for example, depression (see Section 10.5).

So far the bulk of the experimental evidence and theoretical interpretation leads to a dichotomy between active and passive strategies on confrontation with a stressor. The active strategy is associated with predominant sympathetic activation amd the passive strategy with predominant activation of the pituitary–adrenocortical system. Another fundamental dichotomy is that between sympathetic and parasympathetic activation in the face of a stressor. The following section will look at the evidence here. It will be shown that in a range of situations active engagement is associated with sympathetic activation whereas passivity is associated with parasympathetic activation.

6.9 STRATEGIES AND AUTONOMIC MEASURES

6.9.1 Introduction

Behaviour is accompanied by changes in the autonomic nervous system (ANS). What is the relationship between the organization of behaviour and the autonomic response? This section will examine this question.

In terms of humans, Vingerhoets (1985) developed a model of ANS activity somewhat along the lines of the model of Henry. The sympathetic branch of the ANS was associated with active coping, whereas it was argued that: '. . . PNS activity is triggered when people realize that they are powerless, unable to take adequate action, and are submitting to passivity'.

Vingerhoets (1985) notes that three very different psychological states can be associated with a dominance of PNS activity: (1) relaxation; (2) fear; and (3) depression. Thus, one cannot identify the psychological state simply from the PNS activity. Both relaxation and depression are characterized by passivity. Fear can of course be associated with passivity or an active coping strategy; passive fear is associated with elevated PNS activity. As Vingerhoets expresses it: '. . . the most parsimonious hypothesis, concerning the relationship between emotions and ANS activity, is that proneness to action or passivity determines the specific physiological activity rather than the emotional state'. (As part of a passive strategy of control in the face of a

stressor, Fowles, 1982, associates cardiac deceleration with a behavioural inhibition system similar to that proposed by J. Gray. See
Gray, 1987.)

Could there be an adaptive value in an elevated PNS activity during
fear, with its associated reduction in heart rate and, in humans, tendency to fainting? Vingerhoets (1985) argues: 'If the person sees no way
for escape or avoidance, and no other active coping responses are available, the individual feels as if he or she must surrender or give up.
Then, for example, fainting might be an adaptive response'. Immobility
means that the victim is less conspicuous to predators. Vingerhoets
also notes that the threat of excessive blood loss is reduced by lowered
heart rate and blood pressure.

Related to such an analysis is the observation of a role of endogenous
opioids in circulatory control (McCubbin, 1993). At times of stressor
exposure, they exert a hypotensive role. This is seen in humans in,
among other conditions, cases of social helplessness, comparable with
learned helplessness in rats discussed elsewhere (Section 5.8). McCubbin relates it to an opioid-mediated analgesia seen in rats after defeat
(see Chapter 8). The effect on circulatory control appears to be mediated via a vagal parasympathetic excitatory effect accompanied by
sympathetic inhibition. Such an input to circulatory control was said
by McCubbin to arise at times when stressor exposure is 'inevitable,
but neither escapable nor avoidable'. This is in contrast to the sympathetic dominance seen in active avoidance behaviour. However, the
role of opioids should not be seen simply in terms of a rather extreme
situation of the reaction to inescapable stressors. Rather, endogenous
opioids seem to exert a role in day-to-day adaptive interactions with
the environment by providing some kind of brake on excessive sympathetic activity. Thus MCubbin suggests that, in some individuals
showing hyperreactivity and hence cardiovascular risk, sym-
pathoinhibitory opioids might be relatively unresponsive or sluggish in
their reaction. The abnormality could arise at a high level of autonomic
control (see also Section 10.2).

6.9.2 Heart Rate and Strategy

Heart rate is a popular index of autonomic activity. A number of theorists have speculated on the relationship of heart rate to the organization of behaviour.

In a study of wild-living incubating willow grouse (*Lagopus lagopus*)
Gabrielsen *et al*. (1977) monitored a decrease in heart rate on approach
by a human. This could rapidly switch to the opposite response of car-

diac acceleration, corresponding, Gabrielsen *et al.* speculated, to 'when the bird got the impression of being detected'. They remarked that 'the grouse seemed to be very alert in its "frozen" state'. This state might be similar to a form of immobility called *tonic immobility*, also termed *animal hypnosis* (Gallup *et al.*, 1983). It consists of remaining absolutely motionless as a result of motor inhibition and is seen in many different types of animal (e.g. insects, amphibians, birds and mammals). However, Rodgers and Randall (1987a) distinguish between: (1) immobility, as a response to detection by a predator at a distance and which serves the function of camouflage and (2) tonic immobility, which is a response to capture. In chickens, one of the best studied species, tonic immobility consists of lying on the back. The adaptive value is that many types of predator respond to movement of their prey. In rabbits, the susceptibility to tonic immobility correlates positively with plasma corticosteroid levels and negatively with plasma testosterone level (Carli *et al.*, 1979). According to some authors (see Fowles, 1982), the most extreme form of parasympathetic activity (which constitutes the extreme of stress and anxiety) is seen in the vagal death phenomenon, associated with giving up in the face of a stressor.

In a variety of species, heart rate reflects the strategy the animal is adopting rather than exertion *per se* (see also Jaworska and Soltysik, 1962). Active avoidance is associated with a heart rate acceleration in response to a conditional stimulus (CS) predictive of shock (Black, 1971). The passive strategy of freezing is associated with a lowering of heart rate and the switch from this to an active strategy is accompanied by an almost instant increase in heart rate (Obrist, 1976; discussed by Espmark and Langvatn, 1985). The evidence from conditioning studies shows that heart-rate changes conditioned by association with shock reflect the strategy that the animal normally adopts (Cohen and Pitts, 1968; Cohen and Obrist, 1975). Thus, species (e.g. humans, cats, rabbits, rats) which react to a cue predictive of trauma by decreasing motor activity (e.g. freezing) tend to show a conditioned cardiac deceleration. Bruner (1969) found that in restrained cats acquisition of a freezing response to a tone predictive of shock was associated with acquisition of cardiac deceleration. Those species (e.g. monkeys, dogs, pigeons) whose reaction is one of increased motor activity tend to show a conditioned cardiac acceleration. Thus the heart rate changes should be seen as part of an adaptive strategy for coping with the unconditional stimulus (UCS), cued by the CS; although other interpretations are also possible (Powell *et al.*, 1993). For example, an active strategy in response to the UCS involving exertion might be assisted by an anticipatory increased heart rate triggered by the CS (Schneiderman, 1974).

In this context, it is also revealing to look at the effect of chemicals that influence heart rate. Suppose, for instance, that a CS is predictive of the injection of such an extraneous chemical. Schneiderman (1974) discusses an example of this kind, the UCS being injection of adrenaline and the CS being the injection procedure itself. Whereas adrenaline elicited an increase in heart rate, repeating the injection procedure but injecting a neutral substance, physiological saline, elicited a decrease in heart rate. In the terms of Eikelboom and Stewart (1982), conditioning would occur between the injection procedure and compensatory responses to the extraneous chemical. These compensatory responses and thereby the conditional response (CR) also would be opposite in sign to the responses elicited by the chemical itself. Again the conditioned response appears to be adaptive; an acceleration in heart rate to the UCS in an inactive animal is opposed by the conditioned effect.

To return now to the specific stimulus of shock, conditioned heart rate deceleration is vagally mediated (Cohen, 1974). Conditioned acceleration is mediated by both increased sympathetic activity and decreased vagal inhibition. Even within a given rat or dog, in a given experiment, in response to the same CS, heart rate acceleration (on occasions when somatic activity increased as in attempted escape) and deceleration (on occasions when immobility was shown) can be obtained (reviewed by Fowles, 1982). A CS that evokes cardiac acceleration in freely moving rats can provoke cardiac deceleration in restrained rats (Fitzgerald and Teyler, 1970). The cardiac response is associated with *intention* to act or not and is not simply a reaction to movement *per se* (Elliott, 1969; Fowles, 1982; see also Cohen and Obrist, 1975). Evidence that the intention to act is associated with cardiac acceleration is to be found in the observation that action in fact might be prevented by constraint, e.g. curarized muscles, but still the acceleration is seen (Obrist *et al.*, 1974a). Under more natural conditions, any comparable uncoupling of autonomic from somatic activity is clearly of relevance to the development of a criterion of stress, for example, in terms of inappropriate activation. Fowles subsumes the heart rate acceleration to a CS predictive of shock and to that predictive of food (see Chapter 5) under the description of control exerted by a behavioural activating system.

An interesting series of studies by Iwata and LeDoux (1988) reveals the complexity of conditioning in the ANS. They note that the behavioural reaction to a neutral stimulus (e.g. a tone) that was earlier paired with foot shock is the inhibition of ongoing behaviour; the rat takes a freezing posture. This is true, for example, in the case of the rat bar-pressing for food or exploring a novel environment. Iwata and LeDoux looked closely at the autonomic changes that accompany this behaviour, noting that in

earlier studies, in 'freely behaving' rats, the response is one of increased arterial pressure and heart rate. In Iwata and LeDoux's study, the CS (tone) was presented in the animal's home cage. An increase in mean arterial pressure was observed. The reaction of 16 of 19 rats was an increase in heart rate, whereas for the remaining three it was a decrease.

Iwata and LeDoux (1988) investigated whether the effect of the tone and shock reflected an example of associative conditioning in the strictly defined terms. That is to say, was it the fact that the tone predicted shock that endowed the tone with its capacity or was simply a history of tones and shocks, not necessarily paired, sufficient? In other words, suppose the rat was exposed to a series of tones and shocks *randomly* presented as a function of time. Would the tone still acquire a behavioural capacity or is it necessary to pair tone and shock? If random presentation is sufficient, this would be described as a case of 'pseudoconditioning'. Thus a group for which tone and shock were paired was compared with a group for which they were randomly presented. As far as overt reactions were concerned, conditioned rats showed piloerection and hunching on presentation of the tone whereas pseudoconditioned rats 'continued to rest quietly'. As to autonomic reactions, every pseudoconditioned rat showed an acceleration of heart rate to the tone comparable with that of the 16 conditioned rats that showed an acceleration. Both conditioned and pseudoconditioned groups showed an increase in arterial pressure following tone presentation but it was of larger magnitude in the conditioned, compared with the pseudoconditioned, group. Thus the change in arterial pressure reflects an associative process whereas that of heart rate does not.

The fact that some conditioned rats showed a slowing of heart rate whereas no pseudoconditioned rats did, led Iwata and LeDoux (1988) to reason that different processes might underlie the reactions comparing the two conditions. This is in spite of the fact that the mean reactions are not significantly different. Could the fact that some conditioned rats show a slowing whereas no pseudoconditioned rats do, be explained by a mixed sympathetic/parasympathetic activation in the former case but a pure sympathetic activation in the latter? To test this possibility, the effect of selective chemical blockade of either sympathetic or parasympathetic effects on the heart was investigated. In conditioned rats, parasympathetic blockade increased the cardiac acceleration to the tone whereas for pseudoconditioned rats it had no effect. Blockade of sympathetic innervation caused a marked deceleration of heart rate in response to the tone in conditioned rats, whereas in pseudoconditioned rats the tone caused no change in heart rate. Iwata and Le Doux concluded that, for conditioned rats, the CS evokes both sympathetic and parasympathetic discharge. The net result, an acceleration of heart rate, is a reflection of the sympathetic activation buffered by the parasympathetic effect. For the pseudoconditioned rats, the heart rate acceleration is a reflection of a pure sympathetic effect.

In their review of the literature, Iwata and LeDoux (1988) note that some researchers obtain a conditioned acceleration of heart rate and some a conditioned deceleration. Examination of their summary table of results shows that, in each case where acceleration resulted, the rats were freely moving, whereas, in each case where deceleration resulted, rats were restrained. As a possible explanation, Iwata and LeDoux suggested that restrained rats would already have a high baseline heart rate and therefore it would be difficult for sympathetic innervation to increase it still further. The effect of the parasympathetic influence would be more pronounced against such a background. In the terms developed in this chapter an explanation, which would not necessarily be incompatible with that of Iwata and LeDoux, is that restrained rats would only have the freezing strategy to switch in whereas freely moving rats would have the option of an active strategy.

6.9.3 Rebound Effects Within the Autonomic Nervous System

Evidence was marshalled by Anisman (1975) to show that exposure to electric shock leads to activation of catecholaminergic neurons followed by a *rebound* of activity of cholinergic neurons and a decrease of activity in catecholaminergic neurons, an idea proposed by Manto (see discussion in Carlton, 1969). This bias towards cholinergic activity is associated with an increased tendency to show behavioural inhibition, e.g. freezing. Such freezing competes with active avoidance. Administering anticholinergic or adrenergic drugs (and particularly a combination of the two) shifts the animal's tendency towards showing active avoidance responses (Barry and Buckley, 1966; Bignami and Michalek, 1978). Barry and Buckley (1966) and Anisman (1975) suggested that, following exposure to shock, the cholinergic rebound might in large part be responsible for gastric ulceration (see Chapter 10). It would also seem that a parasympathetic rebound might underlie the phenomenon of sudden death following activation on the part of the SNS in sudden trauma (Richter, 1957).

6.9.4 Differentiation Within the Sympathetic Nervous System

For some purposes we speak in general terms of 'sympathetic activation' or a 'catecholamine response'. However, at other times it is necessary to look more closely at these expressions and to differentiate aspects of the response. Although, as has been shown, a response of adrenaline usually parallels the noradrenaline response, there are some situations where this is not so (see e.g. Section 5.11.2). There are hints that plasma noradrenaline rises more at times of control whereas plasma adrenaline is sometimes more sensitive at times when control has been lost.

Discussion of a differentiation of this kind has a rather long history. Ax (1953) exposed reclining human subjects to situations designed to elicit either fear or anger and examined various possible indices of autonomic activity. Being connected to monitoring apparatus, the subjects presumably felt some inhibition about responding overtly so the experiment could associate only mood with physiology. Ax reported that the physiological changes in response to the fear-eliciting situation were similar to those seen after adrenaline injection, whereas in the anger-eliciting situation the responses were similar to those induced by a mixed adrenaline and noradrenaline injection.

Although the emphasis of the present book is the reaction of the animal to aversive stimulation, it is useful to compare reactions in aversive and appetitive contexts. The reaction to an aversive stimulus might not be to the aversive quality *per se* but rather to the demand for action that the stimulus presents. The following section considers this possibility.

6.9.5   Appetitive Behaviour and Autonomic Effects

By associating heart rate changes with the strategy the animal is adopting (or about to adopt) rather than the nature of the stimulus *per se* (Section 6.9.2), the possibility of a more integrative theory of autonomic control emerges. Thus in an appetitive goal-directed situation, there is evidence that heart rate is a reflection of the value of the *incentive* (Toates, 1986) towards which behaviour is directed. For rats working for food or water rewards in a Skinner box, heart rate tends to be an increasing function of the number of hours of prior deprivation (Bélanger and Feldman, 1962; Malmo and Bélanger, 1967; Goldstein *et al.*, 1970), although this is not always so clearly shown (Doerr and Hokanson, 1968). Such results cannot be explained by the vigour of bar-pressing increasing with deprivation and do not appear to be explained by other motor activity (Bélanger and Feldman, 1962). Neither can they be explained by deprivation *per se*, since merely depriving animals of food or water does not increase heart rate. Rather, heart rate elevation depends upon the combination of deprivation and cues predictive of the incentive, such as the lever in the Skinner box or secondary cues associated with the lever (Malmo and Bélanger, 1967). The exact relationship between cues predictive of incentives and heart rate elevation is a complex and revealing one. For example, placing a rat in a Skinner box with the lever retracted can be associated with a higher heart rate than actually having the lever present.

6.10 CONCLUSIONS

On first exposure to a stressor, and in some cases subsequently, both SNS and HPA systems will be activated (Axelrod and Reisine, 1984). Only later, if at all, will one or other system dominate (e.g. the HPA in the case of the submissives in von Holst's study, 1986). Therefore, any dichotomy between SNS and HPA systems is not an absolute but a relative one. Similarly, the active versus passive distinction is not an absolute one; it refers to *tendencies* towards two different strategies. A given animal has the capacity to show either, according to context, but might be intrinsically biased towards the one.

In spite of a few complications, the empirical evidence is usefully summarized by a model that associates activation of the sympathetic system with active strategies. Such active strategies are presumably assisted metabolically by activation of the pituitary–adrenocortical system prior to responding. As shown in the case of tree shrews, the activation of the HPA axis tends to be switched off or at least reduced when the strategy is successful and established. This fits the model of HPA activation in terms of prediction and uncertainty, developed in the last chapter. Passive strategies are more closely associated with activation of: (1) the pituitary–adrenocortical system and (2) the parasympathetic system.

If either passive or active strategies fail, this can be associated with a particular kind of stress and its associated pathology. The subdominant tree shrews shown in Figure 6.3 are displaying an elevated heart rate that is unjustified in terms of the energy demands of their situation. This could form a useful animal model of circulatory disorder. Conversely, the submissive tree shrew is showing the pathology associated with excessive and inappropriate activation of the pituitary–adrenocortical axis (Figure 6.2). Subordinate baboons and the badly adjusted air traffic controllers were associated with chronically elevated cortisol secretion rates and a relatively low rise in cortisol in response to a challenge. Such a rate of secretion of corticosteroids that is *inappropriate* to metabolic demands might provide a useful index of stress.

This chapter has focused upon the endocrine responses to behavioural situations, implying causality in the direction (CNS) → (hormonal response). The next chapter looks at the influence of hormones
on behaviour.

Chapter 7

The Effects of Hypothalamic–Pituitary–Adrenocortical and Sympathetic–Adrenal–Medullary Hormones on Behaviour

7.1 INTRODUCTION

In Chapter 1, the feedback nature of the systems implicated in stress was introduced. Feedback implies two directions of causality. So far, in considering interactions between neuronal and endocrine systems, we have looked mainly at the effects of sensory events and psychological processes, as organized in the central nervous system (CNS), upon endocrine secretions (e.g. Chapters 2, 3, 5 and 6). In Chapters 7 and 8, we look at the reverse direction of causality: the way in which stress hormones influence the brain and behaviour. In this context, where the endocrine events affect the nervous system and thereby behaviour, this would be termed a *feedback* effect. Chapter 7 looks at hormones of the hypothalamic–pituitary–adrenocortical (HPA) and sympathetic–adrenal–medullary (SAM) axes. Chapter 8 is on a closely related theme: the specific topic of stress-induced analgesia. It will look at how this phenomenon is dependent upon hormones and neurotransmitters produced by stressors. Some authors (e.g. Yates and Maran, 1974) are not convinced that the primary role of increased adrenocortical activity on exposure to a stressor is that exerted on peripheral tissue. Rather, they argue that the effect is a behavioural one mediated via corticosteroid action on the CNS. Unfortunately, as interesting as the proposal is, we have no clear evidence on this role that would enable us to be convinced of its primacy. As this chapter will show, at best we have hints as to an adaptive behavioural role of the stress hormones.

Before looking at the evidence that HPA hormones do modulate behaviour via a feedback process, it could be useful to examine the functional value of both feedback in general and specifically the part it might play in the systems under discussion here. When considering a number of motivational systems, it is not difficult to appreciate the functional value of feedback from the consequences of behaviour (Toates, 1986). For example, if an animal ingests a particular diet and is subsequently made ill, it will tend to avoid that diet in future. Clearly, in this case the feedback of consequences that enable the motivational choice mechanisms to readjust can spare future poisoning. Similarly, if the outcome of a fight is defeat, it is clear that avoidance, passivity or submission might be profitably exhibited in any similar future encounter. So there is no difficulty in seeing the value to the animal of a feedback pathway deriving from the consequences of behaviour. Following an encounter with a stressor, there will be behavioural consequences (e.g. defeat in a contest) and endocrine consequences (e.g. elevated corticosterone secretion). The value of feedback based upon the behavioural consequences is clear but what is the functional significance of feedback from hormonal consequences? Alas the answer remains unclear but it is possible to speculate.

Suppose adrenocorticotrophic hormone (ACTH) released by a stressor serves to increase fear, as some authors argue. This could constitute a positive feedback system such that fear would be self-reinforcing. A number of theorists have postulated the existence of positive feedback processes in behavioural control (Section 9.5.3.7). For example, it is claimed that positive feedback, involving natural opioid substances, is implicated in feeding (reviewed by Toates, 1994c; Section 9.5.3.7). Positive feedback could serve to sensitize motivational processes underlying fear, making the animal particularly responsive. What could be the functional significance of feedback from corticosteroid state? Here the hormonal response is slower and of longer duration than that of ACTH. Given that any corticosteroid response is presumed to be organized by the CNS, it is not immediately clear that information fed back to the CNS concerning the hormonal response would be useful. In this sense the system would appear to be different from say, taste–aversion learning, where information on gastrointestinal upset arises in the periphery and carries information that the CNS would not already have. One idea that will be investigated here is that perhaps the magnitude of hormonal feedback as such carries rather little information on its own, but it might act in collaboration with behavioural consequences to lay down a memory (Anderson, 1993). The hormones might selectively consolidate stressor–behaviour–consequence-related memories.

Alas, the investigator into this domain will find the literature full of isolated and contradictory results that often seem to do little more than to highlight the difficulties of interpretation and a multiplicity of apparatus, procedure, dose, route of application, sex, species and strain effects. Rarely is anything but the most superficial, restricted and qualified conclusion able to be drawn. The lack of signposting and the difficulty that authors, even those counted among the pioneers of the field (e.g. De Wied, 1969), have experienced and acknowledged in trying to present any kind of integrative theoretical model makes this journey one to be avoided by the weak-willed.

7.2 THEORIES ON THE ROLE OF HYPOTHALAMIC–PITUITARY–ADRENOCORTICAL HORMONES

There are various theories and suggestions as to the role of HPA hormones in behaviour and, before surveying the experimental results, it can be useful to look briefly at these. Although the theories address different underlying processes, they need not be mutually incompatible. Table 7.1 shows a table of these theories, describing the process underlying any changes seen in behaviour as a result of the action of a hormone on the CNS. Although it is useful to attempt such distinctions, in practice experimental results can lead to an interpretation that is a combination and does not neatly fit any one. For example, a memory can only ultimately be revealed in combination with motivation in a measure of behaviour.

Consider the result that ACTH tends to speed up the learning and slow down the extinction of an active avoidance task (discussed in Section 7.9). In principle, this result could be explained by any of the four processes shown in Table 7.1. The conditional stimulus (CS) might be more strongly attended to (1). All levels of motivation might be increased (2A) or specifically fear motivation could be increased (2B). The animal could show a general increase in all activity (3). Finally, the learning of the relationship (tone) → (shock) could have been consolidated better (4A' over A") or retrieved more easily (4B' or B") or both. However, further experimentation can enable these categories to be teased apart. For instance, if the memory of appetitive learning is

Table 7.1. Possible processes underlying behaviour in which hypothalamic–pituitary–adrenocortical hormone effects are implicated

Underlying process changed by manipulating hormone level (broad category)	Sub-types of possible process within broad category		Behavioural predictions
1. Arousal			Reaction to any stimulus might be changed; learning of anything might be improved; changes might be seen in processing of information (e.g. evoked potentials or EEG changed)
2. Motivation	A. General		Any goal-directed activity (e.g. escape, avoidance, running for food) affected. Effect might not outlast presence of hormone in brain
	B. Specific to fear		Specifically fear-related activities affected. Effect might not outlast presence of hormone in brain
3. Activity			A general change (e.g. increase) in amount of movement seen irrespective of context or stimulus; active avoidance might be better learned than passive avoidance
4. Memory	A. Consolid-ation	A' General	It would be expected that effect of, say, adrenocorticotrophic hormones given at training would be apparent a long time later
		A" Specific to fear	
	B. Retrieval	B' General	
		B" Specific to fear	

also improved by ACTH this favours 4A' or 4B' over 4A" or 4B". If an effect of ACTH injection given prior to a learning task is still seen in improved performance 10 days later this would suggest category 4 rather than 1–3. If the effect is seen only in the context in which ACTH was injected this would favour 4 over 1–3. Possibly a state-dependency memory effect is seen; memories laid down at a time of high HPA activity can be better retrieved in a subsequent state of such high activity. This would tend to suggest a combination of 4A" and 4B". If an effect is seen in any context, this would favour 1–3 over 4.

Before looking in detail at the effect on behaviour of manipulating hormones of the HPA axis, it is necessary to sound a general caution about such hormonal manipulations and apply it to the specific case of the HPA axis.

7.3   GENERAL PROBLEMS WITH MANIPULATION OF HORMONES

Experiments that artificially manipulate the levels of hormones always need to be interpreted with caution. The results might reflect something interesting about the normal organization of the processes underlying behaviour but they might also be simply the outcome of gross disturbances to general metabolism, effects on the whole brain or non-physiological effects at certain brain sites. Particularly, where behavioural differences comparing active versus passive reactions are concerned, caution is in order. One might want to argue, say, that a drug is acting on specific processes to exert 'a bias of specific motivational systems and decision-making towards passivity' but the result might simply be due to the rat being made to feel ill. Thus, it is known that manipulations of corticosteroid level can alter general cerebral extracellular/intracellular sodium ratio and levels of metabolism of amino acids (Bohus, 1970), speed of neuronal conduction and conduction time at synapses (Henkin, 1970; McEwen et al., 1988) and that some steroids can exert an anaesthetic effect (Wimersma Greidanus, 1970).

In considering the HPA axis, there is also the complication of feedback effects between corticosteroids and ACTH. Thus manipulation of either of these can lead to alterations in the level of the other. For this reason, a rigorous categorization of manipulations would need to involve consideration of which of the following four conditions are being investigated (Di Gusto et al., 1971): (1) high ACTH–high corticosteroids; (2) low ACTH–low corticosteroids; (3) low ACTH–high corticosteroids; and (4) high ACTH–low corticosteroids. Not all studies are able to be so neatly categorized.

Complications also arise as hormones other than those of the HPA axis are inevitably involved. For instance, if condition 2 above is achieved by hypophysectomy, other hormones of pituitary origin will also be eliminated with potentially confounding effects. Condition 4 achieved by adrenalectomy eliminates adrenal catecholamines at the same time.

7.4   THE BRAIN, RECEPTORS AND THE HYPOTHALAMIC–
PITUITARY–ADRENOCORTICAL AXIS

ACTH and adrenocortical steroids are able to modulate neuronal activity in the CNS and thereby might have effects through any or all of
1–4 in Table 7.1 (De Wied *et al.*, 1976). Some authors suggest that they
have a variety of effects upon behaviour, acting via memory, perception, learning and motivation (Levine, 1971). As we saw in Chapter 2,
the CNS contains receptors for corticosteroids. How does the binding of
the hormone at these sites affect behaviour? Is it relevant for how the
adaptive behavioural responses to stressors are organized? Panksepp
(1990) speculates on this issue, posing the question: '. . . what is the
normal evolutionary adaptive reason for there being so many glucocorticoid receptors in hippocampal/amygdaloid tissues which have now
been demonstrated to be so remarkably susceptible to stress-induced
injury?' As a clue, he notes that the hippocampus and amygdala play a
central part in the processes underlying aggression and fear. However,
he can do little more than speculate on the role of corticosteroid-
sensitive processes: 'Do they increase, dampen, prolong, shorten or
deepen emotional and related memorial responses?'—but tentatively
suggests that they promote sustained emotionality and thereby increased effort.

McEwen and Weiss (1970) note that any assumption that the brain
monitors the blood level of corticosteroids requires that they enter the
brain in increasing amounts as blood level rises. McEwen and Weiss
showed that the concentration of corticosterone in the cortex, hypothalamus and septum increased in proportion to blood levels over a
physiological range of doses. The capacity of the hippocampus showed
a tendency to saturation over the upper part of the same range.
Corticosteroids penetrate the cell membrane and affect intracellular
processes, e.g. to alter rates of protein synthesis (McEwen and Weiss,
1970). Presumably this could be of moment in the organization of the
processes underlying behaviour. A possible perspective on the role of
the corticosteroid receptors at the hippocampus is provided by noting
that corticosteroids play a part in memory consolidation (Dubrovsky,
1993). There is the possibility that their elevation might play a part in
selectively favouring the consolidation of stress-related memories such
as defeat or victory.

McEwen *et al.* (1986) reported that there was a positive correlation
between (1) binding capacity for corticosterone in the hippocampus and
(2) capacity for acquiring either a passive or active avoidance response
(discussed in Sections 7.8 and 7.9). Using a Morris maze, Oitzel and De

Kloet (1992) found that adrenalectomy caused some disruption of place navigation. In intact rats, antagonists to both mineralocorticoid (MR) and glucocorticoid (GR) receptors also caused disruption. They concluded that MRs are implicated in the evaluation of the situation to be navigated and the response selection whereas GRs are concerned with the consolidation of information in memory.

Woodbury and Vernadakis (1967) report an increase in brain 'excitability' caused by cortisone and cortisol, the effects of corticosterone being more ambiguous. In studies on rabbits, rats and cats that were administered cortisol, Feldman and Dafny (1970) report 'increased brain excitability', an increase in the magnitude of evoked potentials, particularly in regions of the hypothalamus. For cortisone in humans, Michael and Gibbons (1963) report 'a high incidence of euphoria induced by hormone administration' (see also Chapter 10), in some cases addiction to corticosteroids is reported (see Deroche *et al.*, 1993). Corticosterone has positively reinforcing properties; rats will learn an operant task for its administration and will prefer a corticosterone-containing solution over pure water (Deroche *et al.*, 1993).

A novel stimulus tends to cause desynchronization of the EEG response (termed arousal). Repeated presentation of the same stimulus is associated with less desynchronization, termed habituation. Habituation to the repeated presentation of a stimulus, as indexed by the EEG reaction in humans and the startle response of rats to a sudden sound, is slowed by ACTH injection (Levine, 1971; Endröczi, 1972, p. 102). This could be relevant to an aspect of the theory of stress proposed in Chapter 1 that suggests that with repeated presentation benign stimuli and stimuli that make no demands upon the organism tend to become assimilated into a model of the world and thereby do not trigger action. Conversely, stimuli that herald significant events demand continued focused attention. It would fit with the assumption of a feedback loop between hormones and perceptual processes.

Jacquet (1978) reported that in rats injection of ACTH into the periaqueductal grey matter was followed by active signs of fear (escape attempts characterized by jumping) associated with tachycardia. Signs were also seen of an opioid abstinence syndrome (e.g. 'wet-dog shakes', teeth chattering). However, Jacquet raises the point that it is unknown whether the brain is a natural target for ACTH.

Again fitting a feedback model, Arthur (1987) argues that, in addition to their role in general metabolism, corticosteroids exert an arousal effect upon the animal: 'so that it is vigilant and physically ready to take action'. This would locate an effect in category 1 in Table 7.1. Crossing categories 1 and 2, De Wied (1977) argued that ACTH

and similar substances: 'temporarily increase the motivational significance of environmental cues'.

Specifically, he argues that an arousal state is increased. Conversely, implanting hydrocortisone in the hypothalamus of rats increased the rate of habituation. Sensory thresholds in humans tend to
be decreased by corticosteroids and elevated by their loss.

In category 2B, but again suggesting feedback loops, McEwen and
Weiss (1970) propose a motivational role for the action of hormones of
the HPA axis on behaviour. They note the rapid release of ACTH
following exposure to a stressor and suggest that: 'ACTH has general
excitatory effects which potentiate fear-motivated responding'. Somewhat after this effect occurs, the ACTH-stimulated increase in corticosterone secretion is seen and, according to McEwen and Weiss, the
effect of corticosterone (note, an effect specific to *corticosterone*) on the
brain is such as to counter the excitatory effect and restore normality.
Thus, in such terms, ACTH would participate in a positive feedback
loop and corticosteroids in a negative feedback loop. The evidence
which McEwen and Weiss used to support their model was that hypophysectomized rats (i.e. lacking ACTH) were deficient in both active
and passive avoidance tasks. By contrast, adrenalectomized rats:
'showed more pronounced avoidance behaviour than normals'. (The
evidence will be looked at later.)

Weiss *et al.* (1970) suggest that the effects of hormones of the HPA
axis on behaviour can be most clearly seen when fear is mild rather
than intense. McEwen and Weiss (1970) suggest that: 'ACTH and corticosterone are not primarily responsible for reactions to clearly-
signalled, imminent dangers but are more important in affecting the
responses of the animal to what might be called a general level of
anxiety'. McEwen (1970) further specifies this by considering the question of: 'whether the behavioural response is clearly signalled, or
weakly and ambiguously signalled. In the former situation hormonal
factors are not seen, while in the latter strong hormonal effects on
behaviour are observed'. Again this is suggestive of a positive feedback
effect: hormones released by a certain type of stressor potentiate the
reaction to such stressors.

Bohus and de Wied (1980) suggest that 'ACTH and related peptides
maintain fear-motivated responses presumably due to preserving the
motivational value of environmental stimuli'. In such terms, it is possible to envisage at least two possible roles of ACTH. One is in broad
motivational terms. The capacity of any stimulus (which in this case
happens to be specifically that of the CS) to evoke fear is ACTH-
dependent. Alternatively, one might interpret it in learning terms,

such as ACTH is necessary for the animal to learn (and maintain the learned association) that the CS predicts an aversive event.

In explanatory category 3, Endröczi (1972) implies that there is a behaviour-suppressing action of corticosterone, suggesting a negative feedback mode of control. He argues that this is seen in such things as: (1) high corticosterone levels and low exploration; (2) facilitation of passive avoidance learning; and (3) inhibition of active two-way avoidance. Endröczi (1962, p. 43) proposes that the effect of corticosteroids in: (1) facilitating passive avoidance learning and (2) suppressing two-way active avoidance is a specific example of their more general effect in inhibiting *goal-directed motor responses*. In such terms, the effect is not seen as being specifically fear-related. Thus, it was found that, for rats maintained on a schedule of water deprivation, the latency to drink was increased by corticosterone administration. Endröczi (p. 61) reported that, at some sites, the rate of electrical self-stimulation of the brain was reduced by intravenous injections of dexamethasone and corticosterone.

In rats, there is a positive correlation between corticosteroid level and the rate of passive avoidance learning, whereas there is a negative correlation between corticosteroid level and rate of active avoidance learning (Dupont *et al.*, 1971; Endröczi, 1972, p. 120). Of course, correlation does not prove causation; this might reflect an effect of corticosteroids on promoting passivity or it could be a hormonal consequence of the aversive stimulation received. Manipulation of hormone levels is needed and studies of this kind are described in the following sections.

Attempts to explain the role of HPA hormones on behaviour need to take into consideration the principal target of these hormones and by all accounts, as far as corticosteroids are concerned, the hippocampus figures large. The discussion which follows might be usefully illuminated by considering theories on what the hippocampus does and here controversy has raged. In recent years the influential journal *The Behavioural and Brain Sciences* has contained at least five major theories on exactly what it does (O'Keefe and Nadel, 1979; Olton *et al.*, 1979; Gray, 1982; Rawlins, 1985; Eichenbaum *et al.*, 1994) and other reviews have posed the question: is it an inhibitor or a comparitor (Blozovski, 1986)? Toates (1994a, 1995b) suggested a possible resolution of the conflict in terms of seeing the role of the hippocampus as being the instrument of cognitive (Hirsh, 1974) as opposed to procedural control of behaviour. In such terms, it might indeed sometimes serve in an inhibitory role, i.e. to inhibit the behaviour that might otherwise occur in the situation. However, it should not simply be seen as inhibitory; rather it should be seen as serving a role in the inhibition of some responses and excitation of others, based upon a cognitive assessment of the current situation. Such a model raises the possibility that what corticosteroid receptors in the hippocampus are doing is to exert a bias towards cognitive control. Take for instance an animal in a passive avoidance situation. The model would suggest that the hippocampus is responsible for organization of the cognitive representation of the world involving extrapolation to events not physically present in space or time: 'here is safe but over there shock occurs and a move in that direction involves the expectation of shock'. Successful avoidance cannot easily be described as mediated by a response to a particular physically present stimulus except possibly freezing in response to the whole situation and this raises the question of what is the cue to freeze as the animal is in the safe location at the time. 'Don't go there' hardly constitutes a response as such. Rather, successful passive avoidance might be seen as a reaction to a cognition concerning the state of the world at another location.

By contrast, active avoidance can be solved by a response 'if CS then jump'. In two-way active (shuttle-box) avoidance, cognitive control might even tend to impair behaviour as the rat needs to return to precisely the location it has just learned to fear. Indeed, two-way avoidance is superior in hippocampally lesioned rats (O'Keefe and Nadel, 1978).

A line of logic proposed by Grossman (1991) fits part of the argument of the present volume and is as follows. In the tradition of Gray (1982), Grossman associates the septohippocampal system with behavioural inhibition and notes the high density of cortisol receptors located there. He poses the question: 'If cortisol is ultimately secreted in response to incipient noncoping, what might its function be?'. His proposal is that: 'cortisol may keep the organism temporarily more alert to the significance of its environment'. In terms of the present study being alert means exerting full cognitive control but is not synonymous with being in a behavioural inhibition mode of control, although it might be in this state at times. In this context it is also of interest to note that corticotrophic-releasing factor tends to activate the hippocampus (Koob, 1991; Chapter 3).

7.5   HYPOTHALAMIC–PITUITARY–ADRENOCORTICAL EFFECTS ON ACTIVITY AND EXPLORATION

7.5.1   Activity

Weiss *et al.* (1970) found no difference between normal and hypophysectomized rats in a measure of spontaneous activity when placed in a novel environment. De Wied (1969) reported no significant difference in ambulation as a result of administration of ACTH 1–10 to hypophysectomized rats. This result might be interpreted as evidence against the idea that ACTH raises emotionality in some general sense. In a study of activity in rats, Weijnen and Slangen (1970) attempted to tease apart the effect of ACTH and corticosteroids. To do so they used a substance that contains fragments of ACTH and which has similar behavioural effects (a so-called ACTH analogue) but which does not stimulate the adrenals. Ambulation in an open field test was not altered by subcutaneous injection of such ACTH analogues. Ambulation in a Y-maze was drastically reduced by foot shock but there was no difference in the magnitude of reduction as a function of whether the rats were injected with ACTH analogues or not. This result must be seen as possibly running counter to others (see Sections 7.8.2, 7.8.3, 7.9.1 and 7.9.4) that suggest a role for ACTH in increasing anxiety associated with a particular environment. However, as rats had intact pituitary glands, it is possible that sufficient ACTH was present in the placebo-injected controls to have a maximum effect on tagging the environment as fear related.

The diurnal cycle in corticosteroid level was discussed in Chapter 2. Endröczi (1972, p. 80) notes the negative correlation that occurs in rats between corticosteroid level and activity (see also Section 5.11.1). Around the transition from light to dark, activity is high and corticosteroid level low. The correlation might well owe something to suppression exerted on the HPA axis by the animal engaging in such activities as feeding. However, the reverse direction of causality, from hormonal state to behaviour, is suggested by a suppression of exploration caused by exogenous corticosteroids. There are several experimental reports of decreased motor activity in rats as a result of corticosteroid injections (reviewed by Laborit, 1986, p. 142). McEwen et al. (1988) argue that this cyclicity of hormone level causes a parallel cyclicity of 'behavioural state' and draw an analogy with hormones affecting sexual motivation. In other words, the circadian rhythm of corticosteroids serves a role in the co-ordination of metabolic activities both between tissues of the body (including brain tissue) and between such intrinsic events and behaviour (McEwen et al., 1991). According to McEwen et al. (1988), in all mammals studied, whether diurnally or nocturnally active, corticosteroid secretion peaks just before waking. In the case of rats, this rise and fall in secretion might play an important part in the exploration, feeding and locomotory activity that occurs immediately following waking. Corticosteroids are a powerful stimulus to feeding and food-seeking behaviour (McEwen et al., 1991).

7.5.2 Exploration

Placed in a novel environment, rats will tend to explore it. Micco and McEwen (1980) found no effect of adrenalectomy or adrenalectomy plus corticosterone on exploration, suggesting that this axis does not affect fear in any general sense. In rats, Endröczi and Nyakas (1976) examined the effect of ACTH injections on exploration. Although, on initial exposure to a novel environment, exploration levels were not affected, the rate of decline in exploration seen over daily sessions was greatly reduced by ACTH (comparable with the effect on habituation; see Section 7.4). Endröczi (1972, p. 36) reported that, in adrenalectomized rats, exploratory activity was decreased by corticosterone injection. As the rats had intact pituitary glands we do not know whether this was a direct effect of corticosteroids or an indirect effect mediated via ACTH suppression. However, as an effect of dexamethasone was seen at 24–48 h post-injection, it might suggest a direct effect on the nervous system.

In an experiment by Veldhuis et al. (1982), adrenalectomized rats showed a slightly lower tendency to explore a novel environment than did controls, an effect that was corrected by corticosterone but not by dexamethasone. Pretreatment of adrenalectomized rats with dexamethasone 1 h before giving corticosterone abolished the restorative effect of corticosterone. Why dexamethasone blocks the effect of corticosterone is not clear. It has a low affinity for corticosterone receptors in the hippocampus and cannot block cell uptake of corticosterone.

Different populations of corticosteroid receptors in the brain appear to be implicated when comparing, say, exploration and depression of the swimming task (McEwen et al., 1988). In a study on chicks, Sandi and Rose (1994a) raised the possibility that corticosterone serves to increase arousal or motivation but reported no evidence of a change in behavioural responsiveness as indexed by the normally sensitive measure of pecking. However, somewhat paradoxically, in a further study injection of a mineralocorticoid antagonist (MCA), but not a glucocorticoid antagonist (GCA), did affect behaviour (Sandi and Rose, 1994b). The authors noted that control-injected chicks introduced to a new cage normally show a predominant immobility whereas MCA-injected chicks readily investigated a mirror. They also showed a high pecking tendency towards a bead without the habituation shown by control-injected chicks. It was argued that the MCA altered 'the strategies required for the learning process' whereas the GCA affected the formation of memory.

7.6   AGGRESSIVE BEHAVIOUR

A possible role of the HPA activation in aggression was noted by Brain (1971) in the context of an experimental report by Cherkin and Meinecke (1971). These researchers had observed that, if previously aggressive rabbits were anaesthetized and then allowed to recover from anaesthetics in pairs, aggression between them was subsequently much reduced. Animals recovering singly and then put in pairs did not show this effect. Anecdotes were noted of a similar effect in chickens, dogs and cats. Brain suggested that as anaesthetics activate the HPA system possibly this is implicated in the decrease in aggression. If HPA activation is implicated, the effect is not due to this factor alone. Rather it is a combination of HPA activation and the social context that is involved. The result suggests a labelling process influenced by a hormonal consequence of the procedure (e.g. high HPA activity plus presence of conspecific exerts a bias away from aggression).

Leshner (1978) noted that manipulations of the pituitary–adrenal axis have less influence on aggression than those that manipulate androgens and the effects are less consistent. In mice, adrenalectomy is followed by a decrease in aggressiveness which is reversed by corticosterone replacement (Leshner, 1978; Brain, 1980). In some cases, giving intact mice moderate levels of corticosteroids stimulates aggressiveness. However, large doses of corticosterone decrease aggression in mice, intact and adrenalectomized (Candland and Leshner, 1974). Could the effect of adrenocortical hormones be mediated via their effect upon ACTH? Treatment of mice with ACTH over long periods decreases their aggressiveness, an effect that appears to be independent of the effect ACTH exerts on corticosteroids (see Leshner, 1978). Leshner argues that the long-term effect of adrenalectomy on aggressiveness is mediated via ACTH; adrenalectomy is followed by a rise in ACTH levels. Another possibility when considering the route by which corticosteroids exert their effect is in terms of an inhibition of androgens (Brain, 1980).

Opioid peptides in general suppress aggressive behaviour (Miczek *et al*, 1984), although one must always be aware that there are opioid subtypes which might have very different, even opposite, behavioural effects (Cabib, 1993).

7.7   SUBMISSIVE BEHAVIOUR

One role of hormones of the HPA axis on behaviour in mice was neatly demonstrated in a series of experiments by Leshner and associates, in which hormonal state and experience were manipulated (see Leshner, 1980). These researchers were interested primarily in submissiveness as a distinct category of behaviour in its own right. Submissiveness is not simply a lack of aggressiveness. Although the tendencies normally correlate negatively, these behaviours are dissociable. They noted that, although mice do not need to learn *how* to act submissively, the timing of when submission is shown depends heavily upon prior experience. On repeated confrontation between two mice, the latency for the loser to show submission falls very sharply. After four trials, submission was shown even before the winner showed attack. Over the same period, the tendency to show attack normally decreases.

ACTH treatment made at the appropriate time (discussed later) tends to increase submissiveness provided that the ACTH is able to provoke increased corticosterone levels (Leshner and Politch, 1979). If corticosterone level is controlled, ACTH treatment does not affect submissiveness. Treatment with corticosterone increases submissiveness is a dose–response manner. Castration had no effect upon submissiveness, suggesting that androgens play no part in this behaviour. Of course, androgens play an important part in aggression, supporting a dissociation between aggression and submission.

Leshner (1980) notes the similarity between the naturally occurring hormonal consequences of defeat and the artificial manipulation that is effective in biasing the animal towards showing defeat. Following a competitive encounter, both defeated and victorious mice show elevations in corticosterone levels. However, the response of the loser is somewhat greater than that of the winner. The artificial elevation of corticosterone levels seems to bias the animal towards submissiveness and away from aggressiveness. Leshner proposed that: (1) the experience of defeat and (2) the hormonal consequences of defeat (elevated activity of the HPA axis) normally act jointly to exert this bias. In order to test this hypothesis, two forms of artificial manipulation of the hormonal consequences of defeat were studied: preventing the normal consequences and exaggerating them. Mice were hypophysectomized and given fixed amounts of ACTH and testosterone. This prevented the normal rise in ACTH level and fall in testosterone level that follow defeat. This retarded the appearance of submissive behaviour.

On their own, HPA hormones appear not to modulate behaviour in this situation. Rather they act conjointly with the experience of defeat to modify future expression of defeat. Simply giving ACTH or corticosterone does not affect future behaviour. Giving supplementary ACTH or corticosterone immediately after the experience of defeat biases the mouse towards submission up to 48 h later. It was found that treatment with corticosterone alone had the same effect as stimulating the system with ACTH.

Some results that are congruent with those of Leshner *et al.* in implicating a joint hormone–experience role were obtained by Jefferys and Funder (1987). These researchers looked at the immobility response of rats on being placed in water. In an initial 15 min test, the tendency to show immobility was not influenced by prior adrenalectomy. However, the tendency to show immobility on *subsequent* exposure was greatly reduced by adrenalectomy and was restored by dexamethasone. Insofar as the active strategy did not succeed in getting the rat out of the water and the passive strategy enabled energy conservation, the active strategy failed and the passive succeeded. Based upon evidence such as this, one possible interpretation is that corticosteroids seem to be implicated in the consolidation of the memory of a 'failed' strategy and a switch of strategy (McEwen *et al.*, 1986). However, from this result one cannot simply assume that only the HPA axis is involved, as hypophysectomized rats showed a strong tendency to immobility. The solution to what is going on seems to be that there is a certain inbuilt redundancy in the system. Either corticosteroids or opioids of adrenal-medullary origin are capable of exerting modulation on the tendency to exhibit immobility. It is interesting that dexamethasone is able to substitute for the lost corticosteroids in this task (presumably showing an effect mediated through the glucocorticoid class of receptors described in Section 2.3.2.5), by contrast to some others (e.g. forced exposure in a passive avoidance task) where only replacing corticosterone suffices, presumably mediated via the corticosterone receptor population (McEwen and Brinton, 1987).

The studies described in Sections 7.6 and 7.7 on aggression and submission relate to situations that might be commonly encountered in the animal's natural life: defeat and victory. However, most research on the role of HPA hormones on behaviour has employed passive and active avoidance learning under rather contrived laboratory conditions. The next sections describe this.

7.8 EFFECTS OF ADRENOCORTICOTROPHIC HORMONE AND CORTICOSTEROIDS ON PASSIVE AVOIDANCE

7.8.1 Introduction

Passive avoidance refers to a situation in which an undesirable consequence is avoided by not doing something. In the typical passive avoidance situation a rat avoids shock in one location (B) by remaining in another location (A). Successful avoidance involves a process of behavioural inhibition which is mediated by acetylcholine (Blozovski, 1986).

Both ACTH and corticosteroids have effects upon avoidance behaviour. Injections of ACTH could exert their effect on behaviour via corticosteroids whereas the corticosteroid effect could be mediated via its effects on ACTH. However, various procedures suggest that each substance exerts an effect by its direct action on the nervous system apart from any indirect effect via the other hormone (Bohus *et al.*, 1982). There are reports that corticosteroid injection tends to disrupt acquisition of passive avoidance (Bohus and de Wied, 1980). However, Endröczi (1972, p. 97) found that a tendency to passivity was increased by corticosteroid injection.

The reader must be warned that the results are contradictory. Apparently slight changes in procedure can sometimes have major effects on the outcome. For that reason, in both this section and the next (on active avoidance), studies are organized according to the test apparatus used. The present reviewer is unable to reconcile these differences but can merely offer some tentative and possibly contradictory hypotheses, which invite discussion and testing.

7.8.2   Lever-pressing

7.8.2.1   Effect of non-contingent shock

In a somewhat cryptically reported study on rats, McEwen and Weiss (1970) examined the conditioned emotional response (CER): a tone heralds shock and the tone then acquires the capacity to suppress lever-pressing for food. They reported that the capacity of the tone to suppress was not affected by manipulations of the HPA axis but suppression 'to the training box alone' was affected.

In rats, Weijnen and Slangen (1970) examined the CER to a tone. The tone's capacity to suppress instrumental behaviour was not affected by whether the animals were injected with an ACTH analogue (ACTH 4–10). This substance is supposed to have the same effects on the CNS as ACTH but lack a capacity to stimulate the adrenals. Thus, Weijnen and Slangen argued that such studies 'did not bring evidence in support of the hypothesis that ACTH-analogues might modify conditioned behaviour through an influence on a hypothetical "fear motivation" level'. These studies also suggest that ACTH does not help consolidate a Pavlovian association of the kind (tone) → (shock).

In one of the earliest reported studies, Mirsky *et al.* (1953) described an experiment on passive avoidance in monkeys. Subjects were taught a bar-pressing response to obtain a food reward, preceded by a tone. After learning the operant response, subjects were divided into ACTH- and vehicle-injected groups. All subjects were then exposed to Pavlovian conditioning sessions in a different environment, in which the tone was followed by shock. As indexed by running and jumping responses to the CS, both groups formed (tone) → (shock) associations. They were then returned to the operant situation in which a bar-press now delivered both the tone and reward. ACTH-injected animals were reported to perform the response 'rapidly and efficiently', whereas controls 'displayed exaggerated startle reactions when the pressing of the bar caused the tone to sound'. They tended then to avoid the bar, mean scores being very low over subsequent sessions.

Mirsky *et al.* reasoned that ACTH did not prevent the formation of a (tone) → (shock) association. Rather, for ACTH-treated animals, when returned to the context of the original testing situation, as opposed to the environment in which the tone → shock had been experienced, this association was not revealed in behaviour. One possible explanation is that ACTH enhanced learning about the *place* in which shock occurred. ACTH-treated animals might have learned that a location predicted shock or a tone predicted shock in a particular location, whereas untreated animals might have learned a (tone) → (shock) association unqualified by place. As the animals had intact adrenal glands, the effect of ACTH could have been mediated via activation of corticosteroids.

In a study on rats also using a CER procedure, Hall and Honey (1990) found that *context specific* conditioning was revealed after one tone–shock pairing but not after extensive pairings. It would seem that repetition led to a more automatic mode of responding determined simply by the tone (cf. Toates, 1994a,b, 1995b). It might be that, in the experiment of Mirsky *et al.*, which involved 100 tone–shock pairings, ACTH maintained animals longer in a state where context-specific processes were being formed or there might be a species difference revealed here.

O'Keefe and Nadel (1978) suggest that hormones of the HPA axis might be particularly effective in learning about situation-related fear and Endröczi (1972, p. 112) reports a situation-specific effect of corticosteroid administration.

7.8.2.2   Contingent shock

Levine (1971) reported an experiment in which rats were trained to press a bar to obtain water. When the rats were established on this task, an electric shock was administered following such a bar-press. Subsequently, the animal avoids the bar, but gradually returns after some days in order to obtain water. A dose of ACTH given after shock considerably strengthened the animal's tendency to avoid the bar. In a similar study, Levine and Jones (1965) reported that ACTH injections given over a period, before, during and after shock, strengthened the tendency of the rat to refrain from pressing. There was also some suggestion from their results that for uninjected animals, the tendency to refrain from bar-pressing had a positive association with HPA activity, as indexed by adrenal weight.

In general, these studies are compatible with ACTH acting to strengthen either: (1) a cognition of the kind (bar-press) → (shock) or (2) the learning that a certain location, e.g. that of the lever or another location where shock is experienced, is dangerous.

The experiment of Mirsky *et al*. would suggest a rather specific role in learning what is aversive (a specific location), rather than in increasing fear in some general sense. The following experiments might also usefully be interpreted in this light.

7.8.3   Passive avoidance of a location

Weiss *et al*. (1970) studied rats in a passive avoidance test by measuring the latency to leave one compartment (the 'safe') for another. On entering the second compartment, shock was given. The initial latency did not differ when comparing normal, hypophysectomized and adrenalectomized rats. Neither did the number of boluses defecated differ between groups. In a similar study by Guth *et al*. (1971), made over several days of observation, there was no difference in latency comparing ACTH- and vehicle-injected animals. These results seem to run counter to the assumption that ACTH increases fear in some general sense. Presumably rats taken from their home cage and placed in a novel environment would have experienced a significant level of fear. Such procedures greatly increase HPA activation in intact rats (Section 5.3).

In the experiment of Weiss *et al*., following the experience of shock, for all three groups of rats, the latency to leave the safe compartment and to enter the previously dangerous, but now innocuous, compartment was greatly increased. There was a tendency for the hypophysectomized rats to come out most readily and to defecate the least. The adrenalectomized rats tended to come out with the longest latency and defecate the most. It would seem than that, in this situation, an intact adrenal is not necessary for learning about the danger of a certain location. An intact pituitary appears to be necessary.

Following three such tests of the willingness of rats to leave the safe environment, the physical characteristics of the previously dangerous side were changed. This caused a drastic lowering of latency to leave in hypophysectomized rats and less of a reduction in adrenalectomized rats.

Using intact rats and measuring latency to leave the safe compartment, Guth *et al.* (1971) compared two treatments: the effect of ACTH injections given either at (1) the learning experience, i.e. just prior to the single punishing shock or (2) the recall experience, i.e. prior to each test when the animal was on extinction conditions. Both treatments, (1) and (2), caused an increase in latency to leave the safe compartment over the 7 days of observation on extinction conditions. The fact that treatment (1) caused an increased latency several days later suggests a memory interpretation, i.e. as a result of ACTH injection, the memory of shock was better consolidated or better able to be recalled subsequently. The fact that group (2) showed longer latency could be explained by an effect of ACTH in increasing either general fear motivation or memory recall. It is somewhat surprising that a combination of both (1) and (2) did not yield longer latencies than either treatment on its own and this would argue against a state-dependent learning effect.

In an experiment by Smotherman and Levine (1978), mice were shocked for moving within a certain area. Shock had an immediate suppressive effect on movement, which was not enhanced by prior injections of ACTH. Again this result suggests that ACTH does not in a general way enhance fear. However, over subsequent days on extinction conditions, ACTH treatment enhanced the response-suppression effect of shock; mice showed less tendency to move than controls. ACTH seemed to consolidate the motivational significance of the environment and experience. The result is compatible with ACTH acting in combination with the shock experience either to (1) lay down a stronger memory of the shock experience or (2) facilitate recall of the shock-associated memory of the earlier experience. Smotherman and Levine concluded that ACTH *per se* was implicated in the effect rather than ACTH acting via stimulation of the adrenals.

Bohus and de Kloet (1981) and Bohus *et al.* (1982) investigated the forced extinction of a passive avoidance task. The researchers sought to extinguish this behaviour by confining the rats in the 'dangerous' area for a while in the absence of any shock. The index of extinction was whether they were later less reluctant to move from the safe to the previously dangerous location. Such forced extinction was revealed in the rat 'unlearning' its fear; latencies were subsequently like those of unshocked rats.

The effects of adrenalectomy and corticosteroid replacement on such forced extinction were investigated. To be able to look at a direct effect of corticosteroids upon behaviour, rather than an indirect effect mediated via ACTH, a short interval between adrenalectomy and testing was employed. It was assumed that this avoided implicating any boost of ACTH secretion consequent upon reduction of the negative feedback effect of corticosteroids. Andrenalectomy made 1 h before forced exposure to the 'dangerous' area totally disrupted extinction: as compared with sham adrenalectomized controls, adrenalectomized rats were reluctant to move from the safe area when tested 24 h later. Thus, whereas an intact adrenal is not necessary for learning about the danger of an area (see study by Weiss *et al*. above), it is necessary for 'unlearning' about danger, i.e. that a once dangerous area is now safe. Injection of corticosterone to adrenalectomized rats prior to forced exposure prevented the disruption of extinction from appearing.

For explaining the effect of adrenalectomy on forced exposure, this result is compatible with either: (1) a general increased fear level revealed at the time of testing or (2) a specific failure to learn by forced exposure that the previously dangerous side is now safe. Further investigation would appear to favour the second interpretation. Adrenalectomy performed 1 h after forced exposure had no effect upon extinction when the rat was subsequently tested (Bohus and de Wied, 1980). From this result it would seem that a *combination* of: (1) experience of the safe area and (2) the presence of corticosterone at that time is necessary for extinction to occur. In cognitive terms, relabelling the previously dangerous area as safe requires such a combination.*

As if the situation was not sufficiently complex already, a note of caution is sounded by Borrell *et al*. (1983), who implicated adrenal catecholamines in the passive avoidance learning situation described in this section.

7.8.4 Step-down Passive Avoidance

Keyes (1974) used a step-down apparatus to investigate the role of ACTH in memory. In the step-down passive avoidance task, the rat is

---

* The experiment argues against one possible theory of the action of corticosteroids, that their action is due to an emotion congruency (state-dependent) effect (see also earlier discussion in this section); it might otherwise have been argued that memories established at a time of high HPA activation are recalled better in a similar hormonal state. Note that, for rats learning in the forced exposure, experience was best when rats were injected with corticosterone 1 h before exposure. However, they were tested 24 h later, when presumably there would be little or no corticosterone left in the system. Rats receiving sham injections did not learn in spite of the fact that the endocrine state at exposure and testing would presumably have been closer than for the injected rats.

placed on a platform slightly above the level of a grid. If the rat steps down on to the grid it will receive shock to the feet. After such an experience, the latency to step down increases, indicating learning about the nature of the aversive stimulus. It is known that giving electroconvulsive shock immediately after the step-down experience tends to disrupt learning; on the subsequent day, the step-down latency is lower than that of controls. However, a so-called reminder can assist recall. By this is meant that if, between learning and recall the rat is given a shock to the feet (in a different apparatus and not contingent upon its behaviour), the shock can assist recall on subsequent exposure to the step-down task (i.e. latency is increased). Keyes showed that an ACTH injection is just as effective a reminder as foot shock and suggested that: '. . . retrieval agents are effective not because they have physical properties similar to the training stimulus, but rather because they reinstate an internal physiological state, motivation, that is similar to that present during training'. Keyes notes that foot shock is not an effective retrieval agent for an appetitive task. So the explanation is not in terms of a general process such as increased arousal. Rather, Keyes argues, foot shock is not part of the internal state associated with an appetitive learning task. By contrast elevated ACTH would have been part of the motivational complex at the time that the rat was consolidating its memory of the step-down response and its consequence.

7.8.5   Taste–aversion Learning

Taste–aversion learning refers to learning that harmful consequences follow ingestion of a particular substance. The consequences might be experienced up to several hours following ingestion and still learning can occur. Learning is revealed by a subsequent tendency to ingest none or relatively little of the substance. Taste–aversion learning is usually treated as a special class of learning with rather peculiar properties not only in assimilation but also recall (Garcia, 1989; Dickinson and Balleine, 1992) but, as its strength is indexed by the rat *not* doing something that it previously did, it would appear to have features in common with the passive avoidance situations described earlier in this section.

   Hennessy *et al.* (1976) found that a toxic dosage of lithium chloride (LiCl) caused a rise in plasma corticosterone concentration, presumably mediated via activation of ACTH. Injection of dexamethasone 2.5 h before LiCl severely reduced the rise in corticosterone concentration. It was assumed that it did so by inhibiting ACTH activation. All animals exhibited an aversion after the experience, as indexed by a greatly reduced ingestion. However, dexamethasone injection reduced the strength of the aversion, i.e. such animals ingested more than saline-injected controls. Hennessy *et al.* concluded that normally elevated ACTH levels as a result of toxicosis would help to consolidate the memory of the taste and its association with untoward consequences. They found that giving ACTH just before extinction sessions somewhat prolonged extinction and suggested that: 'The administration of ACTH prior to recovery sessions can be viewed as a reinstatement of part of the stimulus complex associated with LiCl induced illness'.

Sandi and Rose (1994a) investigated passive avoidance learning in chicks; following exposure to a noxious (bitter) tasting substance, chicks tend to suppress their spontaneous pecking behaviour directed to the object (even though there were no long-term negative gastric consequences involved in the design). This avoidance lasts for a long period of time but, if the substance is diluted, the memory tends to fade more quickly. In the bird brain, Sandi and Rose note: (1) the high density of corticosteroid receptors in the intermediate medial hyperstriatum ventrale and hippocampus and (2) that these regions are associated with the memory that underlies passive avoidance. They note that experiences such as tasting a noxious substance trigger the HPA axis and raise the question of whether exogenous corticosteroids might enhance a weak memory.

An enhancing effect of intracerebral corticosterone injection in a certain dosage range given 15 min before training was revealed in a recall test 24 h later. Sandi and Rose also investigated whether corticosterone could influence retention revealed at 24 h post-testing if it was administered after training. Avoidance was facilitated in chicks injected up to 60 min post-training. The effect was not due to an aversive consequence of the injection *per se* becoming associated with either the bead or the act of pecking. Pecking at a water-coated bead was not reduced by corticosterone injection.

To find out about the receptor type involved in mediating the result, the effect of injecting both an MCA and a GCA was examined. The latter injection, but not the former, cancelled the effect of the corticosterone implicating specific GRs. Sandi and Rose suggested that corticosterone: 'is affecting one of the intermediate stages in long term memory', although somewhat surprisingly protein synthesis inhibitors had little effect upon the memory. The authors suggested that injected corticosterone serves to enhance memory such that chicks trained on a relatively mild test substance 'experience the weak training situation as if they were trained with a stronger stimulus'.*

7.8.6 Conclusions

Several of the results discussed in this section suggest that ACTH is involved in consolidation or retrieval of memory, or both. Specifically, the memories that are consolidated seem mainly to be those related either to dangerous *locations* (Sections 7.8.2.1 and 7.8.3) or to learning (response) → (outcome) cognitions, where the outcome is aversive (Section 7.8.2.2). There is evidence that ACTH does not strengthen (CS) → (aversive stimulus) associations (Sections 7.8.2.1). However, the result of taste–aversion learning might force a broadening of this description of the range of situations in which ACTH can be shown to have an effect on increasing passive avoidance. In principle, the effect of ACTH on the rats in the taste–aversion study might have been via their learning to stay away from the location of the spout. However, when learning occurs over long delays between taste and consequences, it tends to be specifically about the quality of taste rather than the location where the substance was ingested (Pelchat *et al.*, 1983). Only a test of the animal's reaction to the taste of the substance applied to the mouth (Berridge and Grill, 1984) would enable it to be known whether ACTH plays a part in consolidation of a memory that helps steer the rat away from the taste or the location.

7.9 ACTIVE AVOIDANCE

In an active avoidance task, the animal can avoid a noxious stimulus by acting in a certain way (e.g. locomotion from A to B or lever-pressing). Van Delft (1970) concluded that 'neither ACTH nor corticosteroids seem to be essential for the acquisition of an avoidance

---

* Sandi and Rose (1994b) found that at certain doses either MCA or GCA injected 15 min before training impaired retention measured 24 h later. Sandi and Rose also tested whether injecting either of the antagonists 5 min after training affected recall 24 h later and found that it did not. These results would appear to be compatible with a state-dependent learning effect, i.e. if the animal learns something in one state (in this case in the presence of the antagonist) it is more difficult to recall in a different state but easier if tested in the same state. However, injecting the antagonist prior to both training and the recall test did not lead to a recovery of memory. Again this result would cast doubt on what might otherwise seem a viable theory of the action of corticosteroids: that in states of fear the presence of corticosteroids might facilitate those memories that were assimi-lated at a time of fear and high HPA axis activity.

response'. However, there is evidence that both can affect acquisition of an active response, as is discussed in this section.

7.9.1   Lever-pressing

Mirsky *et al.* (1953) reported an active avoidance experiment on monkeys. A tone CS was sounded just before a shock to the grid floor of the cage was given. The monkey could avoid the shock by pressing a lever during the 4 seconds of warning CS tone, which they rapidly learned to do. After reaching a criterion of accomplishment at this task, extinction conditions were imposed, i.e. shock no longer followed tone presentations. Corresponding to the time of imposition of extinction conditions, animals were divided into two groups: ACTH- and vehicle-injected. Extinction was rapid in the ACTH-treated group but responding persisted in the vehicle-injected controls.

This report of ACTH speeding up extinction of an active avoidance task in monkeys appears to be at odds with reports on rats (described shortly) that ACTH prolongs extinction. As the animals had intact adrenal glands the effect of ACTH on promoting extinction could have been exerted via corticosteroid activation. A result of Mirsky *et al.* on passive avoidance in monkeys (Section 7.8.2.1) also appears to be at odds with results on rodents. These differences might indicate a species difference or might be explained in terms of differences in experimental procedure. Thus, in Mirsky *et al.*'s active avoidance experiment the monkey was required to lever-press whereas in the rat experiments, the animal was required to shuttle from one location to another. If it is the case that ACTH specifically codes spatial information a possible resolution of the difference emerges. Presumably, monkeys in the experiment of Mirsky *et al.* learned temporal associations between the tone and shock and also spatial associations between the location (the Skinner box) and shock. If, under extinction, extraneous ACTH strengthened the latter association, it might have: (1) promoted passivity and (2) detracted from the associations between (a) tone and shock and (b) lever-pressing and shock termination. The latter would need to have been reinstated to promote lever-pressing. Such an account would dovetail with the argument presented for the passive avoidance result of Mirsky *et al.*

7.9.2   One-way Avoidance

In an experiment on one-way avoidance in rats, in which the rat was required to move from one compartment to another to avoid shock, it was found that hypophysectomized, adrenalectomized and normal rats did not differ from each other in their rate of learning (Weiss *et al.*, 1970). This result is perhaps surprising. However, one-way avoidance is already a relatively easy task to learn (Bolles, 1970), which, it would seem, can be made no easier by hormones.

Suppose a rat is placed in a situation where it has been shocked in the past. By opening or blocking an escape hole, the experiment can be arranged such that active avoidance is either possible or not. If active avoidance is not possible, then the tendency is for freezing to occur. Adrenalectomy impairs both active and passive tendencies. The active behaviour is restored by adrenaline and the passive tendency restored by giving corticosterone (Bohus *et al.*, 1987a).

Weiss *et al.* (1969) found that adrenalectomized rats persisted with a one-way active avoidance task for longer under extinction conditions than did controls. Conversely, hypophysectomized rats extinguished faster than controls. These results as well as those for passive avoidance, described earlier, led Weiss *et al.* to conclude that ACTH increases, and corticosterone reduces, fear-motivated behaviour. However, the effect was most evident when fear was mild rather than severe. This led them to conclude that 'the pituitary–adrenal system plays a rather subtle role in fear responding, probably influencing the rat's general level of arousal or emotionality'. Conflicting results might have arisen from researchers looking at ceiling effects.

That adrenalectomized rats persist longer than controls in active avoidance can be interpreted in either of the terms advanced earlier for the effect of corticosteroids on passive avoidance. Adrenalectomy might increase fear level in a general sense. Alternatively, corticosteroids might be needed for learning that what was once dangerous (the side where the animal is situated when the tone occurs) is now safe.

7.9.3 Jumping

In a pole-jumping avoidance task (on presentation of the CS, the rat must jump on to a pole to get away from an electrified grid), van Delft (1970) found a negative correlation between basal levels of corticosterone prior to training and the number of responses made in a session. This result is compatible with corticosteroids exerting a bias towards passivity but the correlation on its own does not prove it.

For normal rats with intact adrenal glands, extinction of the active avoidance task of jumping on to a pole was slowed up by subcutaneous ACTH injection (van Wimersma Greidanus and de Wied, 1971).

Evidence that at least one site of action of ACTH is on the CNS is derived from the observation that a similar effect is obtained by intra-cerebral injection of minute amounts of ACTH. The slowing up of ex-tinction on the pole-jumping task by ACTH is true even in rats bearing intracerebral cortisone implants, which otherwise have the effect of speeding up extinction (Bohus, 1970). Because of the speeding up of extinction by hydrocortisone implants, Bohus reasoned that an active inhibitory process underlying extinction is sensitized by cortico-steroids. In a somewhat similar apparatus, Bohus and Lissak (1968) found that cortisone speeded extinction and adrenalectomy slowed it.

Kovacs et al. (1976) examined the effects of corticosterone treatment on extinction of a task in which rats had learned to jump on to a ledge to avoid shock. Whereas low doses speeded up extinction, a large dose retarded it. Kovacs et al. found that the low doses increased hypoth-alamic serotonin content whereas the large dose decreased it. This is suggestive that the effects of corticosteroid manipulation might at least in part be mediated through brain serotonin levels. Van Wimersma Greidanus and De Wied (1969) implanted corticosteroids in the brain of rats (in some thalamic regions) and found that this speeded up the extinction of a pole-jumping avoidance task.

As an example of how elusive the effects of ACTH can be, consider an experiment reported by Weijnen and Slangen (1970). They devised an experiment that would seem to be rather similar to the pole-jumping task. A box was equipped with a grid floor and a retractable jump-on ledge. A CS predicted foot shock, which could be avoided by the rat jumping onto the ledge. After successfully executing this response and thereby avoiding the shock, the ledge was retracted from the apparatus, causing the rat to fall back to the grid floor to await the next CS. At presentation of the CS, the ledge re-emerges into the box. Extinction of this task was not altered by injection of an ACTH analogue (ACTH 4–10). Why ACTH did not affect this task, in contrast with the results for the task where the rat is required to move one-way from one chamber to another and for the shuttle-box (see next section) and pole-jump avoid-ance, is unclear. Superficially, the tasks would seem to be very similar; the CS is the cue for danger at the present location and for a move to somewhere else as a safe goal to be reached. If the effect of ACTH is to increase fear in a general sense or more specifically fear of a particular location or fear of the CS, then the results are inexplicable. If the effect is to label a location, other than that presently occupied, as safety-related, then it is not clear why ACTH does not tag the ledge in this experiment. Possibly the emergence of the safe platform simultaneously with the presentation of the warning CS could be implicated.

7.9.4   Two-way (Shuttle-box) Avoidance

Pagano and Lovely (1972) found that rats tested at 2–3 h before lights out, when the intrinsic rhythm of ACTH is at its peak, learned shuttle-box avoidance better than those tested at 1–2 h after lights on, when the rhythm is at its trough. This result has implications for the effect of exogenous ACTH: an enhancement of acquisition was seen in rats tested at the trough but not at the peak. Presumably, a ceiling effect is evident at the peak.

In two studies it was reported that, in neither intact (Murphy and Miller, 1955) nor adrenalectomized (Miller and Ogawa, 1962) rats, was the acquisition of two-way shuttle-box avoidance speeded up by the injection of ACTH prior to learning. However, in both cases the extinction of behaviour is extensively prolonged by such injection (Murphy and Miller, 1955; Miller and Ogawa, 1962; Smith, 1973; Endröczi and Nyakas, 1976; de Wied, 1977; McEwen et al., 1986). In neither case is extinction affected by injection of ACTH during the course of extinction whether or not it was also injected at the time of training. In summary it seems that ACTH serves a conservative role in strengthening the assimilation of an aversive association in such a way that it is resistant to subsequent disconfirmation. The result argues against a state dependent effect; retention is not better if the hormonal context of the extinction conditions are similar to those of acquisition.

Reports show that learning an active avoidance response in a shuttle-box is impaired in rats lacking the adrenohypophysis (de Wied, 1969) or whole pituitary gland (Appley, cited by Levine, 1971; de Wied et al., 1976; de Wied, 1977; Bohus and de Wied, 1980). An injection of ACTH restores their learning ability. Bohus and de Wied (1980) found that, provided that injections of ACTH are made prior to training for avoidance, hypophysectomized rats acquire the task normally. However, if after acquisition of avoidance behaviour, the supply of exogenous ACTH is stopped, the animal makes progressively fewer avoidance responses with the result that it receives an increasing frequency of shock. Bohus and de Wied argued that '. . . the behavioural effect of ACTH-like peptides is of a short term nature which does not extend beyond the actual presence of the peptide in the body'.

The effect of loss of ACTH is not mediated via a loss of corticosteroids, as adrenalectomy does not impair such behaviour. Treatment of hypophysectomized rats with the synthetic corticosteroid substance, dexamethasone, does not improve their acquisition of an active avoidance task (Bohus and de Wied, 1980). Thus, Bohus and de Wied, as well as Smith (1973), conclude that the effect of ACTH on avoidance behaviour is mediated via its action on the CNS. Use of ACTH analogues lacking any effect on the adrenal gland restores the learning ability of adrenalectomized rats (de Wied, 1969).

Evidence suggesting that the role of ACTH in active avoidance learning is to be understood in terms of learning the significance of the CS or its context is provided by Bohus and Endröczi (discussed by Bohus and de Wied, 1980). These researchers found that ACTH facilitated learning provided that the rat had made at least one avoidance response at the time of ACTH administration. Responding between trials was actually *decreased* by ACTH (although de Wied, 1969, reported the opposite effect), which is what might be expected if ACTH increases fear of the apparatus and promotes freezing or increases the salience of the CS. However, it might be that the inter-trial effect was mediated by elevated corticosteroids. Using a one-way avoidance task, Bohus and Lissak (1968) found that cortisone decreased inter-trial responding and adrenalectomy increased it.*

It is known that rats with lesions to the hippocampus acquire shuttle-box avoidance more readily than controls (Antelman and Brown, 1972). These authors suggested that as such rats have elevated levels of secretion of ACTH, their superior performance might be attributed to increased fear resulting from this elevated secretion. Also they argue that hippocampal rats are like ACTH-injected rats in the sense that their inter-trial responding is elevated, although this is at odds with the report of Bohus and de Wied (1980). To test this hypothesis, Antelman and Brown examined the capacity of the CS to inhibit an appetitive task (see also Section 7.8.2.1). The lesioned animals showed greater suppression, in keeping with the fear hypothesis. However, as was discussed in Section 7.8.2.1, other researchers, using intact rats, have not found an effect of ACTH on conditioned suppression.

A possible, and not mutually exclusive, explanation for the superior learning of hippocampals is that intact rats learn about the CS in its spatial context, whereas the hippocampal rat, being deficient in spatial

---

* There are reports that in intact rats, acquisition of active avoidance is not markedly altered by corticosteroid administration (McEwen *et al.*, 1986), a similar effect being shown for one-way, platform jumping avoidance response (Bohus and Lissak, 1968). Adrenalectomy leaves avoidance acquisition intact. However, the stage of learning at which the manipulation of corticosteroids is made might prove crucial. In rats, Endröczi (1972) studied the effect of corticosterone on active avoidance in a shuttle-box. Corticosterone administration given at the beginning of training did not affect speed of learning. Similarly, it has little effect when animals were at near 100% performance. However, in the middle stages, where performance was at about 40–60%, corticosterone produced a suppression in the number of conditioned responses shown.

mapping skills (O'Keefe and Nadel, 1978), learns more about the CS itself, out of context (Toates, 1995b). As noted by Antelman and Brown, the notion that the hippocampal rat's behaviour can be explained by elevated fear as a result of elevated ACTH levels runs into some difficulty with the observation that hippocampal animals are deficient at learning a passive avoidance task; additional processes need to be postulated to explain this. Also it cannot explain why hippocampal rats are not similarly superior at one-way avoidance, although possibly the ease of this task means there can be little room for improvement (Section 7.9.2).

Encröczi (1972, p. 44) reported that, for adrenalectomized rats showing 100% efficiency in a two-way active avoidance task in a shuttle-box, hydrocortisone implants in the preoptic region, among other brain regions, facilitated extinction. Other researchers obtain a similar effect: administration of corticosterone, in contrast to the effect of ACTH, speeds up the extinction of shuttle-box avoidance in rats (de Wied *et al.*, 1976; McEwen *et al.*, 1986). One might have supposed that such opposite actions could be explained simply in terms of the negative feedback effect of corticosterone upon ACTH. Such a factor appears to play a part, but the effect is seen also in hypophysectomized rats. In mediating this effect, corticosteroids appear to have a direct role on the CNS. Laborit (1986, p. 142) associates the role of corticosterone in speeding up extinction with engagement of a behavioural inhibition system (see Section 6.8) and ACTH with a behavioural activation system. However, the role of ACTH in passive avoidance is not compatible with this interpretation.

7.9.5   Conclusions

In theorizing about specific motivational or learning roles of a hormone, the investigator has to be careful that the effect of any extraneous substance is not mediated via a route such as debilitation or activation. This would seem unlikely here as ACTH tends to increase passivity in a passive avoidance task (Section 7.8.3) and to retard extinction (i.e. increase activity) in an active avoidance task (Section 7.9.4). Also ACTH analogues that are effective at retarding extinction of an active avoidance task do not alter general activity in an open-field test (Weijnen and Slangen, 1970; Section 7.5).

In the three situations of: (1) acquisition of active avoidance, which under certain conditions seems to be better consolidated by ACTH; (2) extinction of active avoidance, which (as a more general and reliable effect) is slowed down by ACTH; and (3) the period of immobility in passive avoidance, which is increased by ACTH, the effect of ACTH helps the animal avoid contact with the stressor (Di Gusto *et al.*, 1971; Archer, 1979). Di Gusto *et al.* conclude that, in general, '. . . high ACTH–high glucocorticoid levels reliably serve to prolong learned fear-motivated responses'. However, the means by which this occurs (e.g. better recall of a stimulus) remains to be established. There is some evidence to suggest that, rather than fear being increased in a general sense, the salience of particular environmental cues predictive of trauma is increased by ACTH.

Di Gusto *et al.* (1971) noted two studies (on shuttle-box avoidance by Levine and Brush, 1967, and on bar-press avoidance by Wertheim *et al.*, 1967) in which injection of corticosteroids enhanced performance. In both cases, the injection was made at a time after the response had, fully or to some extent, been acquired. In another study, that of jump-up avoidance reported by Bohus and Lissak (1968), behaviour was not influenced by cortisone injections and these were made prior to ac-quisition. Di Gusto *et al.* concluded that corticosteroids exert a direct action that enhances fear-motivated responding provided that the cop-ing response has at least been partially learned at the time of injection. By contrast, they conclude that 'The catecholamines, on the other hand, appear to enhance such performance at least *until* the relevant coping response has been at least partially acquired'. They also con-cluded that corticosteroids speed up extinction in a shuttle-box but do not affect passive avoidance.

In several experiments, it has been found that corticosteroids speed up extinction of an active avoidance task (Bohus and Lissak, 1968). They also decrease inter-trial responding whereas adrenalectomy in-creases inter-trial responding. Bohus and Lissak suggested that corticosteroids suppress fear. One problem with this interpretation is why any suppression of fear is manifest in a change in behaviour in extinction and inter-trial learning but not in learning the avoidance task itself (Bohus and Lissak, 1968).

7.10 APPETITIVE SITUATIONS

7.10.1 Introduction

As was shown earlier (Section 5.11), hormones of the HPA axis are also implicated in appetitive and consummatory behaviour. In principle, information on learning and extinction of appetitive tasks might also cast useful light on theories of the action of HPA hormones. Indeed, consideration of such studies is necessary in any attempt to tease apart the possible explanations described in Section 7.2.

7.10.2 Acquisition

Bohus and de Wied (1982) reported that hypophysectomy has rather little effect upon appetitive learning tasks. Any slight effect might be attributable to general metabolic, rather than psychological, effects. Guth *et al.* (1971) examined the latency with which thirsty rats left a small compartment for a larger compartment where water was available. This latency fell slightly over daily sessions but was not altered by giving ACTH prior to the test. Miller and Caul (1973) suggested that the effect of ACTH on appetitive tasks is a fragile one compared with aversively motivated behaviour.

Miller and Caul noted the effect of ACTH in improving acquisition of an aversively motivated task (although, as discussed earlier, this is revealed only under certain conditions) and the difficulty of teasing apart explanations based upon fear and memory. To address this issue, they looked at the effect of ACTH upon an appetitive task in which rats had to perform a discrimination between black and white alleys to gain reward. At doses said to enhance the learning of aversively motivated tasks, no effect of ACTH on learning this task was seen. The authors concluded that: 'Our results clearly give no support to the notion that ACTH is involved in memory processes'. This might need to be qualified as *non-aversively associated* memory processes.

In mice, Micheau *et al.* (1981, 1985) found no effect of intraventricular injections of corticosterone on the learning of an appetitive task, lever-pressing for reward in a Skinner box. However, when a discrimination task was added to this, an effect was found, consisting of better learning. Mice were taught to discriminate between two stimuli, one signalling availability of reward and the other unavailability. The effect was seen principally in the corticosterone-injected animals showing a greater tendency to withhold responding in the presence of the cue signalling non-reward. This result is interesting in the context of the earlier discussion (concerning extinction of aversively motivated behaviour) of a possible role of corticosteroids in inhibition of responding.

7.10.3 Extinction

The results discussed earlier suggested that the effect of ACTH is to increase fear or the salience of particular fear-related stimuli and that of corticosteroids is to decrease it. There is some evidence that fear is a state comparable with frustration arising from failure of an expected reward to appear (Gray, 1987; see also Section 5.11.2). In such terms the effects of ACTH and corticosterone on extinction of appetitive tasks is of interest.

At this point, before comparing the results for extinction, it can be useful to consider some similarities and differences between appetitive and aversively motivated behaviour. In an appetitive situation, information concerning a change made by the experimenter is always immediately available to the subject (e.g. on extinction conditions, on arriving at the goal box, food is no longer there). Presumably, to risk anthropomorphism and enter the head of the rat, the stronger the motivation and the better the learning, the more evident is the change. For aversively motivated behaviour, the opposite is the case. On extinction conditions, in a passive avoidance task, the moment the animal responds, information on the change in environment (e.g. the chamber that was previously shock-associated, no longer is) is available to the animal. However, the more highly motivated it is to stay in the safe location or the better it has learned about danger, the longer it will take to be in a position where the information on changed circumstances is available. Similarly, on extinction, in an active avoidance task, the animal who successfully avoids is, by definition, not around at the previously dangerous location to perceive that there has been a change in the world and it is no longer dangerous.

Levine and Jones (1965) reported a preliminary study indicating that ACTH did not have an effect upon the extinction of an appetitive task. Weijnen and Slangen (1970) reported that injections of an ACTH analogue (ACTH 1–10) had no effect upon the rate of extinction of an instrumental task learned for water reward. However, Levine (1971) reported that injection of ACTH delayed extinction of bar-pressing for water. Similar effects have been reported with food and sexually rewarded behaviour (Garrud et al., 1974; reviewed by de Wied, 1977; Bohus and de Wied, 1980).

For intact rats, there is a report that the rate of extinction of an appetitive task (running a maze for food) is unaffected by injections of corticosterone (Micco et al., 1979). The explanation that the authors offered is the possibility that target areas in the brain would already be saturated with corticosterone. There are reports that corticosteroids speed up extinction of appetitive tasks (Garrud et al., 1974; de Wied, 1977), an argument being that their action is mediated by receptors located in the limbic mid-brain area (de Wied, 1977). Micheau et al. (1985) reported that corticosterone injected into the hippocampus speeded the extinction of an appetitive task. This would be comparable with the effect on aversively motivated behaviour and would lead to the suggestion that corticosteroids are implicated in revising a strategy, possibly via exerting cognitive control (Toates, 1994a,b, 1995a,b; Chapter 9). However, there is also a report of the opposite result: that, specifically for adrenalectomized rats, corticosterone can prolong extinction of an appetitive task (Micco et al., 1979); adrenalectomized rats extinguished faster than controls, an effect that was countered by corticosterone injections. To set the discussion in context, it is worth noting: (1) that Micco et al. found that hippocampal lesions prolong responding under extinction conditions; (2) that corticosterone has a selective affinity for pyramidal neurons of the hippocampus; and (3) one effect of corticosterone uptake by such cells is an inhibition of their spontaneous responding. On the stength of this, Micco et al. suggest that the hippocampus serves a role in behavioural inhibition of unreinforced responses. Such an interpretation accords with the model of Gray (1987) and with that of cognitive control (see above).

7.11 CATECHOLAMINES AND BEHAVIOUR

Depletion of brain catecholamines impairs acquisition of active avoidance and speeds up its extinction (Endröczi and Nyakas, 1976). This is what would be expected on the basis that catecholamines seem to have a central role in the control of goal-directed behaviour (Chapters 3, 5 and 6).

Researchers have looked for effects of manipulation of adrenal–medullary hormones on fear-motivated behaviours, with somewhat inconclusive results. There are a significant number of reports of a disruption of behaviour with their removal but also some reporting no effect (see Smith, 1973). In humans, there are reports that injections of adrenaline tend to amplify any prevailing emotion.

Di Gusto et al. (1971) concluded that injection of adrenaline on its own did not affect fear level. However, if the elevated adrenaline levels occur at a time when noxious stimuli are present, such indices as defecation and choice of a familiar compartment rather than a novel compartment, indicate increased fear. Rats injected with adrenaline spent less time than controls in a compartment that had earlier been associated with shock. (Such results would fit with Schachter's theory of emotion, suggesting it arises as a function of both peripheral autonomic arousal and cognitions; Schachter and Singer, 1962.) In spite of such evidence, from the studies reviewed by Di Gusto et al. injected adrenaline has little or no effect on avoidance tasks, either in acquisition or extinction. As they note, such studies are open to the interpretation that, in addition to increasing fear, elevated adrenaline levels might lead to debilitation. A further interpretation is that increased fear might occur, but accompanied by a bias towards immobility.

Using dogs in a shuttle-box task, sympathectomy carried out before training had a retarding effect upon learning. However, if it was carried out after a criterion of acquisition had been achieved and before extinction conditions were imposed, no effect on extinction was seen (see Di Gusto et al., 1971). Such a result is compatible with a model in which behaviour becomes automatized with experience (see Chapters 1 and 9).

7.12   CONCLUSIONS

The reader was led to believe that this area would be something like the start of a *Times* crossword, blank spaces and highly cryptic clues, and I trust that by now he or she does not feel cheated.

Table 7.1 showed four possible modes of action of hormones of the HPA axis on behaviour: that these hormones affect arousal, motivation, activity or memory. In the context of avoidance learning (where most data have been generated), Weiss et al. (1970) suggested that ACTH increases mild fear and corticosterone decreases it. Evidence compatible with this view was discussed (Section 7.9.2), but also reservations were expressed. In Section 7.6, evidence that either ACTH treatment or adrenalectomy is followed by a decrease in aggressiveness and moderate doses of corticosteroids increase aggressiveness could be construed in compatible terms; an increase in fear might bias away from aggressiveness. However, the evidence that ACTH does not increase submissiveness unless it is able to provoke increased levels of corticosteroids (Section 7.7) would argue against the idea that ACTH accentuates fear and corticosteroids diminish it. Leshner's evidence (Section 7.7) that a combination of the *experience* of defeat and elevated corticosteroids biases towards future submission suggests not a direct role of HPA hormones on motivation but a modulation of the significance of events. The finding that the tendency to immobility on first being placed in water is not influenced by prior adrenalectomy (Section 7.7) would again argue against a role of HPA hormones in modulating fear in any general sense. That the subsequent tendency to show immobility was reduced in adrenalectomized rats suggests a role of HPA hormones in consolidating the strategy of immobility. Perhaps then the strongest hint as to the role of the HPA hormones is in terms of the consolidation of earlier experiences and their utilization in the current situation or the replacement of earlier strategies by alternatives.

The evidence that ACTH prolongs extinction of both aversive and (more tentatively) appetitively motivated tasks might suggest that its role is that of *maintaining* (once established in the learning phase) the significance of particular stimuli as the goals to action. Thus, in the appetitive task, the bond is between lever-press or the box itself and reward, whereas in avoidance learning the association is between a location and shock. The fact that corticosteroids tend to speed up extinction of both aversively and appetitively motivated tasks suggests a role in the *revision* of the cognitions underlying goal-directed behaviour in the light of experience. For example, in the aversive class, this would be consolidation of the new experience of no shock received in a previously dangerous area and in the appetitive case it would be that of no food in a situation where food was previously received.

Chapter 8

Stress-induced Analgesia

8.1 INTRODUCTION

Noxious stimuli normally trigger the pain system which leads the animal to take appropriate action, e.g. favouring an injured limb, flinching or jumping in the case of a rat exposed to electric shock. However, evidence shows that the reaction to such stimuli can depend upon context. This chapter looks at the context of stressors in its effect upon an animal's reaction to certain noxious stimuli.

Chapter 1 introduced the topic of central nervous system (CNS) *states* and their role in the production of behaviour. The present chapter is concerned with two such states, fear and pain, and their interaction. Engaging in one particular activity is often incompatible with doing something else and the nervous system involves processes of reciprocal inhibition at both the motor output level (see Gallistel, 1980) and the motivational level (Dickinson and Dearing, 1979; Ludlow, 1980; McFarland, 1985; Toates, 1986). There seems to be something like (1) positive affect/motivation states and (2) negative affect/motivation states with a mutual inhibition between them (Dickinson and Dearing, 1979). At least within the positive affect/motivation state there is evidence of a 'common pool' and for substitution, e.g. a cue paired with morphine can excite the sexual motivation state (Mitchell and Stewart, 1990). However, there can also be inhibition between two systems associated with appetitive behaviour; the existence of thirst motivation inhibits feeding motivation (Toates, 1974, 1979). The present chapter looks at inhibition between two aversively motivated states, fear and pain.

The object of this exercise is not to understand pain *per se*, although any insights here might, of course, be relevant and valuable, but rather to understand the processes underlying stress in the context of the reaction to noxious stimuli. Data on pain have proven to be illuminating to the study of stress and offer valuable insight for the construction of general theories of stress. It will be argued that the relationship between pain and fear is potentially relevant to the issue of strategies of behaviour. Chapter 1 introduced the idea of different strategies of action that close the feedback loop. The present chapter looks at the consequences for the pain system of recruiting either active or passive strategies.

The term *analgesia* (sometimes more accurately termed 'hypo-algesia') refers to a process that reduces the pain reaction to potentially nociceptive stimuli by specifically blocking nociceptive input at some level. Under some conditions, prior exposure to a stressor induces analgesia (Maier *et al.*, 1982; Amit and Galina, 1988), termed *stress-induced analgesia* (SIA), and is seen in response to a noxious stimulus applied a short period of time after the stressor exposure. Cold-water swimming is a potent stimulus for analgesia (Amit and Galina, 1986). Also some appetitive situations (Chapter 5) that are associated with activation of the hypothalamic–pituitary–adrenocortical (HPA) system lead to SIA. However, not all stressors induce analgesia. Some stimuli traditionally described as stressors (e.g. ether) fail to do so.

There is evidence that the inhibition from fear to pain is but one example of a broader range of inhibitory inputs to the pain system.

It is argued by some authors that certain procedures that would not fit the definition of 'stressful' employed here (e.g. vaginal stimulation) produce an analgesia comparable in some ways to that induced by stressors (see Watkins and Mayer, 1982; Rodgers, 1989). Pleasantly reported vaginal stimulation in human females, which apparently induces analgesia (Komisaruk and Whipple, 1986), might be seen to have in common with certain stressors that it is behaviour directed to a goal for which nociception would interfere with goal attainment. In mice, Fentress (1976) reported decreased responsiveness to noxious stimuli at a time when the animal was engaged in appetitive behaviour. A period of prior food deprivation or presentation of a particularly palatable food seemed to increase the magnitude of the inhibition, suggesting the possibility of an opioid basis associated with the hedonics of taste (Toates 1994c), though we cannot be certain that such procedures eliminate all 'stress-type' reactions.

SIA might seem counterintuitive; by lay logic, surely stressful situations are likely to increase pain. Furthermore, as Amit and Galina note, suppression of pain in a stressful situation might seem paradoxical in the context of the evolution of pain mechanisms. However, the empirical evidence is unambiguous and, on examination, an 'evolutionary logic' can become apparent, as follows.

Depending upon the exact stimulus and the context, the response to a noxious stimulus might be local, e.g. removal of a limb from a thorn, or involve the whole body, e.g. inactivity to favour a damaged limb. However, in various situations accompanied by tissue damage, survival depends upon the ability to take action (e.g. to flee, fight or freeze) in response to threats. At such times to stop and to react to tissue damage might be maladaptive in the face of the animal's need either to fight or to distance itself from a threat. Hence a process of analgesia is recruited at certain times. As a textbook example, students of pain are told of soldiers sustaining serious wounds in battle but who complained of little pain (Melzack and Wall, 1984). Apparently, only later, in hospital, did they perceive pain.

Although the index of SIA is usually an increase in latency of the local reaction of tail-flick away from a hot object, the evidence suggests that its locus of initiation is in the brain rather than peripheral (Hayes et al., 1978). Thus decreases in vocalization and struggling tend to mirror the increases in tail-flick latency (Hayes et al., 1978; Rushen and Ladewig, 1991). In humans, subjective reports of pain reduction correspond to the behavioural measures in rodents (see Fanselow, 1991; Hayes et al., 1978). Furthermore, on exposure to certain stressors, endogenously released opioids appear to dampen activity in the HPA system (Rushen and Ladewig, 1991). Thus it is justified to view the basis of this phenomenon as being a change in central state. Pharmacological interventions that alter central states affect SIA (Fanselow, 1991).

In other words, under some conditions, the motivational systems of, on the one hand, aggression and fear and, on the other hand, pain might be in competition. A theoretical model that assimilated such ideas is that of Bolles and Fanselow (1980), known as the perceptual–defensive–recuperative model. Part of the data base for this model was the observation that animals do not invariably react to tissue damage; their reaction depends upon the motivational context. Earlier, Bolles (1970) had argued that animals are innately equipped to perform species-specific defence reactions (SSDRs), in the case of the threatened rat to fight, flee or freeze. Conditional stimuli (CS) associated with the unconditional stimuli (UCS) that elicit SSDRs can acquire the capacity to elicit SSDRs. If analgesia is part of the defence system, then it follows logically that those stimuli that evoke SSDRs will also evoke analgesia (Fanselow and Sigmundi, 1986).

Shock and stimuli paired with shock evoke both defensive reactions and analgesia. In rats, exposure to natural predators, dorsal constraint (consisting of the experimenter grasping the animal around the back and sides) and exposure to the odours of stressed conspecifics tend to evoke: (1) freezing and (2) opioid-mediated analgesia (Lester and Fanselow, 1985; Fanselow and Sigmundi, 1986). This provides support for the assumption of the perceptual–defensive–recuperative model of fear and pain that a set of stimuli will evoke both SSDRs and analgesia.

As just noted, the issue of inhibition mediated through analgesia might be broader than the reactions to fear-evoking stimuli. It is not difficult to see a possible adaptive value in inhibiting responses to tissue damage at times when the animal is engaged in such goal-directed activities as mating (Rodgers and Randall, 1987b). Hence Rodgers and Randall suggest the term *environmentally induced analgesia* to subsume the stress-related phenomenon under the broader rubric of effective stimuli; but by convention 'stress-induced' is the term favoured in the literature.

8.2   THE BIOLOGICAL BASES OF STRESS-INDUCED ANALGESIA

Stressors cause the release of opioids, which mediate at least part of SIA (see Grau, 1987 for review; Amit and Galina, 1988). Endorphins are released from the pituitary concomitantly with adrenocorticotrophic hormone (ACTH) (Amir *et al.*, 1980; Chapter 2). Additionally, a stressor can cause the release of endorphins within the brain itself. In some situations, endorphins and ACTH might act in a co-ordinated way in the reaction to potential stressors (Amir *et al.*, 1980). Traditionally, to test whether the SIA seen in a particular situation was opioid mediated, opioid antagonists were administered. If the effect was abolished, it was concluded that it was mediated by opioids. If it survived, the conclusion was that some non-opioid mediation was implicated. Such experiments indicated the presence of both opioid- and non-opioid-mediated analgesia.

Watkins and Mayer (1982) discuss four processes underlying analgesia: neural–opioid, hormonal–opioid, neural–non-opioid and hormonal–non-opioid. However, these four categories are not necessarily mutually exclusive; a given case of analgesia might be simultaneously mediated by more than one of them. For instance, analgesia arising from CNS activity depends upon hormones of adrenal origin, which exert a role in the synthetic pathway involved in the formation of neurotransmitters (Sutton *et al.*, 1994; see also Section 2.4). As some forms of analgesia are blocked by naltrexone and some are not, one dichotomy is described by the terms 'naltrexone sensitive' and 'naltrexone insensitive' (Sutton *et al.*, 1994). Exposed to 100 inescapable shocks, there is evidence for a naltrexone-sensitive analgesia after two shocks ('short-exposure effect'), a naltrexone-insensitive SIA after five to 40 and a naltrexone-sensitive SIA after 80–100 ('long-exposure effect') (Sutton *et al.*, 1994).

Application of naloxone blocks the analgesia following front foot shock (Watkins and Mayer, 1982). Watkins and Mayer asked whether such analgesia could be mediated by opioids released from the pituitary or sympathetic–adrenal–medullary systems. Hypohysectomy did not reduce front-paw-shock-induced analgesia, whereas adrenalectomy and sympathetic blockade increased it; although see later discussion for a qualification. Thus neither pituitary β-endorphin nor opioids derived from the sympathetic nervous system seem implicated here. The amount of β-endorphin released from the pituitary appears to be of insufficient amount to lead to SIA (Sutton *et al.*, 1994). Hence, opioid pathways within the CNS seem to be implicated. Further evidence revealed the existence of pathways of descending inhibition (triggered by front paw shock) running from the brain down the spinal cord. Opioid-based inhibition is exerted on afferent information at its first synapse in the cord (Watkins and Mayer, 1982; Lewis *et al.*, 1989). As naloxone applied at a spinal site was selectively effective in reducing analgesia, a spinal site for the opioid synapse is implicated.

Dexamethasone has a similar effect to naloxone on reversing analgesia seen in long-duration stress exposure. This might seem to implicate opioids of pituitary origin, as dexamethasone blocks the release of both ACTH and β-endorphin from the pituitary. However, the situation is more complex than this; ACTH through its effect on the adrenal cortex is another candidate (Sutton *et al.*, 1994). MacLennan *et al.* (1982) found that such opioid-mediated analgesia was blocked by adrenalectomy and restored by corticosterone replacement. The role of corticosteroids might possibly be one of acting conjointly with β-endorphin. However, Sutton *et al.* (1994) found evidence to suggest that the reason adrenalectomy is followed by a reduction in SIA is that corticosterone plays a part in the synthetic pathway of one or more neurotransmitters involved in SIA. The picture is further complicated by the finding that enkephalin-like peptides coreleased from the adrenal medulla (along with catecholamines) play a part in the analgesia following prolonged stress (Lewis *et al.*, 1982).

Grau (1987) argues that there is reason to doubt whether the HPA axis is able on its own to produce an analgesic effect. The logic is as follows. The opioids that are proposed as the basis of this effect, β-endorphin of pituitary origin and enkephalins of adrenal origin, elicit only a weak analgesia when tested at physiological levels. If the axis cannot on its own produce analgesia, how does it play a part? Grau's suggestion is that it influences the gain of the opioid system, i.e. it exerts an amplification effect. In this case, the hormonal–opioid effect is not independent of the neural–opioid effect but interacts with it in an amplification mode. He suggests that adrenal enkephalins and/or β-endorphin (presumably of pituitary origin) might act multiplicatively with intrinsic spinal opioids. Another factor is, as noted earlier, the evidence of Sutton *et al.* (1994) suggesting that corticosteroids have a role in the synthesis of neurotransmitters involved in producing SIA.

8.3   THE FACTORS THAT INDUCE ANALGESIA

8.3.1   Social Factors

Miczek *et al.* (1982) measured analgesia by the tail-flick test, following exposure of intruder mice to attack in the home cage of another animal. Initially, the intruder responded to the aggression of the resident with active attempts at defence. On failing, this strategy gave way to the mouse's species-typical passive posture of defeat. The degree of analgesia increased as a function of the number of bites received from the resident. However, Miczek *et al.* argued that it was the tendency specifically to show defeat *behaviour* in response to the bites that was closely correlated with analgesia; the number of bites *per se* (and, presumably, noxious stimulation received) was not such a good predictor. The analgesia was blocked by naloxone, indicating its mediation by opioids. The attacking mice did not show analgesia, even though they were exposed to some bites from the intruder. As Miczek *et al.* note, stress, as broadly defined, is not enough to explain such analgesia, as residents show an elevation in pituitary–adrenal activity in the course of attacking: 'Apparently, the special biological significance of the defeat experience, and not simply the experience of being stressed, is critical to the occurrence of opioid-like analgesia'. Such defeat-induced analgesia is particularly strong in animals lacking fighting experience (Miczek, 1980), suggestive of its association with an unambiguous defeat strategy.

Williams *et al.* (1990) attempted to create a seminatural situation within which to study SIA. They exposed intruder rats to defeat by an aggressive alpha resident. The intruders were tested 24 h later in the presence of odours (specifically bedding) from the alpha colony. An increase in freezing tendency and analgesia were seen. Analgesia depended upon a combination of an earlier experience of defeat and the presence of alpha colony odours.

Rodgers (1989) notes the frequency of finding non-opioid-mediated analgesia in situations of activity. He argues:

> . . . functional relationships may exist between opioid analgesia and passive defence and between non-opioid analgesia and active defense. More specifically, in the context of murine social conflict, early non-opioid analgesia would function to prevent the disruption of fight/flight reactions by noxious input whereas late opioid analgesia would inhibit reflexive responses to pain that would seriously compromise the efficacy of the immobility defense.

Thus stimuli, natural or unnatural (e.g. a brief foot shock), that elicit flight/fight induce non-opioid analgesia. Stimuli, natural (capture) or unnatural (e.g. body pinch), which elicit tonic immobility induce opioid analgesia (Rodgers and Randall, 1987b).

In such terms, if active agonistic interactions (assisted by non-opioid-based analgesia) fail, the mouse switches to a passive strategy, assisted by opioid-mediated analgesia; although note the reservation expressed in Chapter 6 regarding the view that passive strategies are simply an option to switch in when active strategies fail. Rodgers reported that this state resembled tonic immobility (Section 6.9.1). In the case of social conflict in mice, Rodgers and Randall (1988) cite evidence showing that extended exposure to a stressor is the precondition both for the organism to learn that it has no control over the stressor and for activation of a 'long-exposure' (see earlier) opioid-mediated analgesia. (As noted, in rats there is also evidence for a short-exposure opioid response; Grau, 1987; Maier, 1989; Sutton *et al.*, 1994.) In this way, for the special case of intraspecific aggression in mice, Rodgers and Randall propose qualifying the description of when opioid-mediated analgesia is experienced, over and above that of 'defeat' (see last section).

Figure 8.1 shows a summary of Rodgers and Randall's (1987b) argument. The perception of danger (for example, odours from a conspecific

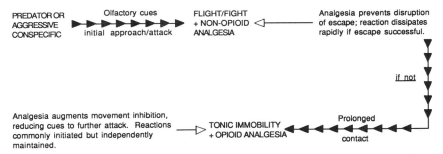

Figure 8.1.   Model of stress-induced analgesia proposed by Rodgers and Randall (1987b, figure 2)

on entering novel territory arouses: (1) motivational mechanisms of active defence and (2) non-opioid analgesia. The function served by such analgesia is to prevent disruption of either flight or defensive attack. If active mechanisms fail and prolonged (but passive) contact ensues the function of the opioid analgesia which this stimulates is to 'eliminate involuntary cues (i.e. reflexive responses to tissue damage) which might provoke further attack'.

8.3.2   Artificial Stimuli

As this section will show, analgesia induced by artificial stimuli such as electric shock fits a similar pattern to that induced by natural stimuli. Short uncontrollable shock seems to tap into the processes underlying active defence, whereas longer-term uncontrollable shock seems to mimic defeat with its associated passive strategies. Certain of the evidence both from natural (last section) and artificial (this section) stimulation fits with the notion of an association between active defence and a non-opioid form of analgesia. However, it should be noted that some analgesia is seen even in decerebrate and deeply anaesthetized animals (Maier, 1989), an unlearned effect mediated at the spinal and brainstem levels (Sutton *et al.*, 1994). It would seem that, in part, analgesia, whether opioid- or non-opioid based, is an immediate consequence of the sensory stimulation of shock. Later, analgesia depends upon such things as conditioning and appraisal of the situation as controllable or not (Maier, 1989; Sutton *et al.*, 1994).

Maier *et al.* (1982) noted that the parameter of controllability versus uncontrollability influenced an organism's reactions to a potential stressor and investigated its role in SIA. Analgesia was measured by the tail-flick test, the latency for a rat to move its tail away from a hot object. Rats subjected to escapable shock were compared with yoked rats unable to influence shocks. As a control, a third group was simply restrained but not exposed to shock. When tested 30 min after shock, the escape group were found to have a slightly longer latency than the restrained controls, but the yoked group had a much longer latency than the escape group.

In a similar vein, Sumova and Jakoubek (1989) argue that, in their experiment, opioid-based SIA, caused by a warning signal of forthcoming inescapable shock, is associated with situations where active coping is not possible. (Interestingly, in humans performing cognitive tasks, an opioid-mediated analgesia was associated with a *failure to cope*, termed inefficacy; Bandura *et al.*, 1988). Lewis *et al.* (1980) reported that their rats subjected to intermittent stress and showing an opioid-based analgesia 'appeared behaviourally depressed'. Further evidence also points to an association between the 'passive behavioural control system' and the opioid-mediated system of analgesia (see also Section 6.9). Thus the cholinergic antagonist scopolamine strongly lowered opioid-based, but not non-opioid-based analgesia (Lewis et al., 1983; Terman et al., 1984). That this was a central effect, presumably involving a CNS synapse, is suggested by the result that methyl-scopolamine, which has only a peripheral cholinergic antagonistic effect, failed to affect analgesia.

The stressor commonly employed in studies of analgesia is shock to the feet. The resultant analgesia is termed foot-shock-induced anal-gesia (FSIA). Whereas shock to the front feet (FFS) causes an opioid-based analgesia, shock to the rear feet (RFS) causes a non-opioid-based form. FSIA can be classically conditioned. The cage within which shock was given can serve as a CS and shock as the UCS. Conditioning is tested by exposing the rat to the cage (CS) in the absence of shock (UCS), and a conditioned analgesia is obtained. A CS paired with either FFS or RFS causes an opioid-based analgesia (Watkins and Mayer, 1982). Like the FSIA following the UCS, this analgesia is neu-ronally rather than hormonally mediated (Watkins and Mayer, 1982). Conditioned analgesia seems (at least usually) to be opioid mediated (Maier, 1989).

A difference in response depending upon which feet are shocked might appear slightly bizarre but there is a well-established precedent in the literature for a distinction in behavioural outcome based upon site of stimulation and this might similarly be interpreted in terms of strategy. For rats running in an alley of a maze, FFS is response suppressing (apparently, switching in a passive control system) whereas RFS is not; the rat's reaction to FFS is to decelerate whereas that to RFS is to accelerate forwards (Fowler and Miller, 1963). Also the reaction to a CS paired with shock is one of freezing (Fanselow and Lester, 1988). Thus, as for social contexts discussed earlier, the opioid-based SIA would seem to form part of a behavioural system of passivity (cf. Gray, 1987). The fact that the reaction to a CS paired with RFS is different from the reaction to the shock itself is a further instance of a general principle that the conditional response (CR) need not resemble the unconditional response (UCR) (Bindra, 1978; Fanselow and Lester, 1988).

Grau (1987) discusses the parameters that distinguish neural– and hormonal–opioid analgesia. A brief exposure to shock can elicit a neural–opioid analgesia. A more extensive series of uncontrollable shocks (e.g. 60 or more shocks), which the animal learns are uncon-trollable, leads to hormonal–opioid analgesia. This analgesia, seen after inescapable shock, which takes some minutes to develop, can be reversed by opioid antagonists and is blocked by procedures which disrupt secretion of β-endorphins by the pituitary. McCubbin (1993) notes that there is relatively little opioid-based analgesia seen in response to a single brief but unbroken foot shock as compared with the reaction to multiple intermittent shock. The suggestion that 'this may reflect the role of multiple trials in the extinction of coping attempts' implies a switch to a more passive mode of control in the case of opioid analgesia.

Hormonal–opioid analgesia is evident in the cases of acupuncture, prolonged shock of all four paws and immobilization (Watkins and Mayer, 1982). It is disrupted by removal of the pituitary or adrenal. There is a tendency for opioid-mediated analgesia that is insensitive to hypophysectomy to be found in short-duration experiments (e.g. 3 min exposure to shock), whereas that which is sensitive to these disruptions to be found in longer duration (e.g. 30 min of intermittent shock) experiments (Lewis et al., 1980; Terman et al., 1984).

In addition to analgesia shortly after exposure to the stressor, another hormonal–opioid effect is also seen, that of sensitization (Grau, 1987). That is to say, following shock exposure that elicits opioid-based SIA, a brief exposure to shock (inadequate in itself to induce such analgesia) can reinstate analgesia 24 h later. Evidence for the hormonal basis of this effect is provided by the observation that both initial analgesia and reinstatement are blocked by dexamethasone which inhibits activation of the HPA axis.

Grau (1987) looked at the conditions which give rise to opioid and non-opioid analgesia. The non-opioid analgesia is seen immediately after shock but its effect is transient and soon dissipates. Its magnitude depends upon the intensity of the shock. Although it can be seen within 1 min of shock, the opioid analgesia is of longer duration than the non-opioid. Grau then developed a theoretical model to explain the magnitude and duration of SIA. He reasons from the premise that the duration of SIA depends upon not simply the parameters of the physical shock itself but 'according to our hypothesis, the dissipation of analgesia is also determined by the rate at which the memory of the aversive event decays'. The fact that non-opioid analgesia is transient suggests that only a strong memory is sufficient to trigger it and dovetails with the finding that non-opioid analgesia is sensitive to the magnitude of shock. The relatively long-lasting nature of opioid analgesia suggested that a weaker memory trace was sufficient to stimulate this form. However, as Grau notes, considering the strength of memory representation in this way does not give insight as to why conditioned analgesia should be opioid based. At this point the theory

leads to consideration of a contemporary understanding of the processes forming memory and the notion of activation of memory. Grau
found that a distracting stimulus presented immediately after shock
reduced the extent of SIA and argued that the distractor displaced the
memory of the shock from the active phase.

Grau does not address the issue of why there should be a difference
depending upon which pair of feet are shocked. It is not clear why such
a difference should be associated with differences in the strength of
activation of memory. However, a difference in reaction does follow
logically in terms of a difference in strategy recruited in the two shock
conditions, as does the opioid basis of conditioned analgesia. The model
proposed here might be compatible with features of Grau's model. For
example, suppose a short shock: (1) strongly arouses a memory into an
'active' store (Lewis, 1979) and (2) recruits an active strategy. If the
shock is controllable, its termination will coincide with performance of
behaviour. However, even for an uncontrollable shock there might be
some coincidence between behaviour and termination (see also discussion in Section 5.9). As has been argued elsewhere (Toates, 1995b),
there is probably a process by which successfully performing behaviour
can trigger removal of a memory from the active state. Such an approach dovetails with the conclusions of Fanselow and Lester's (1988)
analysis that nociception itself is not what triggers analgesia; although
see Maier (1989). Indeed, such a process would seem to be illogical and
maladaptive. Rather, as they argue: 'it is that the stimuli that lead to
antipredator defences also lead to analgesia'.

Differences in results between subjects when compared between different laboratories in the relative weight of opioid and non-opioid analgesia might depend upon genetic and experiential differences, an as
yet largely unexplored area (Brush and Shain, 1989).

8.4   FUNCTION SERVED BY STRESS-INDUCED ANALGESIA

In the natural environment, the so-called stress hormones will perhaps
be released mainly in times of conflict. During a threat to the integrity
of the animal or to its resources, the adaptive value of postponing
attention to wounds is not difficult to envisage. Considering active
defence, Amit and Galina (1986) note that when an animal pursues a
particular goal then persistence might be adaptive in spite of a signal
indicating tissue damage. As an example, consider an animal that has
wounded its prey but none the less sustained an injury in the process.
To attend to the wound by, say, licking it or by retiring from the scene

could be counter-productive. The task needs completion. On termination of the encounter, it is presumably adaptive to attend fully to the
signal arising from noxious stimulation, e.g. to rest, to lick a wound or
favour an injured limb.

If an animal cannot sustain active defence, passivity might be the best
strategy and one function of SIA would therefore seem to be to assist the
animal at times of immobility. A defeated animal may be better able to
remain in a passive submission posture if it does not attend to wounds.
Immobility in mice can sometimes serve to deflect the interest of a
predator. Rodgers (1989) notes an association between opioid analgesia
and motor inhibition. He also notes that exogenous application of morphine and β-endorphin is able to elicit a catatonic-like state.

Rodgers and Randall (1987a) suggest that considerations of function
are relevant to answering the question—Why two types (opioid and non-
opioid) of analgesia? Flight and tonic immobility are mutually exclusive
reactions and logically it might prove impossible for a given neurochemical to be associated with both. Also a difference in the properties of two
different classes of substances might be implicated in the different time
course of non-opioid (less than 10 min) and opioid (40–60 min) analgesia.
In evolutionary history, successful active escape or attack might have
been quicker than successful tonic immobility.

The type of stressor that can induce SIA might point to its function.
Amit and Galina (1986) suggest a cognitive component of the effective
stressors. The situations considered, e.g. passive submission, attack
and predation, all involve goals, assessment and decision-making.

8.5 APPETITIVE SITUATIONS AND STRESS-INDUCED ANALGESIA

Throughout the present study, both aversive and appetitive situations
have been considered for insight into stress, and analgesia is another
example of where it is useful to study both. Certain appetitive situations that are considered to be stress-evoking elicit SIA (Tazi et al.,
1987a). Given that depriving a rat of food and exposing it to cues
associated with food is potentially stress evoking by the criterion of
HPA activation (Chapters 5 and 9), researchers have looked at the
influence on SIA of: (1) prediction over food delivery; (2) control over
food delivery; and (3) the ability to engage in drinking, as measured by
tail-flick latency.

The increase in tail-flick latency over the session was greater for
animals in the 'no prediction' condition as compared with the 'prediction' condition. Similarly, the increase for a group having no control

over delivery was greater than that of a group having control. When a water-spout was made available, rats were able to be dichotomized into schedule-induced polydipsia positive, i.e. showing polydipsia (SIP pos) and schedule-induced polydipsia negative, i.e. not showing poly-dipsia (SIP neg) (see also Chapter 9). SIP neg rats were found to have higher pre-session tail-flick latencies than SIP pos rats. SIP neg rats were found to be like rats not having water available in that tail-flick latency increased during the session. By contrast, for SIP pos rats with water available, tail-flick latency decreased over the session and be-tween sessions. SIP pos animals were tested without water on day 10 and a significant increase in post-session latency was seen.

Given that schedule-induced drinking reduces tail-flick latencies and that SIP neg animals had higher tail-flick latencies than SIP pos, Tazi *et al*. (1987a) suggested that: '. . . the intriguing possibility that endogenous pain-suppressing systems could play a role in the motiva-tion of this behaviour'.

Some insight might therefore be obtained by looking for common features between SIP and active coping strategies (flight, flee, lever-press) on confrontation with a stressor.

8.6   A PARALLEL AMONG THE REACTIONS TO STRESSORS

As noted at the start of the chapter, SIA, apart from its intrinsic inter-est, offers the possibility of insights into broader issues of stress. Cen-tral states manifest in SIA are also revealed in other indices of stress. A certain parallel among events initiated by stressors has been noted by a number of authors (McCubbin *et al*., 1984; Grau, 1987; Murison and Overmier, 1993). This section forms an appropriate place to look at the phenomenon of SIA in the context of other consequences of apply-ing stressors.

Grau (1987) describes a similarity between the acquisition of opioid analgesia and learned helplessness. According to him, the learned helplessness hypothesis might describe: '. . . the conditions under which the pituitary–adrenal axis sensitizes the opioid analgesic sys-tem. That is, the axis may only increase the gain in the opioid system after the organism has learned that the aversive event is uncontroll-able'. McCubbin *et al*. (1984) describe an opioid-based analgesia to prolonged inescapable shock but not to escapable shock or to that ap-plied to the rear paws only. Further, they report that exposure to such a stressor is also followed by a deficit in a one-way avoidance task (Section 7.9.2). Opioid blocking reverses these effects.

Murison and Overmier (1993) were interested in seeing how the reaction to one stressor would influence the reaction to another applied later, in terms of: (1) behavioural; (2) nociceptive; (3) immunological; and (4) gastrointestinal reactions to the second. The message to emerge from the study was that the reaction to a stressor as reflected in the four aspects depends upon: (1) the qualitative nature of the stressor and (2) the history of stressor exposure to which the animal had been subjected.

Murison and Overmier (1993) note that prior repeated exposure to shock exerts a bias towards freezing behaviour and a relatively large corticosterone response when the rat is subsequently given an open-field test. They discuss a result of Fanselow (1980) showing that there is an attenuation of the effect if the initial shocks are administered in a different environment from that in which the rat is later tested. This shows the role of associative factors. Further, they note that the effect of such a series of shocks of the kind that would induce an opioid-based analgesia is also manifest 24 h later as a deficit in an escape/avoidance shuttle-box task (Section 7.9.4). This is commonly termed 'learned helplessness'. The effect of intermittent uncontrollable shocks on subsequent escape/avoidance behaviour depends partly on the presence of cues in the test situation which were also present at the time of initial stressor exposure. Such learned helplessness is not found 24 h after a single long shock, this being the kind of stressor that produces a non-opioid analgesia. Neither is it found if the shocks are escapable or if 'safety from them is predictable'.

The analgesia following a series of intermittent shocks is reversible with naloxone, suggesting that it is mediated by opioids. It is also blocked by scopolamine, indicating a cholinergic involvement and by disruption of the HPA axis, implicating a role of this axis. Murison and Overmier suggest, on the grounds that the analgesia is blocked by pentobarbital and not seen in decerebrates, that it is dependent upon higher nervous activity. The opioid-based analgesia seems to depend upon the animal learning that the shock is uncontrollable. The analgesia following a single relatively intense shock is not affected by naloxone, suggesting that it is not a form of opioid analgesia. By contrast to opioid-based analgesia, the non-opioid form does not depend upon learning, it being an immediate unconditional reaction to the shock.

Murison and Overmier (1993) go on to note that the opioid form of analgesia (but not the non-opioid form) can be reinstated by priming shocks that would themselves be inadequate to produce analgesia (i.e. inadequate in the absence of the shock session 24 h or more earlier).

They suggest that such opioid-based reinstatement depends upon associative processes (although whether this is the most appropriate expression has been questioned by Grau, 1987), that is to say a similarity between induction and test phases in terms of 'psychological–environmental context'. (There is evidence from a memory study for such a process of reinstatement by reminder cues, reviewed by Lewis, 1979.)

By analogy with analgesia, Murison and Overmier (1993) then go on to consider the effects of prior shock on immunomodulation (see Chapter 4). For instance, this might be implicated in the result that exposing young rats to uncontrollable shock increases their susceptibility to tumours when adult. In another study reviewed, adult rats were injected with tumour cells 3 h after shock exposure. When exposure was to a shock stimulus of the kind that would trigger an opioid-based analgesia, rats showed reduced survival time. By contrast, those exposed to a stimulus that would trigger a non-opioid form of analgesia did not differ in survival time from unshocked controls. Evidence entirely compatible with an opioid mediation of the effect upon the tumour cells was that a comparable effect upon mortality could be obtained simply by injecting morphine and omitting the shocks.

Having seen evidence of a commonality in three indices of the effects of prior shock, Murison and Overmier (1993) then looked to see whether the commonality could be extended to the role of stress on gastric ulceration. Specifically, they investigated the role of prior exposure to shock on later development of gastric ulceration in response to the stressor of restraint in water. Rats were subjected to a session of exposure to either predictable or unpredictable foot shock and then, 45 h later, to restraint stress. There was evidence of an amplification effect of prior shock exposure on the subsequent development of ulcers to restraint. Unsignalled shock had a greater effect than signalled shock. Animals exposed to uncontrollable shock showed a greater degree of ulceration in response to restraint tested even up to 30–60 days after prior shock exposure. However, the effect is not seen if exposure was to either an escapable shock or to a shock accompanied by signalled safety.

Further experiments looked at whether it is possible to get a proactive effect of stressor exposure on subsequent restraint ulceration when a single long shock is used. In so doing, Murison and Overmier (1993) compared the situation of giving the shock: (a) immediately upon being placed in the apparatus or (b) at the end of a period of confinement. Condition (a) produced an effect comparable with exposure to 80 short shocks whereas condition (b) resulted in no proactive effect. Murison and Overmier suggest that in condition (a) there is backward conditioning between exposure to the apparatus post-shock and the shock. This might well be so but the result does not allow this interpretation to be distinguished from, for example, conditioning between the apparatus and the consequences of the shock (e.g. a rebound parasympathetic discharge to the stomach; see Sections 6.9.3 and 10.7.5).

Murison and Overmier (1993) also investigated whether the proactive effects of, for one group, 80 5 second shocks and, for the other group, one 400 second shock (given early in period of exposure to apparatus), are affected by blocking opioid processes. Preliminary studies indicated that opioid blocking prior to the shock exposure disrupted the proactive effect of the 80 5 second shocks. By contrast, the effect of the single 400 second foot shock is not disrupted by opioid blocking. Again, evidence compatible with an opioid mediation is shown by the result of giving an injection of morphine on its own. It was found that this can mimic the exacerbating effect on ulceration that would be produced by shock exposure of the kind that would normally recruit an opioid-based analgesia.

8.7 CONCLUSIONS

Although it might prove dangerous to stretch the argument too far and some curious results remain to be explained (Foo and Westbrook, 1994), some evidence emerges to suggest that the varieties of SIA are to be understood at least in part in terms of different stimuli setting the scene for different strategies to be implemented. However, it is as well to recall that there are basic unconditional analgesic reactions to shock (Maier, 1989). In defending a model in which central emotional reaction mediates SIA, Fanselow (1991) qualifies this by observing that the emotional response to the UCR of shock must be different from that shown to the CS predictive of shock. This is because the analgesia is different. Whether one uses Fanselow's terminology or thinks of the emotional state as being the same with different reactions switched in according to context, is perhaps a matter of semantics.

When associated with analgesia, it might be that stressors such as rotation and immobilization, which are said by some (Hayes et al., 1978) to constitute a 'non-noxious stressor', might none the less be fear-evoking (Bolles and Fanselow, 1980) and recruit a passive strategy. Certain stressors, e.g. ether vapours and horizontal oscillation (Watkins and Mayer, 1982), fail to elicit analgesia and it is tempting to suggest that they do not permit recruitment of a clear strategy.

If analgesia is used as an index of stress, this reveals certain parallels with other effects of stressors. The dichotomy between active and passive reactions to a threat (Chapter 6) appears to be reflected, respectively, in non-opioid- and opioid-mediated analgesia.

Stimuli that induce freezing (e.g. a CS predictive of shock, presence of a predator) tend to elicit opioid-based analgesia. The common property of aversive stimuli and exposure to certain appetitive situations in activating the HPA system is also reflected in SIA.

The conclusion is that SIA depends upon a central state that modulates the reaction to tissue damage in the overall interests of survival. Understanding the two aspects, opioid and non-opioid analgesia, might be helped by an understanding of passive and active controls exerted in reaction to a stressor. That SIA is part of an integrated reaction to a particular situation of threat is further suggested by the existence of an anti-analgesia system (Wiertelak *et al.*, 1992). This antagonizes the opioid-based analgesia system described in this section and is recruited by cues of safety (e.g. a stimulus that predicts no shock). It would seem to be part of a system promoting attention to tissue damage when the animal is in a safe location. This factor might help explain an otherwise anomalous *hyper*algesia reported by some researchers in the safe period following termination of a CS that would be expected to trigger an immediate analgesia (see Grau, 1987).

There are factors yet to be interpreted. For example, in snails, exposure to warmth causes an analgesia that is blocked by naloxone whereas cold exposure causes a non-opioid analgesia (Kavaliers, 1987). By analogy, in rats and mice, a warm-water swim induces a mild opioid analgesia whereas a cold-water swim induces a non-opioid-based analgesia (O'Connor and Chipkin, 1984). The similarity is striking and suggests a general functional significance. In line with the trend observed in this chapter one might suggest that the warm environment encourages passivity and a cold one activity. However, the differential effect might arise from events intrinsic to the temperature regulation system.

Recently, a role for adenosine in SIA has been suggested (Minor *et al.*, 1994b). Injection of adenosine or its analogue can create a state of helplessness and analgesia. This state is also associated with a lack of interest in positive incentive objects (cf. Wise, 1994). Therefore if adenosine is importantly implicated in SIA it would suggest the existence of rather different states when comparing the analgesias induced by aversive and appetitive stimuli (Section 8.1).

Evidence reviewed in Chapter 5 suggests that normal social interactions are affected by a background level of endorphin release and indeed that their frequency can be altered by naloxone injection. This is in contrast to reports in the literature on SIA, where evidence of no such background level of endogenous opioid or naloxone influence has been found (Jacquet, 1980).

Chapter 9

Ethology Pure and Applied— Issues of Animal Welfare

9.1 INTRODUCTION

The scientific study of animal welfare has assumed great importance in recent years, with ethological evidence being at the core of the discussions. In this context, stress is of central relevance to the welfare, suffering and husbandry of domestic animals, the topic of the present chapter. The relationship between 'pure' and applied stress research is a reciprocal one: 'pure' ethologists and psychologists are sometimes able to illuminate applied issues, whereas applied research has provided much of the impetus for reconsidering motivation theory (Wiepkema and Van Adrichem, 1987; Hughes and Duncan, 1988a,b; Toates and Jensen, 1991; Jensen and Toates, 1993). The evidence cited in this chapter is the result of such cross-fertilization.

9.2 CRITERIA OF WELFARE AND DISTRESS

9.2.1 Definitions of Stress and Welfare

In discussing issues of welfare, it can be useful as one guide among others to consider the definition of stress suggested by Fraser and Broom (1990), in terms of a reduction in fitness (Section 1.3.11). For example, a change in housing conditions might elevate the secretion of corticosteroids and thereby inhibit reproductive capacity and compromise the immune system. In principle, it might be possible to extrapolate to a more natural context, use this as a frame of reference and thereby to obtain some measure of just how much such a procedure would lower fitness. In so doing, one might be able to argue that the animal's welfare was lowered. However, as always these theoretical tools need to be handled with caution. For example, it might be misleading to argue in such a situation that welfare had been fully restored by, say, giving multiple vaccinations, as this would not address the environmental stressor at the root of the problem (Fraser and Broom, 1990, p. 274).

After reviewing the evidence from veterinary science and practice, Fraser *et al*. (1975) propose the definition of stress as: 'An animal is said to be in a state of *stress* if it is required to make abnormal or extreme adjustments in its physiology or behaviour in order to cope with adverse aspects of its environment and management'. Fraser *et al*. argue that one could not expect to find a unitary state within the animal corresponding to stress, just as one would not find a single entity called 'disease' that could be located on a single-dimension scale. No one behaviour or endocrinological index would invariably be present. Neither should a clear boundary between 'normal' and 'abnormal' be expected. They argue that whereas a general all-embracing definition of what is abnormal might not emerge, none the less there appears to be a good consensus that certain particular cases in domestic animals (discussed later) constitute abnormal behaviour.

Fraser *et al*. (1975) note that the definition covers an environment that makes excessive demands upon an animal but how about cases of understimulation, of 'boredom'? They argue that such situations are covered by the definition as, '. . . animals in monotonous and restricting environments seek out opportunities for exercise and stimulation'. Wemelsfelder (1990) notes that, placed in a situation which, by human criteria, would be described as 'boring', animals can react with either active strategies (e.g. pacing) or passive strategies (e.g. giving up, lethargy). This might prove to map on to the active/passive dichotomy developed in Chapter 6.

Novak and Suomi (1988) propose tentatively a set of criteria for establishing the psychological well-being of captive non-human primates, as follows:

(a) The primate is in good physical health; (b) it exhibits a substantial range of the species' behavioural repertoire and, if individually housed, does not display high levels of bizarre, stereotyped, or disorganized patterns of behaviour; (c) it is not in a chronic state of distress; and (d) it is able to respond effectively to environmental challenges.

Although acknowledging the difficulties of definition, these authors suggest that if evidence of two of these four criteria a–d are present, this would be evidence for psychological well-being.

Wiepkema and Koolhaas (1993) suggest that transient conflict can be indicated by displacement activities (see below), but should be seen as being within the bounds of normal behaviour. However, if the conditions remain chronic, implying a failure to resolve underlying conflict, a welfare problem is indicated. Transient conflict behaviour (e.g. displacement activity) can give way to stereotypy.

9.2.2 Corticosteroids

One commonly used criterion of stress is an elevation in corticosteroid levels. Quite often, the literature contains the implicit or explicit assumption that, if an animal is able to confine its plasma levels of corticosteroids to within a relatively low range, it is showing coping in the face of a stressor and thereby positive welfare (Broom, 1991; Dantzer, 1991; Le Moal and Simon, 1991; Mason, 1991; Section 9.5.3.8). Barnett (1987) argues that: '. . . a sustained elevation of free (biologically active) corticosteroids arguably provides *prima facie* evidence of a real or potential risk to welfare'. He notes that such elevation is associated with a loss of body protein, a reduction in reproductive capacity, increased metabolic rate and suppression of the immune system (see Chapters 4 and 10). He contrasts such undesirable consequences of chronically elevated corticosteroid activity with the innocuous short-term activation accompanying, for example, physical exercise. Barnett notes the clear practical application of stress criteria; pigs housed in certain solitary environments show a sustained activation of the hypothalamic–pituitary–adrenocortical (HPA) axis.

As Fraser *et al.* (1975) point out, common sense might suggest that, in social crowding, animals are exposed to too much social stimulation whereas in isolation they are exposed to too little. However, both of these situations can lead to an increase in activity of the HPA axis in rodents. In the terms advanced in this book, either situation could correspond to disparity between actual and desired states, to fruitless attempts to resolve disparity and consequent HPA activation. Sigg *et al.* (1966) found elevated adrenal weight in isolated mice; although logically crowding and isolation might be regarded as opposite ends of a dimension, the terms 'under-stress' and 'over-stress' to describe such situations could be inherently misleading. Fraser *et al.* argue for the use of 'stress' to refer to a pathological extreme, irrespective of whether it arises from too much or too little stimulation, a point also argued by Ödberg (1993).

There is, however, a paradox in the use of corticosteroid levels as a frame of reference for good welfare in that rats will learn an operant task for their administration and prefer to drink a corticosteroid-containing fluid over pure water (Deroche *et al.*, 1993). Thus, although a restrained level of corticosteroids might be an index of good welfare, one cannot necessarily suppose that the animal tracks its level of corticosteroids and adopts strategies that serve to restrain them. It might even learn such strategies *in spite of*, rather than because of, the resulting low corticosteroid level.

It needs to be stated that, although excessive levels can bring dangers, through their metabolic effects a basal level of corticosteroids plays a positive part in biological function. Animals lacking corticosteroids show a reduced survival in the face of stressors (Dallman, 1991). Therefore, from functional considerations, one should not necessarily expect to see a process that simply motivates an animal to lower its level of corticosteroids. Given that an optimal range of corticosteroids exists (Sapolsky, 1991), from functional considerations one might expect to see an evolutionary pressure to maintain corticosteroids within such an optimal level.

9.2.3   Catecholamines

Techniques designed to reduce stress in domestic animals can raise some interesting and paradoxical issues. For example, reserpine, a substance that depletes catecholamines, is sometimes used to sedate chickens undergoing stressful experiences (Freeman, 1971). By such indices as blood pressure and heart rate, the birds are indeed less stressed, and might survive better. However, it should be noted that: (1) catecholamines are associated with active coping strategies (see Chapter 5 and discussion on toughening in Chapter 10) and (2) by CNS depletion of catecholamines, reserpine tends to induce depression in some human subjects (Veith, 1991). There are therefore potentially dangers in basing conclusions concerning welfare upon isolated autonomic indices.

9.3   STRESS AND THE BEHAVIOUR OF SICK ANIMALS

The behaviour of sick animals is a topic that interfaces with that of stress. This section will consider an integrative review 'Biological basis of the behaviour of sick animals' presented by Hart (1988) and discuss its relevance to the topic of stress.

Hart (1988) starts by noting that most things written on adaptation and function concern healthy animals. However, he adopts a functional perspective on the behaviour of animals ill with protozoan, bacterial and viral infections. The behaviour of infected animals is characterized by such terms as depression, lethargy and a loss of the motivation to feed and drink. Grooming is greatly reduced and the amount of time spent sleeping increases. A pattern of such behaviour, accompanied by fever, is commonly interpreted as a sign of infectious illness. The pattern is not confined to one species but is seen in a variety, including humans. Hart's argument is that such a pattern of responses is not to be interpreted as an incidental product of illness but rather, in collaboration with the immune reaction, as a highly adaptive pattern that plays a crucial part in recovery.

On initial infection, there is: (1) activation of part of the immune system; (2) increased body temperature; and (3) lowered plasma iron concentration, having the effect of inhibiting the growth of pathogens (Hart, 1988). Hart argues that depression and anorexia form part of a behavioural mode of control that has the effect of raising body temperature and lowering plasma iron concentration. Rather than fever being an undesirable side-effect of the infection and something that forms a target to be combatted, it should be viewed as an adaptive response.

As part of the immune response (Chapter 4), bacteria and viruses cause leucocytes to secrete a product that has the effect of inducing fever. Such a product is termed an endogenous pyrogen, several of which are released. The one that Hart focuses upon is interleukin-1 (IL-1), whose role is not only that of raising body temperature but also lowering plasma iron and zinc concentrations. As was discussed in Chapter 4, IL-1 also activates the HPA system. Hart suggests that the corticosteroids released in this way help the animal to meet its energy demands. As was noted in Chapter 2, corticotrophin-releasing factor (CRF) serves both as a neurotransmitter in the CNS, implicated in activation of the sympathetic branch of the autonomic nervous system (ANS), and as a neurohormone that initiates the sequence of the HPA system. As was discussed in Chapter 4, IL-1 seems to activate this substance.

As part of the reaction described, an elevated body temperature arises from, in effect, pyrogens raising the set-point (Toates, 1975) of the temperature regulation system, this being true even in lizards (Cabanac and Gosselin, 1993). Depending upon the species, the actual elevation of body temperature is achieved by both autonomic (e.g. shunting blood from the periphery) and behavioural (e.g. curling up, sleeping) means of heat production and conservation. Inhibition of grooming presumably serves to reduce heat loss by allowing the animal to remain immobile. In addition, for oral grooming, the inhibition reduces heat loss that would otherwise be accelerated through moist skin. Clearly, it reduces water loss. Anorexia is not so easy to explain and, like all such functional explanations, any explanation presented is difficult to verify. Indeed, it might seem counterintuitive to cut down on food intake at a time when energy is needed to maintain an elevated body temperature. However, as Hart (1988) notes, an animal that is unmotivated to feed is one unmotivated to move in the pursuit of food, which might otherwise increase heat loss from the body. Also, a sick animal is one most probably at a strong disadvantage in escaping from predators. Some of the effects described are summarized in Figure 9.1.

Hart (1988) argues that the practical relevance of the perspective he develops is that the animal, human or otherwise, should be treated in such a way as to allow temperature to be maintained at the elevated set-point. Antipyretics should only be used if the elevation in temperature reaches dangerous limits. Force feeding should only be employed if lack of nutrients is threatening and any nutrients supplied should not contain iron.

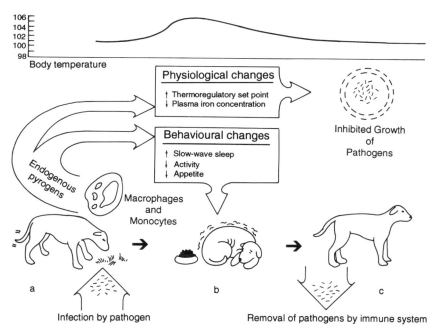

Figure 9.1. Representation of the sequence of an acute infectious illness as proposed by Hart (1988). (a) Exposure to pathogens, (b) behavioural changes characterizing sickness and (c) recovery. (Reprinted from Hart, 1988. Copyright 1988, with kind permission from Elsevier Science Ltd, The Boulevard, Langford Lane, Kidlington OX5 1GB, UK)

There is some evidence for an anticipatory process at work in this system. As was introduced in Chapter 4, simply exposing an animal to a stressor induces a rise in body temperature. Singer *et al.* (1986) speculate that this is mediated via IL-1. They also speculate that such a rise in body temperature should be viewed in functional terms. Thus, a stressful situation is one of potential injury and infection, and a rise in body temperature could play an adaptive part against any infection (see also Cabanac and Gosselin, 1993, for a comparable effect in lizards).

9.4 BEHAVIOUR, ITS CAUSES AND ITS CONSEQUENCES

The study of animal behaviour in an applied setting has a reciprocally beneficial effect on the more 'pure' study of animal behaviour and the development of explanatory models of behaviour. A number of basic issues in behavioural science have been raised in an applied context and behavioural models are of potential importance to husbandry practice. This section considers a few such issues.

9.4.1 Representations and Expectations

Chapter 1 claimed that animals create expectations regarding the state of the world and their actions upon the world. In arguing the case for welfare considerations, Poole (1992) associates frustration with the failure to reach goals. Good welfare involves provision of facilities (e.g. a safe and secure nesting site) such that goals can be realized. According to this analysis, a limited amount of uncertainty might be introduced into the environment to defend against the emergence of boredom, apathy and presumably in certain species something analogous to depression.

Wiepkema (1990) discusses 'gakeln', a particular call made by laying hens. Hens emit this call when, for example, they have learned to expect food at a given time of day and in a particular location and then the food does not appear. Prior food deprivation intensifies the call. The call is also heard when a laying hen, on attempting to use her laying nest, finds that entry is blocked. Gakeln is also exhibited when hens go to a location associated with dustbathing, consisting of a tray containing sand, but when the tray is inaccessible. Wiepkema suggests: '. . . that hens perform "gakeln", when they expect some goal situation, but experience an unforeseen change and/or a blocked goal situation. The call's intensity appears to reflect the strength of the expectation and/or the significance of the goal'. It might therefore be argued that a positive contribution to welfare would be made by providing an environment that minimizes the occurrence of frustrated expectations.

9.4.2   A Need to Behave?

Do animals have a need to perform certain behaviours? This question, involving definition of what is meant by the term 'need', is one that has occupied the attention of applied ethologists and others (Toates and Jensen, 1991; Jensen and Toates, 1993). By intuition some behaviours such as feeding are the reflection of a need which if not met will lead to pathology.

Some would argue that one can classify motivations according to whether they are internally driven (e.g. feeding) or externally driven (e.g. predator avoidance) and only the former class is associated with needs (Hughes, 1980, 1988). Thus it is possible to imagine, for example, an environment in which animals are never given a trigger to perform species-typical predator avoidance but do not suffer as a result of not performing it. However, caution is required in drawing such a distinction, both in its theoretical and applied aspects (Toates and Jensen, 1991; Jensen and Toates, 1993). For example, some environments might inadvertently provide the stimuli for fear-motivated behaviour without the opportunity to take appropriate action. Indeed, Duncan and Poole (1990) discuss the 'extreme alarm' caused to laying hens in battery cages by the use of bristle brushes to remove dirt. It would seem that the brush in some way simulates a predator against which the hen has no avoidance strategy.

Behaviour has consequences, both internal (e.g. proprioceptive feedback from muscles) and external (e.g. gain of food). Examination of these factors has assumed some importance in discussions of animal welfare. In an influential and controversial article, Baxter (1983) noted:

> If the motivationally significant consequences of a behaviour can only ever be brought about by allowing the animal to perform behaviour, it would be as well to describe welfare requirements as the need to perform behaviour. An example of this would be if the factor reducing motivation was proprioceptive feedback from motor patterns characteristic of the behaviour.

However, Baxter places emphasis upon such *external* consequences of behaviour as the construction of adequate nesting rather than the performance of behaviour *per se* as being important for welfare, even suggesting the principle, in theory at least, that '. . . both productivity and welfare could be accommodated without the animal ever performing behaviour'.

In spite of Baxter's (1983) speculative suggestion, there is a growing feeling within applied ethology that the performance of species-typical behaviour has some intrinsic motivational and welfare value for the animal over and above its obvious functional consequences, e.g. for feeding, a factor additional to the gain of nutrients (Toates, 1986, 1987; Hughes and Duncan, 1988a,b; Toates and Jensen, 1991). Normally, such activities as gaining food would necessitate the performance of species-typical behaviour. However, as will be discussed later, if such behaviour is unable to be expressed or impeded, then behaviour can appear in an out-of-context form. In other words, animals seem to have a *behavioural* need to behave in certain species-typical ways.

In this context it is interesting to note that when rats are presented with an operant task for the reward of intravenous nutrients of water, successful performance of the behaviour is associated with recruiting such auxiliary activities as licking and chewing the lever at the time of pressing (reviewed by Toates, 1981, 1986). Conversely, rats for which the daily fluid needs are seemingly taken care of by intravenous or intragastric infusion continue with a considerable amount of consummatory behaviour (Nicolaidis and Rowland, 1975). This suggests that the state of normal satiety is achieved as a result of a combination of various inputs, e.g. taste, oro-motor feedback, stomach filling and postabsorptive consequences. There might well be an important lesson here for understanding stereotypies.

The notion of a need to behave might give some insight into what are termed *redirection activities*. Given that the environment does not afford the opportunity for certain species-typical actions to be performed, they will appear in a distorted, out-of-context form. For example, housing chickens in an environment not conducive to normal pecking can increase the frequency of pecking at conspecifics whereas simple environmental manipulations that facilitate normal pecking can reduce the incidence of destructive pecking (Blokhuis and Van der Haar, 1992). Keiper (1969) found that so-called spot-picking, repeated touching of a bird's bill on a particular spot on the body or the cage, could be reduced by requiring the bird to perform some pecking to obtain food. A class of behaviours for which the notion of behavioural need might provide some explanation is considered in the next section.

9.5 BEHAVIOUR WITHOUT AN OBVIOUS GOAL

9.5.1 Introduction

Behaviour is sometimes inexplicable in terms of the motivational processes that guide an animal in its normal commerce with the environment, to feed, drink, mate, explore, build nests and sleep, etc. When behaviour is inexplicable in this way, seems bizarre or, in the extreme, self-destructive, stress is sometimes invoked as an explanation. The animal is said to be behaving in an abnormal way because it is stressed, although in some cases one might argue that stress arises from the behaviour. In some cases, a lack of opportunity for species-typical behaviour seems to cause bizarre behaviours (see Wiepkema and Koolhaas, 1993). Wiepkema and Schouten (1992) discuss stereotypies (see below) and injurious behaviour, whereby animals inflict damage on conspecifics or themselves. For example, calves for which the technology of nutrient provision does not require or allow sucking of a teat are often observed to engage in extensive cross-sucking of conspecifics. Veal calves also engage in sucking each other's ears, navel and penis, associated with urine drinking (Wiepkema, 1985). Pigs engage in biting the tails of their pen mates which causes serious damage and is a major economic factor in pig production (Wiepkema, 1985). Wiepkema and Koolhaas (1993) note that a failure of the environment to allow for the animal to perform its species-typical foraging behaviour can play a crucial role. Offering pigs a substrate in which to root or hens one to scratch and peck can reduce the behaviours of tail biting and feather pecking, respectively.

Although the term 'abnormal' is widely used, its precise meaning is commonly left unspecified. There are two quite distinct meanings and it is important not to confuse them (Mason, 1991). On the one hand, the term can be used to mean 'away from the norm', meaning unlikely to be seen. As Mason notes, whether stereotypies fall into this category depends upon the frame of reference for normality. Although they might never be seen in the wild, they might constitute the norm for a group of intensively housed animals. On the other hand, abnormal might be used to mean maladaptive or pathological. Again whether stereotypies qualify here depends upon the frame of reference. The whole situation might be maladaptive relative to another environment, but might be rendered no less so by the performance of stereotypies.

9.5.2 Displacement Activities

The principal topic of later discussion in this chapter is stereotypies and one possible route to understanding them might be through displacement activities. The term 'displacement activity' is used to refer to an activity that appears to be out of context, i.e. irrelevant to the ongoing, apparently goal-directed behaviour within which it appears (Maestripieri *et al.*, 1992). Examples include cleaning of the bill or feathers by birds within a sexual or agonistic context. Self-maintenance activities such as grooming and preening commonly form a large part of an animal's displacement activities. Yawning and auto-grooming are well represented in primates. Cabib (1993) suggests that in stressed animals displacement activities are due to sensitization of the mesoaccumbens system. Furthermore, the kind of displacement activities seen in 'natural' conditions in rats (typically, grooming, sniffing and gnawing) correspond to what is seen (in exaggerated form) in pharmacologically induced stereotypies (see Section 9.5.3.13).

Traditionally, displacement activities have been thought to be triggered in situations of motivational ambivalence, either arising from the simultaneous existence of two incompatible motivational tendencies or the frustration of a failure to reach an appropriate goal as a result of thwarting. There are certain behavioural situations that might appear to have something in common with displacement activities and which might give a lead in finding a relationship between stress and displacement activities (Levine and Billington, 1991). For instance, loud sounds can induce searching for food and chewing in rats, rabbits and guinea-pigs. Pinching of the tail in rats, mice and cats is followed by consummatory behaviour, an analogous effect being seen even in the giant slug *Limax maximus* and the mollusc *Aplysia* (reviewed by Levine and Billington, 1991).

Maestripieri *et al.* (1992) review the hypotheses that have been evoked to explain displacement activities. Some authors propose that tension accumulates at a time of conflict and the displacement activity is a means of discharging this tension. Others suggest that there is a mutual inhibition between two competing tendencies and this allows a third candidate for behavioural control to gain expression. A third idea is that conflict and thwarting are conditions of high arousal and this state permits other activities to emerge.

Exactly how one characterizes a displacement activity is not always clear. They were once described as: (1) occurring in the absence of appropriate external stimulation and (2) different from the same general class of behaviour when it is performed in an appropriate context. However, more recent evidence shows that these characterizations are often inaccurate. For example, displacement grooming shows evidence of being influenced by the normal causal factors that underlie grooming. Also behaviour shown as a displacement activity can often be apparently identical to the same behaviour exhibited in its appropriate motivational context. Thus, displacement activities need to be defined not by their morphology but by their context.

Maestripieri *et al.* (1992) suggest that displacement activites might be used as an index of the emotional state of an animal. Given the assumption that they occur at times of internal conflict, they are commonly assumed to have emotional connotations. Indeed, Maestripieri *et al.* suggest that they are consistently accompanied by autonomic activation.

Maestripieri *et al.* place displacement activities into the broader context of the social life of primates. They note the growing awareness within ethology of the rich opportunities that social interaction provides for primates to utilize cognitive capacities. Within a cognitive context, they also approve of the assumption that emotion is associated with a comparison involving the confirmation or disconfirmation of an expectation about the external world (see Section 1.3.5). Complex social interactions are likely to involve the frequent appearance of emotion based upon such comparisons, arising from, for example, conflicting motivations (e.g. to move away or stand one's ground), thwarting and interruption. From their review of the evidence, Maestripieri *et al.* conclude that, in primates, displacement activities are more commonly seen in situations that would be described as stressful. In rhesus macaques, *Macaca mulatta,* observed at a feeding site, auto-scratching is most frequently seen in individuals of middle rank. Their status is seen as being one of ambivalence and frustration as opposed to the dominants who can monopolize the situation and the subordinates who stay out of the way. Maestripieri *et al.* suggest that displacement activities in the context of aggression reflect ambivalence about the future strategy, to withdraw or to advance in anger or reconciliation. Assessment of social status and establishment of commensurate boundaries on the first encounter between two individuals is likely to be a situation of high ambivalence and stress. In macaques, such a situation is accompanied by a high frequency of auto-scratching, auto-grooming and yawning.

Maestripieri *et al.* (1992) discuss various possible functions served by displacement activities, such as a communication of intentions and a means of distraction (a form of deception). It is perhaps not difficult to appreciate the functional significance of being able to interpret displacement activities, e.g. signs of ambivalence that might herald fight or flight. However, it is not so easy to understand in such terms their emergence as part of the response repertoire of the animal showing them. The function might be both extrinsic and intrinsic to the animal exhibiting them or, to commit an ethological heresy, they might have no functional significance in themselves. In the present context of stress, as with other aspects of behaviour discussed earlier in the present volume, a logical question to ask of displacement activities is whether there are immediate intrinsic consequences for the animal performing them. For instance, are there indices of stress that are reduced in some way by their performance? There is little or no hard evidence of this. Maestripieri *et al.* cite the result that in cross-grooming, the groomed animal releases endogenous opioids (see Section 5.2). However, it would be dangerous to extrapolate from this to auto-grooming as the social context is totally different. They also raise the possibility that displacement activities might provide a focus of attention away from some kind of noxious stimulus.

As far as the present study is concerned, displacement activities are of interest as a possible index of stress. In the context of stress, they are of relevance in providing additional data for developing a broad theoretical model that might begin to explain the kind of disturbed behaviour that is of most concern in applied ethology. In this domain, the focus of attention is primarily on what might appear to be a grossly exaggerated form of displacement activity, termed stereotypy, discussed in the next section.

9.5.3 Stereotypies

9.5.3.1 Introduction

A type of repetitive behaviour said to occur under conditions of stress is termed 'stereotypy'. Examples include repetitive chewing and jumping movements. Veal calves housed in small wooden boxes show 'tongue playing', which consists of the animal rolling its tongue in and out or swaying it from side to side. Tethered sows engage in bar-biting and sham chewing (Cronin, 1985; Wiepkema, 1985). 'Stereotypy' is often used to describe such behaviour, for which a stress concept is thought to provide, in principle, part of the explanation. Stereotypies have been defined as actions: 'that are fixed in form and orientation and serve no obvious function' (Dantzer, 1986). Dantzer argues that the term should be applied only to: '. . . repetitive sequences of activities that consist of a few fixed elements carried out at a higher-than-normal rate and occurring in nearly the same order in successive cycles'.

Some authors refer to stereotypy as a response or class of behaviour in its own right but, as Cooper and Dourish (1990) point out, any behaviour when done to excess and out of context can constitute a stereotypy. So stereotypy is more correctly used as a *description* of behaviour rather than a category in its own right. Exactly how one defines 'stereotypy' raises issues at the core of the classification and explanation of behaviour. For instance, Teitelbaum *et al.* (1990) note that, in our normal classification of behaviour, something such as feeding is described in terms of its end-point: food ingestion. In making such a classification, one does not need to specify the exact motor act employed. In the case of stereotypies, there is no such end-point and so description must rest upon the motor act itself. However, a somewhat different emphasis is placed by Isaacson and Gispen (1990). The implicit assumption of a disruption in a *negative feedback system* as underlying stereotypy is made. They note that stereotypy does not require the assumption of a repetition of identical motor responses. In the spirit that a response should be defined in terms of its outcome, they write:

> . . . behaviours, even though varied, that all lead to the same, less-than-optimal results or consequences should be regarded as stereotyped. Therefore, we will regard stereotypy as a reduction in an individual's usual abilities *to change* ongoing behavioural patterns or strategies subsequent to changes in environmental events so as to produce optimal consequences.

Can understanding stress illuminate stereotypy? Performance of bizarre repetitive behaviour is sometimes thought to relieve stress. Is an animal showing repetitive behaviour stressed and does the behaviour play a part in reducing stress levels? On close investigation, such questions are not easy to answer. In discussing stress and stereotypies, we must not forget the caution of Robbins *et al.* (1990): '. . . accepting the idea that non-specific states such as stress or activation can produce stereotyped behaviour does not necessarily entail support for the notion that the stereotypy regulates that state'. We shall look at some examples of disturbed behaviour and the kinds of theoretical models that might be applied to them. Alas there are only part explanations throughout, tentative suggestions as to factors that might, under some conditions in some species, yield some explanatory value.

9.5.3.2   Stereotypies and the hypothalamic–pituitary–adrenocortical axis

A clue to the function of stereotypies might be gained by examining pituitary–adrenal hormones and trying to tease apart causal influences and feedback effects (Dantzer, 1986). For example, Delius *et al.* (1976) found an increased frequency of headshaking, described as a displacement activity, in pigeons injected with adrenocorticotrophic hormone (ACTH). Ödberg (1989) investigated the jumping stereotypy commonly shown by caged voles. Thwarting this response by lowering the lid of the cage was associated with a rise in corticosteroid levels.

There is some indirect evidence on the behavioural–HPA axis relationship, derived from placing animals on schedules in which small amounts of food are delivered at intervals of 60–90 seconds or so (discussed in Chapter 8). The assumption is commonly expressed that the schedule is frustrating and stress-evoking in the periods between food delivery. A well-known phenomenon in the psychology literature is that of 'schedule-induced polydipsia' (SIP), excessive water intake by rats and other species rewarded with small pellets of food on such a schedule.

Dantzer et al. (1981) found a positive correlation between a rat's tendency: (1) to engage in schedule-induced drinking and (2) to acquire rapidly active avoidance in a two-way shuttle-box. Also rats inclined towards SIP exhibit less freezing on being confronted with an aggressive resident male. This suggests that SIP correlates with other tendencies to show active coping strategies.

9.5.3.3 Stereotypies and endogenous opioids

One popular focus for experimentation and explanation on the causation of stereotypies is the endorphins. These also form a focus for researchers trying to understand the bases of attachment behaviour and separation distress (Section 5.2).

If endorphins are connected with stereotypies, then broadly two possible interpretations could be given. First, their secretion could be a function of the performance of behaviour; suppose the animal behaves so as to maintain an optimal level of endorphins. This would make their role analogous to that suggested in the context of social behaviour in Chapter 5. Perhaps the animal showing stereotypies has a chronic need to elevate its endorphin levels.

Rushen et al. (1990) noted the large individual differences in the tendency to exhibit stereotypies and classified a group of pigs into either high or low stereotypers. Immediately following feeding, when stereotypies are shown at their highest frequency, an opioid-based hypoanalgesia is exhibited. However, they found that pigs showing a high level of stereotypies were more responsive to a noxious stimulus than the low stereotypers. One might have expected the converse, i.e. that if stereotypies served to boost endogenous opioid activity, animals exhibiting a high level would be relatively unresponsive to noxious stimuli. Rushen et al. found that naloxone only slightly reduced stereotypies. They noted that their subjects were experienced stereotypers and that naloxone exerts a stronger effect if used earlier in the developmental history of stereotypy acquisition.

Alternatively, natural opioids might form an excitatory link in a neural circuit underlying the generation of stereotyped behaviour, in which case opioid antagonists might be expected to reduce their performance. Cronin *et al.* (1985) injected tethered sows with the opioid-antagonist naloxone and found a dramatic reduction in the frequency of the animal's principal stereotypy. The shorter the period of time that the sow had been performing the stereotypy, the stronger was the effect of naloxone. There was some tendency for the sows to acquire new forms of stereotypy on giving up the old.

Mason (1991) notes that: (1) injected opioids tend either to cause or to accentuate stereotypies; (2) injected opioids increase persistence; and (3) endogenous opioids are released at times described as stressful. Injection of the dopamine (DA) agonist apomorphine has been found to lead to an increase in the stereotypies of sucking and licking in cattle, sheep and pigs (see Broom, 1987; see also Section 9.5.3.13). Rushen *et al.* (1990) found that naloxone shortened the bout length of a given session of behaviour and thereby increased switching between activities and decreased persistence. They suggested a role for opioids in giving behaviour its persistence, a positive feedback effect (Section 9.5.3.7). The effect of naloxone on stereotypies might thereby be understood in terms of decreasing bout lengths of their performance (Ladewig *et al.*, 1993).

There is evidence that the effect of opioids on stereotypies might be mediated via the DA system (Cabib *et al.*, 1984). Opioid receptors exist at the terminals of dopaminergic neurons in the nigrostriatal and mesolimbic systems, implicated in reactions to a stressor (Cabib, 1993). Exposure to a stressor can enhance the stereotypies induced by injection of the dopaminergic agonist apomorphine and this enhancement is eliminated by the opioid antagonist naltrexone.

9.5.3.4   Individual differences

The existence of high and low stereotypers was noted in the last two sections. This section further explores this topic. Individual differences in stereotypies are large, the evidence for this being reviewed by Ödberg (1987). A positive correlation has been found between adrenal weight and the frequency of stereotypies in fowl. In tethered sows, hyperactivity positively correlates with levels of stereotypies, a similar result being found by Ödberg for voles.

Tethered sows show either high or low levels of stereotypies and Schouten and Wiepkema (1991) suggested that this might be interpreted in terms of differences in coping style (Chapter 6). They investigated a possible relationship between differences in resistance to tethering and differences in tendency to stereotypies. A significant negative correlation was found between the time spent in stereotypies and the time spent in offering resistance to tethering. This suggested that:

> . . . those sows that resist first tethering most are the ones that experience and register the uncontrollability of their situation most drastically and for this reason are most inclined to develop a state of helplessness characterized by giving up any overt behaviour that may calm them down.

High stereotypers had a lower heart rate prior to and during tethering than did low stereotypers. Tentatively the authors suggest that high resisting/low stereotyping sows might be showing a predominant sympathetic reaction whereas the low resisting/high stereotyping sows might be showing a predominant parasympathetic reaction. Dantzer and Mittleman (1993) raise the tentative possibility that acquisition of stereotypies represents a shift from a dominant sympathetic to parasympathetic control. Adapting this to the terms developed in the present study (Chapter 6), stereotypy would be seen in terms of switching from an active to a passive control system.

9.5.3.5   Welfare implications

Simple environmental changes are sometimes able to reduce the frequency of stereotypies (Ödberg, 1987). However, such animals might be experiencing poorer welfare as a result of the change. A suggestion that some stereotypies serve a useful function was provided by a result of Wiepkema (1987). (Wemelsfelder, 1990, argues a similar point: that stereotypies reflect acquisition of at least some control over behavioural output.) In veal calves, a significant negative correlation was reported between the frequency of tongue playing and the incidence of abomasal (stomach) ulcers; although the generality of this finding has been doubted (see Ladewig et al., 1993). This relationship was not observed between biting/licking and abomasal damage. On the basis of this finding, Wiepkema suggested that different stereotypies might be associated with different aspects of stress occurring simultaneously in a given animal. Wiepkema argues: 'If we assume that ulcers are also unwished and have a negative meaning with respect to animal welfare, then the question arises as to which calves are in the worst state—those with stereotypies or those with ulcers?

As Ödberg notes, equally interesting are the animals that do not display repetitive behaviour. In the context of the argument developed to explain stereotypies, one would need to propose something about the make-up of such animals. In the terms of Wiepkema (1985, 1987), do they not contain representations of *Sollwert* comparable with the other animals? Do they tolerate mismatch? Do they experience mismatch but fail to 'hit upon' the coping strategy of performing stereotypies? Such failure might leave them in greater distress than their conspecifics showing stereotypies.

Wiepkema and Koolhaas (1993) claim: 'If we consider stereotypies as behavioural "scars", that have their origin in former behavioural "wounds", then we have to conclude that we should never keep animals in such a way that they have to rely on the development of such "scars", be they behavioural or physical'.

Wemelsfelder (1993) suggests that stereotypies represent a state in which *active control* over behaviour has been relinquished. By such active control, she means control based upon such processes as planning and anticipation. As such, she sees stereotypies as being necessarily indicative of a state of negative welfare, being associated with such states as boredom and depression. She argues:

> ... the development of stereotyped behaviour in captive animals signifies *the gradual impairment of the capacity to interact with the environment*. Behaviour acquires an increasingly rigid and mechanical character; it is determined more and more by immediately available environmental stimuli and loses its innovative, anticipatory nature.

In some respects, this matches the argument being advanced in the present study, as will be shown later.

9.5.3.6   The explanation of stereotypy

In the terms of the present study, possibly a useful starting point in trying to understand stereotypies is to consider them not as some bizarre instance of pathology but rather as the outcome of perfectly adaptive processes being placed in an abnormal context. There are multiple determinants of behaviour that interact in complex and subtle ways to produce what is seen as normal behaviour. It is not difficult to imagine opportunities for abnormality to emerge from slight changes in the weightings of one or more of these factors. It is perhaps not too surprising that placing constraints upon such complex control systems, imposing parameter changes within a negative feedback system, as is bound to be the case in intensive farming or a zoo environment, will produce profound changes in behavioural output. Indeed, perhaps the surprise with behaviour is that it is so near to normal for most of the time (Toates, 1990). Having said this, it does not necessarily give us much insight into exactly why stereotypies appear where and when they do or the form that they take but it does give a rational framework for considering them. So, to introduce the topic of explanation of stereotypy, it might prove useful to review briefly the kinds of process that are determinants of so-called normal behaviour under normal conditions.

Appetitive behaviour often involves sequences of actions each of which changes the external world in some way such as to bring the animal nearer to the consummatory object (Timberlake, 1993). Completion of one phase, e.g. finding food, is a necessary prerequisite to the next, e.g. shell-opening. Appetitive behaviour is commonly described as more flexible than consummatory behaviour (Tinbergen, 1969) and indeed both the natural habitat and the laboratory operant situation can reveal a rich variety of appetitive forms. However, there are certain species-specific patterns apparent (Breland and Breland, 1961). For example, a pigeon pecking a key for water does so differently from one trained for food (Moore, 1973). Apparent flexibility is often based upon certain preferred forms of behaviour and even lever-pressing, the model of arbitrary responding, is perhaps not quite as arbitrary as is sometimes supposed (Bolles, 1988). Operant tasks are usually best performed when species-typical behaviour can be recruited to solve the problem (Bolles, 1970, 1988; Toates, 1981). A number of authors have suggested that stereotypies can arise when appetitive behaviour gets stuck at a certain stage, unable to proceed to the next stage. A similar logic might be employed in the case of unsuccessful escape behaviour as escape and avoidance unambiguously are best elicited when the animal is able to recruit species-typical responses (Bolles, 1970; Rachlin, 1976, p. 357; Masterson and Crawford, 1982).

Moving on now to consider the consummatory behaviour phase of normal behaviour, this phase is controlled by external stimuli, acting in a so-called 'data-driven' or 'bottom-up' mode, whose effect is potentiated or depotentiated from top-down influences (Gallistel, 1980). For example, feeding and drinking are complexly determined by the taste properties of available fluids/nutrients and the nutrient/hydrational state of the animal. In addition, proprioceptive feedback from the motor acts of licking, chewing and swallowing would seem to play some part in this behaviour, not only in its moment-by-moment mechanics but also in its motivation and affective consequences (Oatley and Dickinson, 1970; Toates, 1981, 1986, 1994c; Berridge and Fentress, 1985). Reinforcement might well consist to an important degree in a combination of the food and species-typical behaviour performed in its consumption (Toates, 1981). The capacity of incentives to engage behaviour will depend in part upon the consequences of past commerce with them. In one of the more dramatic examples, a food might be shunned if it is associated with gastrointestinal illness. A food can be favoured if it is associated with recovery from illness. These effects are mediated by a modulation of the taste reactivity of the food as a result of the consequences of ingestion (Garcia, 1989). In a similar way, it would seem that a complex of external and internal factors is involved in aggressive behaviour, e.g. complex representations of the environment, comparisons of incoming information with expectations and hormonal sensitization (Archer, 1976). In addition, aggressive behaviour *per se* has consequences for physiological state (see Section 5.9).

Mason (1991) notes three respects in which the so-called abnormality of stereotypies in fact resembles aspects of non-stereotyped behaviour:

1. Normal behaviour might sometimes appear to be invariant and resistant to change. Examples include grooming and displays.
2. Over time, behaviour can develop an autonomy from the stimuli that elicited it originally. At the outset, only a specific stimulus might elicit behaviour but later a wider range of stimuli might suffice.
3. It is sometimes difficult to interpret behaviour in terms of goal direction. Examples include (a) Dickinson's (1985) demonstration of a switch from actions to habits, with repetition and (b) the working of animals for food in the presence of free food.

These points will be returned to as the discussion progresses.

Addressing a similar point, Ödberg (1978) describes as 'extremely puzzling' the difference between recently acquired and well-established stereotypies. He describes three developmental stages:

1. An animal attempts to escape from a frustrating situation by behaving in a certain way. At this stage, behaviour can be inhibited by anxiolytic drugs.
2. The behaviour becomes automatic or 'fixated' but is still only evident in the original frustrating situation.
3. Behaviour becomes 'emancipated', meaning it is performed even outside of the frustrating situation.

Drugs seem unable to inhibit stereotypies in stages 2 and 3. Possibly this sequence might be less puzzling if one were to show that such developmental stages to some extent are to be found in 'normal' non-stereotyped behaviour. This section will present the evidence for this.

Mason and Turner (1993) consider some hints that can be obtained from looking at non-stereotyped behaviour and which might give insights into stereotypies. For example, the nature of the external environment might be such as to elicit the same behaviour repeatedly; an animal might be constantly exposed to a releaser. As an example, an okapi housed in a zoo developed a paw-raising stereotypy. It was housed next to an inaccessible female and paw-raising formed part of the courtship sequence. This might be seen as the animal getting locked into a part of the appetitive sequence. Similarly, a captive pine marten developed a scent-marking stereotypy. In a natural environment it would be expected to re-mark previously scent-marked locations, which presumably it would occasionally encounter in the course of daily activities. However, confined in a cage, it repeatedly and inescapably encountered the same scents.

It is as if the animal gets stuck at one stage of executing a programme of action that might, in association with a wider range of activity, normally be appropriate in a similar context. As Ödberg (1986) writes: 'It is as if in some individuals a programme is present inducing the animal *to do something to act'*, and 'Waiting while doing nothing seems to be a difficult thing to do!'

Thus, although stereotypies appear to lack any kind of goal or purpose it is worth asking whether they might be understood as developing out of purposive behaviour. Are they an exaggeration of behaviour that once could be understood as directed towards a goal? Dantzer (1986) and Ödberg (1987) develop the argument that stereotypies often emerge after other attempts at extrication from a stressful situation have failed. Mason (1991) concludes that, 'The stereotypies of some captive animals develop from what appear to be intention movements of escape'.

Stereotypies commonly emerge in situations: (1) where the range of activities shown by the animal is low (Dantzer, 1986) and (2) of thwarting and frustration, when actions that would correct an apparently undesirable situation are unavailable or prove ineffective. Wiepkema (1987) notes: '. . . a crucial point seems to be the impossibility of performing species-specific programs in order to reach a relevant goal situation (often the intake of food) . . .'. For example, stereotypies are likely to appear when (1) an animal has been deprived of food and (2) is in a situation associated in some way with feeding but where food is unavailable or inaccessible (Dantzer, 1986). By the index of corticosterone secretion, it is known that such situations are stressful (Chapter 5).

Consider what happens when sows are tethered. The animals' first attempts are ones of escape and the showing of aggression. This is followed by passivity, which in turn is followed by the emergence and increase in frequency of stereotypies. Ödberg (1987) argues that at the stage of passivity: '. . . the animal is left without answers in a total lack of control of his own life. But then? As not to act is unbearable, the animals starts again doing something (stage 3) and some movements must be rewarded in some way so that they are repeated, even without reducing the original mismatch'. Similarly, Wiepkema and Schouten (1992) describe the sequence following tethering in pregnant sows. Unsuccessful pulling and biting of the chain that secures her and pushing against the restraining bars of the enclosure are followed by changes in this pattern such that it becomes ritualized, stereotyped in a way that is peculiar for the individual. This suggests that the stereotypy develops out of an attempt to produce behaviour with some extrinsic goal involved. Such behaviour as pecking the floor by hungry chickens as a stereotypy (Savory and Maros, 1993) might suggest a similar interepretation.

In other words, the behaviour might form part of a normal motivational control system which is recruited in appropriate circumstances but the end-point fails to be achieved. The animal is then unable to disengage from the behaviour in the light of failure. In the terms of Wiepkema (1987), behaviour has failed to eliminate the mismatch between *Sollwert* (the way the world should be) and *Istwert* (the way the world really is). This is a similar argument to that of Archer introduced in Chapter 1. In control theory language, such a situation is termed 'open loop' (Toates, 1975; see Section 1.3.9). Another possibility is that the extrinsic loop might be open but another loop intrinsic to the animal might realize positive feedback (discussed later). Another way of saying this might be that there is a purely intrinsic consequence of behaviour described as 'reinforcement' (discussed later).

Mason and Turner (1993) also consider the absence of the normal consequences of behaviour:

> The factors that usually act to terminate behaviour are consummation, that is, the reaching of the goal of the behaviour; an accumulation of the costs of the behaviour, such as fatigue; and behavioural competition, where a second behaviour is elicited or becomes higher in priority, so that it replaces the first. Behaviour could recur to an unusual extent if any of these factors failed to have their usual effect.

For example, the pacing stereotypy of a captive dingo was interpreted in terms of a failure to reach conspecifics on the other side of a fence. They also consider a failure of sufficient food to satiate an animal in intensively farmed animals.

Mason and Turner (1993) also review instances of situations in which consequences of an action occur such that the behaviour might be expected to 'move on' in sequence but the animal carries on regardless, as if the situation had not changed. For instance, caged hens have been observed to continue to pace against a door even though it has been opened. Young mink occasionally and briefly continue with a prefeeding stereotypy even following food delivery and amphetamine (AM)-injected rats continue to lever-press in a food rewarded task even after food has been delivered.

Although the conditions that provoke the appearance of stereotypy (e.g. food restriction, thwarting, environmental poverty) are termed stressful, in rats there are some conditions traditionally described as such that do not arouse stereotypy, e.g. immobilization, exposure to cold, inescapable electric shocks and severe food deprivation (Robbins *et al.*, 1990). It is worth asking what these situations have in common. One entirely *ad hoc* speculation that might be worth raising is that under normal conditions there is not an obvious active, species-typical behaviour involving repetition that is potentiated by these states and situations (except possibly severe food deprivation and then only in the context of food-related cues). By contrast, in situations where stereotypy is most often evident, repetition might form a natural reaction in the situation. This could then become exaggerated in stereotypy.

Mason and Turner (1993) suggest that one factor that would predispose to stereotypy is increased weighting being given to central control as information from the environment becomes less important in determining behaviour (discussed in more detail in Section 9.5.3.10). They suggest that a number of factors would lead to increased central control. The fixed action patterns beloved of classical ethologists are an example of behaviour that can run off in a 'relatively unvarying' form even without prior experience. Examples include some courtship rituals in birds and mammalian swallowing. Another situation that Mason and Turner describe is that of behaviour patterns that start out being flexible but then become automatized with repetition. Examples are commonly given from human skill learning situations: 'Eventually one movement in a sequence comes to follow another without conscious, volitional control or prompting by environmental cues, and the form of each movement becomes very predictable from one occasion to the next'. It would seem, in other words, that, with sequences, the weighting given to proprioceptive feedback from one component in a sequence as a cue to trigger the next can increase with repetition. Mason and Turner give the example of the 'short latency of attack' strain of mouse (Section 6.3) as being one particularly prone: (1) to switching into the proprioceptive mode of control; (2) to paying less attention to environmental cues; and (3) to the development of stereotypies.

Broadly speaking, attempts at explanation can appeal to events either: (1) in an individual motivational control system (e.g. in association with a feeding tendency, stereotypies might be an exaggeration of a normal means of increasing the release of digestive juices or promoting stomach motility) or (2) processes that are not specific to a given control system (e.g. any stereotypy might be a means of reducing corticosteroid levels). These might turn out not to be mutually exclusive levels of explanation but are a convenient first attempt at bringing a classification to a bewildering area.

As stereotypies commonly (although by no means always) occur in the context of feeding (Rushen et al., 1993), there is reason to suppose that events intrinsic to the feeding motivational system might in some cases form part of their causation. For example, it was suggested that such behaviour as cross-sucking might have important consequences for the digestion and absorption of nutrients from the gut (Toates, 1987). Stereotypies are sometimes more frequent after, rather than before, feeding (Wiepkema and Schouten, 1992). Possibly extensive oral stimulation, involving the mechanics of sucking, could be explained in terms of an increased release of digestive hormones or simply enhanced transit of nutrients along the alimentary tract (cf. Deutsch, 1979). In such cases it could be misleading to try to understand such stereotypies in terms of a broader stress concept as their causation and even an adaptive value would seem to be intrinsic to the feeding control system (Rushen, 1993). In infants, a variety of hormonal changes (e.g. release of cholecystokinin (CCK), increase in plasma levels of insulin) follow the activity of sucking (Uvnäs-Moberg and Winberg, 1989). Some of these might be expected to have specific effects upon the feeding control system (e.g. CCK) and possibly a more general sedative effect (Uvnäs-Moberg and Winberg, 1989). Plasma somatostatin levels (a hormone possibly released at times of stress) are lowered by sucking. In calves observed following the taking of a meal from a bucket, de Passillé et al. (1991)) found increased blood levels of CCK and insulin in animals having access to a dry teat. This suggests a functional value of such behaviour in terms of the assimilation of nutrients.

The development of some stereotypies in pigs (chain-related activity, excessive drinking) is increased by food restriction (Terlouw *et al.*, 1991a). Terlouw *et al.* draw attention to species differences. In carnivores, a clear appetitive phase might usually precede the consummatory phase and stereotypies occur largely before feeding. In an omnivore such as the pig, appetitive and consummatory phases would normally tend to be interspersed and it might be expected that consummatory behaviour would excite appetitive behaviour. Thus, given restricted feeding, if the pig is still not satiated at the time of finishing available food, one might expect to see stereotypies then. As was pointed out to me by K. Malm (pers. comm.), large cats tend to adopt pacing stereotypies, whereas with grazing animals the form is more closely associated with ingestive movements. One might see this as each animal getting locked into an early stage of its natural 'food-getting behaviour'. An argument along these lines was presented by Morris (1966), who noted that captive animals often: '. . . either devise ways of making more variable appetitive behaviour available to themselves or they abnormally increase the amount of fixed consummatory activity'.

Mason (1991) reviews abnormal behaviours shown in association with feeding. In farmed mink, pacing tends to occur at a maximum rate just prior to feeding, as do rooting, bar-biting and head-weaving in pigs. Possibly these could to some extent be understood in terms of the arousal of an appetitive motivational state by cues predictive of, say, food but prior to food delivery. The animal then proceeds to perform behaviours (increased general activity, rooting) that would be appropriate for the gain of food. Superstition might play some part; the animal might perceive a causal link between behaviour and reward, even where none exists.

At least some stereotypies might reflect an exaggeration of behaviours expected to occur to some extent at the times in question. For example, pigs show such stereotypies as sham-chewing, chain manipulation, drinker playing and polydipsia when being fed at intervals (Dantzer and Mormède, 1983b). Possibly such species-typical 'food-getting' behaviours as nosing, playing, nibbling and chewing, reported by Dantzer and Mormède to be those commonly directed at the chain, represent priming by a combination of a hunger signal and the performance of feeding. Other behaviours, e.g. sham-chewing, might be explicable in terms of a continuing motivational state, primed by feeding (note that opioids both stimulate, and are released by, feeding (Fantino *et al.*, 1986; Lieblich *et al.*, 1991)), which is then strengthened by beneficial consequences (e.g. digestion and postdigestive assimilation of nutrients).

In the context of the argument developed earlier, on active and passive strategies (Chapter 6), there is some suggestive evidence that stereotypies should be seen as an active strategy (although see also Section 9.5.3.4 for a counter argument) in that acetylcholine seems to have an inhibitory effect upon them (Randrup and Munkvad, 1970). Thus, stereotypy is increased by anticholinergics and slightly antagonized by cholinergics. Randrup and Munkvad suggest that normal behaviour is the outcome of a balance between the various amines, a balance which is disturbed in stereotypy. (Note, however, that under some conditions anticholinergic drugs inhibit stereotypies; Scheel-Krüger and Randrup, 1968).

9.5.3.7 Reward, reinforcement and positive feedback

The question is commonly posed (e.g. Mason, 1991) as to whether performing stereotypies is *reinforcing* or *rewarding* to the animal. These expressions derive from psychology where their use is occasionally such as to mean all things to all (wo)men. There are regular appeals for the sanitization of the vocabulary (e.g. White, 1989). Adapted to issues of applied ethology, their use becomes even more open to liberal interpretations that are often not as precise as might be desired, the present author not always being immune to this temptation (Toates and Jensen, 1991). Sometimes 'reinforcing' is taken to mean little more than, 'based on my own feelings, I would suppose the animal enjoys doing it'. It is worth considering terminology closely.

The terms 'reinforcement' and 'reward' were developed in the context of animals' commerce with external objects such as food and water and they do not necessarily easily translate into something that by definition has no extrinsic consequence. The use that the present author will employ is that something is rewarding if it can induce forward locomotion such that, in a spatial dimension, the animal is attracted to the object or cues associated with it (Schneirla, 1959; White, 1989). Reinforcement is slightly more problematic and can be used to describe either an experimental *procedure*, that of making something (e.g. food) contingent upon a response, or an internal *process*, that of strengthening a response that immediately preceded in time the reinforcing agent (Bindra, 1978). The latter use will be employed here.

In such terms and bearing all cautions in mind, the distinction between reward and reinforcement can be clarified by the example of an animal trained to earn intravenous drug (e.g. morphine) and then the behaviour extinguished (Bozarth, 1987). Suppose the animal is standing in a corner scratching and a free priming injection is given. The tendency is to resume lever-pressing. In this case, the drug would be rewarding as it promotes forward locomotion to an associated cue. However, unless the frequency of showing *scratching* increased, one would not describe the gain of drug as reinforcing. When the drug is applied contingent upon a lever-press and the frequency of lever-pressing increases, the gain of drug could be described as both rewarding and reinforcing.

The conventional use of 'reward' is problematic when it is applied to stereotypies as they could hardly serve to bring the animal nearer to themselves. However, intravenous drug reward suffers from a similar conceptual difficulty and in this case reward can be defined in terms of the animal seeking out an environment associated with intravenous infusion (Bozarth, 1987). The nearest one can get to an analogous situation for stereotypies might be to see whether an environment associated in the past with their performance is attractive compared to one not so associated. However, this raises the conceptual and practical problem of how two such environments equal in other respects could be designed. An attempt at this was made by Cooper and Nicol (1991) using bank voles. They found a slight preference for a barren environment in which stereotypies had been performed as compared with a relatively enriched one.

Also suggestive of a rewarding or even purposive aspect to stereotypies (at least in the acquisition stage) is the observation that placing naive animals near to others showing stereotypy can produce a tendency to stereotypy in the naive subjects (Dantzer, 1986; Cooper and Nicol, 1994), suggesting the possibility of imitation. In other situations imitation can be interpreted in terms of achiving some end-point (cf. Fiorito and Scotto, 1992). For instance, there are cases of animals showing imitation in performing an instrumental task for the gain of food (Heyes and Dawson, 1990). Duncan *et al.* (1993) refer to a study on sows in which they claim, 'that the noise from chain-chewing neighbours was additive to the effect of food restriction on performance of stereotypy'. This suggests an analogy with intravenous drug reward, where the sound of a cue previously paired with reward can initiate responding in rats (Stewart *et al.*, 1984).

As far as reinforcement goes, if such a process operates it would mean that a consequence of the behaviour itself has a strengthening effect upon the tendency to repeat the behaviour. The effect would presumably be feedback from muscles although conceivably it could be a collateral of motor outflow. On this basis, one would expect to see an increase in frequency of stereotypies over time (Mason, 1991), which is indeed what is commonly observed. However, even defined in that way, the word 'reinforcement' is not entirely without problems. Food is positively reinforcing as a variety of different behaviours can be strengthened by making its appearance contingent upon a behaviour. Such a use does not obviously translate to stereotypies as by definition each stereotypy would have to be said to be reinforcing itself. Also, by comparison with more conventional situations, to be confident that a reinforcement process is implicated one would need to remove the reinforcing agent (e.g. food) and observe a decline in frequency of behaviour (extinction). How one could do this in the case of stereotypies without rendering a pathological preparation is unclear. By extrapolation from studies where species-typical behaviour has been circumvented in gaining food or water (Section 9.4.2), it might seem reasonable to argue that a part of what constitutes reinforcement derives from the performance of such behaviour *per se* (Glickman and Shiff, 1967). What one might do is try to identify particular consequences to the animal of such feedback and to block these.

Hughes and Duncan (1988a) speculate that repetitive motor patterns might '. . . serve to stimulate the release of brain opioids which may reduce pain and suffering in stressed animals. The performance of such stereotypies may thus be reinforced'. So to consider extinction conditions, if an endorphin agonist was given, one might expect a reduction in the frequency of stereotypies. For an antagonist, one might expect an immediate increase in frequency, possibly followed by a decrease as the behaviour extinguishes.

Injection of the opioid antagonist naloxone is followed by immediate cessation of the stereotypy rather than a compensatory increase followed by a decline that normally characterizes extinction of, say, food- or water-reinforced behaviour (see Mason, 1991; Dantzer and Mittleman, 1993). This might prove to be insightful as to the nature of any reinforcement from stereotypies as rapid extinction is a characteristic shared with behaviour motivated by electrical self-stimulation of the brain (Trowill *et al.*, 1969). Extinction can be more or less protracted with other reinforcers depending upon exactly what is the nature of the reinforcement process and its time relation to the act being reinforced (Trowill *et al.*, 1969). In the case of electrical stimulation of the brain, unlike the inevitable delays with food or water reward, any reinforcement presumably follows instantaneously after responding, a feature that might well contribute to certain of the peculiarities of this behaviour (Trowill *et al.*, 1969). It would seem logical that any reinforcement deriving from stereotypies might also follow very rapidly after the behaviour. Electrical self-stimulation of the brain has traditionally been portrayed as evidence for pleasure centres in the brain. However, a dissenting voice is sometimes heard suggesting that the behaviour has more in common with the compulsiveness of stereotypies rather than the euphoria derived from food or orgasm and that the electrode is tapping into *forcement* regions of the brain rather than reinforcement regions (Atrens, 1984).

If stereotypies are the outcome of a reinforcement process such that their performance increases the tendency to perform them, this would seem to constitute a positive feedback. A number of authors (e.g. Rushen *et al.*, 1990) have suggested the existence of positive feedback, and the model of Robbins to explain AM-induced stereotypy involves such a process (Section 9.5.3.13). In this context, Hughes and Duncan (1988a) proposed the model shown in Figure 9.2. Motivation arises from organismic variables (e.g. energy and fluid levels). Consummatory behaviour has a negative feedback effect upon these variables and upon motivation directly. Appetitive behaviour exerts a positive feedback effect upon motivation. (Although the figure does not show it, just in the very short-term, consummatory behaviour can in some cases also exert a

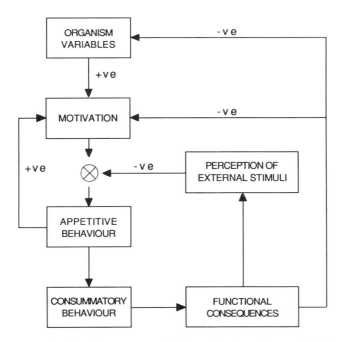

Figure 9.2. Hughes/Duncan model of motivation. (Source: Hughes and Duncan, 1988a, *Applied Animal Behavioural Science*, **19**, 352–355, figure 2)

positive feedback effect.) According to Hughes and Duncan, in abnormal contexts, the positive feedback effect from appetitive behaviour to motivation can become uncoupled from its normal consequences (which exert negative feedback) and the animal can get into a loop from which it cannot easily escape. However, there is evidence that in some cases appetitive behaviour can also exert a negative feedback effect on behaviour (Terlouw *et al.*, 1991a).

Somewhat along the lines of the Hughes/Duncan model, Dantzer (1986) suggests a: '. . . positive feedback mechanism in which sensory factors that normally guide behaviour trigger a behavioural sequence that becomes self-organized independent of further environmental guidance or any particular motivational state'. If the analysis offered here is logically acceptable, positive reinforcement and positive feedback would seem to be virtually indistinguishable. Dantzer concludes that stereotypies: '. . . do not gain strength because of any rewarding properties but simply because of (1) the positive feedback of sensory stimulation engendered by these motor acts on the neural systems that control them and (2) the progressive sensitization of these repeatedly activated neural systems'. Dantzer also argues that stereotypies do not reduce activation but are the expression of such activation.

In the broader context of motivation, positive feedback underlying behaviour has been suggested (McFarland and McFarland, 1968; Houston and Sumida, 1985; Toates, 1986) and it was argued that such a process would, under normal conditions, provide stability to ongoing behaviour in the face of competition. There might well be opioids as a link in the positive feedback effect (discussed by Toates, 1994c), thereby if, say, feeding caused the release of opioids and these then strengthened feeding tendency, behavioural persistence of feeding would be gained. Under normal conditions, any such positive feedback would be expected to be short-lived as negative feedback consequences (e.g. nutrient gain, full stomach) would later be expected to exert a dominant feedback influence.

Parenthetically, as Mason and Turner (1993) observe, it is worth noting that reinforcement in the conventional sense (e.g. food) given occasionally might reinforce powerfully some stereotypical behaviours.

9.5.3.8   The coping hypothesis

The term 'coping', which is popular in the stress literature, has been introduced already (Section 1.3.10). Rather like 'reinforcement', it is open to a wide variety of interpretations. Thus, it defies precise definition and operationalization but generally implies that, by its behaviour, an animal is able to exert an adaptive influence on the environment, external, internal or both. The term would seem to overlap with what is meant in the psychology literature by both positive reinforcement (e.g. gain of food contingent upon behaviour) and negative reinforcement (e.g. contingent termination of a loud noise). However, this does not mean that the terms are necessarily synonymous. Thus, a behaviour might have coping consequences without necessarily being learned as a result of such consequences or extinguish as a result of their omission. Also some authors (Barnett *et al.*, 1985) refer to both behavioural and physiological coping serving a common end, suggesting a possible parallel with, for example, autonomic and behavioural temperature regulation.

In the language of physiology, is there a change in physiological state induced by stereotypies? Is there a homeostatic function for them in maintaining something within acceptable bounds? According to their analysis in terms of neural processes, Robbins *et al.* (1990) suggest: 'If then some of the sequela of activation, such as schedule-induced polydipsia or behaviour evoked by hypothalamic electrical stimulation, are indeed "coping responses", then their performance might be expected to lead to elevated DA turnover in prefrontal cortex, their prevention presumably having the opposite effect'.

In stress, a coping strategy is commonly seen to be one that prevents the conservation-withdrawal pattern and associated HPA activation from appearing (Ödberg, 1989; Wemelsfelder, 1990). Seen in such terms, recent analyses (Mason, 1991; Cooper and Nicol, 1993; Ladewig *et al.*, 1993; Rushen, 1993) have proven inconclusive in finding an unambiguous consequence of performing stereotypies that might be described as coping or reinforcing, although in some cases restraint of corticosteroid level is found. To reiterate the caution just expressed, the relationship between such effects and any possible reinforcement process is not necessarily a straightforward one.

Possibly a reduction in corticosteroid level might exert some strengthening effect on preceding stereotyped behaviour. By analogy the delayed gain of nutrients seems to provide a strengthening of feeding tendency that arises from incentive motivational processes (Toates, 1986). There are reports of beneficial consequences seen in some restricted cases, e.g. in tethered pigs, heart rate is lower in animals showing a high frequency of stereotypies as compared with a low level (Wiepkema and Schouten, 1992), although any such effects need to be treated with caution in terms of inferring causal links (Ladewig *et al.*, 1993).

If stereotypies reduce stress in a situation otherwise characterized by lack of control, they would presumably be expected to lower the level of pituitary–adrenal activity. There is a report suggesting that tethering in sows is accompanied by a sharp rise in plasma levels of β-endorphin which subsequently fall over 2–3 days to near or even below normal levels (Wiepkema and Schouten, 1992). This corresponds to acquisition of stereotypies and is suggestive that they constitute a strategy that inhibits the HPA axis. Mason (1991) reviews evidence from domestic fowl and sows indicating a negative correlation between tendency to show stereotypies and corticosteroid level. She argues: 'Examples of correlations between stereotypies and physiological signs of coping include some behaviour patterns of domestic fowl: pacing is associated with a fall in corticosteroid levels . . .'. However, Dantzer (1991) cautions against the view that stereotypies maintain cortico-steroid levels within bounds.

Some rather speculative evidence that stereotypies might dampen stress levels was obtained by Jones et al. (1989). Stereotypies can be induced in rats by injection of d-AM (see Section 9.5.3.13), and two possible interpretations of this are as follows. The stereotypies might have no functional significance and simply represent an aberration in the nigrostriatal dopaminergic pathway caused by the injection. Alter-natively, d-AM might be stress evoking and stereotypies serve to re-duce stress. By the criterion that d-AM causes an elevation of corticosteroids, it might be termed a stressor. Jones et al. investigated the effect of caudate–putamen lesions, which sharply reduce ster-eotypies. Such lesions also prolonged the corticosteroid response. Cor-relation does not prove causality and results obtained from a lesioned animal injected with an unnatural agent are to be viewed with caution. However, this result might indicate something relevant regarding a functional significance of stereotypies.

As noted in Section 9.5.3.2, the phenomenon of SIP has been studied in the context of the HPA axis. SIP would appear to have certain similarities to stereotypies, including the fact that it takes time to develop (Toates, 1971). Acquisition time appears not to be simply a reflection of learning the schedule. Rats with prior exposure to the schedule in the absence of water still take time to acquire the habit when water is subsequently made available (Toates, 1971), suggesting the possibility of some kind of intrinsic reinforcement derived from licking itself.

An important caution is in order in discussions of SIP and the HPA axis (Ladewig et al., 1993): SIP is associated with a large influx of water to the body fluids, which would be expected to suppress vas-opressin secretion. This might then lower the input to the HPA axis but not be considered indicative of a reduction in stress.

Mittleman *et al.* (1988) firmly attached the idea of SIP being a coping response to its association with the HPA axis: 'It must be demonstrated that (1) exposure to the scheduled delivery of food increases plasma corticosterone above basal levels and that (2) exposure to the food schedule combined with the occurrence of drinking must reduce plasma corticosterone levels'. Some authors do indeed report that SIP is associated with a reduction of pituitary–adrenal activity, as indexed by plasma levels of corticosterone (Brett and Levine, 1979), although on closer examination the results are somewhat contradictory and permit no straightforward conclusions (reviewed by Dantzer and Mittleman, 1993). In the experiment of Brett and Levine, when water was subsequently made unavailable, corticosteroids returned to their pre-session levels. A reduction in corticosterone level was seen as soon as 10 min after exposure to the schedule (Brett and Levine, 1981). They suggest that: '. . . psychological factors involving unspecified reward properties of the drinking behaviour—perhaps arousal-reduction itself or some other reinforcer that leads indirectly to arousal reduction—are responsible'. When the available drinking fluid was rendered relatively unacceptable, by an earlier pairing with nausea, so that only small amounts were taken, still there was a suppression of plasma corticosterone level (Brett and Levine, 1981).

Dantzer *et al.* (1988a) dichotomized rats into those showing SIP (SIP pos) and those not showing it (SIP neg). SIP pos rats showed a decrease in plasma corticosterone level over the course of a feeding session with a water spout available. SIP neg rats showed an increase over the session. The groups were virtually indistinguishable in a subsequent session without water available, both showing an increase in corticosterone level.

Mittleman *et al.* (1988) investigated individual differences between rats and found a clear negative correlation between plasma corticosterone and water consumption in a SIP test. A similar negative correlation was found when plasma corticosterone level was manipulated chemically. As the authors note, such results are compatible with the coping hypothesis of SIP. However, another of their results did not lend support to the hypothesis. Exposure to the food schedule with water available was associated with an increased level of corticosterone whereas exposure without access to water was not associated with an increase in plasma corticosterone to above basal levels.

Dantzer and Mormède (1981, 1983b) observed pigs that exhibited schedule-induced chain pulling on a schedule of intermittent food presentation. Over the session, this behaviour was associated with a decrease in pituitary–adrenal activity as indexed by plasma corticosteroid levels. When there was no chain-pulling facility in the food-delivery set-up there was no such pre-session to post-session decline. Dantzer and Mormède (1983a) argue that such behaviour constitutes a '. . . very effective means for the animal to dissipate its tension or anxiety'. However, the HPA axis activation accompanying extinction was not ameliorated by the presence of a chain to manipulate (Dantzer and Mormède, 1983b).

Terlouw *et al.* (1991b) compared high and low stereotyping pigs, finding no difference in plasma cortisol levels. Removing the chain, the object with which stereotypies were performed, was not associated with an elevation of cortisol level.

To summarize, the results are somewhat confusing and the evidence does not allow clear conclusions. The suggestion that is perhaps made most frequently in the literature is that such behaviour as SIP is an example of a coping response in that it lowers activity in the HPA axis. Alternatively, or in addition, low levels of activity in the HPA axis might give a bias to active strategies one of which is SIP.

9.5.3.9　Arousal

Closely related to notions of coping and reinforcement is that of arousal (see Section 1.2.2.2). The common and implicit assumption is often made that stereotypies reduce arousal, anxiety or frustration. However, as some authors (Dantzer, 1986; Frith and Done, 1990; Robbins *et al.*, 1990) discuss, in the context of both humans and non-humans, the opposite argument is also commonly advanced: that the performance of motor patterns in a dull environment provides some much-needed sensory stimulation. Arousal might sound then like an unsure anchor for a theory of stereotypy but we cannot entirely dismiss the possibility that both of these could be true; from either side behaviour might serve to move arousal level towards an optimum.

9.5.3.10　Tight organization: the Fentress model

An influential paper by Fentress (1976) proposed a model of behaviour that appears very relevant to understanding stereotypies, as Fentress describes characteristics of normal behaviour that would seem to lend themselves to the development of stereotypy. Fentress described observations on various species showing that under certain conditions behaviour gains an autonomy from stimulus input, corresponding, he argues, to a shift from peripheral to central control. This is particularly so for tightly organized, relatively inflexible, species-typical behaviour that commonly has a high frequency of occurrence. An example is grooming of the face in mice, which shows some autonomy from sensory input from the face. Fentress suggested that the: '. . . actual execution of rapid movements during grooming can serve to isolate the "grooming system" from both dependence upon and sensitivity to interruption by sensory factors'.

Fentress describes observation made on a Cape hunting dog (*Lycaon pictus*). The dog exhibited repetitive locomotor patterns in its cage, tracing out a figure eight. At a stage when the behaviour was well established, a chain was placed at a height of 0.8 m at the middle point of the figure eight. The animal's immediate reaction was to alter its path to avoid the chain. However, after external conditions were changed in such a way as to produce a higher frequency of pacing, the animal reverted to its original trajectory, with the outcome of colliding with the chain. Subsequently, when the chain was lowered to the ground, the animal's trajectory included a jump, reacting as if the chain was still present. In other words, the animal's behaviour seemed to be organized centrally in the sense of taking cognizance of stimuli that were once present but no longer. External disturbances (e.g. noise of zoo keepers) tended: (1) to increase speed of movement and (2) to cause a reversion to behaviour appropriate to the continuing presence of the now absent chain, a reversion to 'a previously established central motor programme'.

A similar conclusion arose from Fentress's (1976) observations of captive voles. Environmental manipulations were made in that some objects were removed and others introduced. On attempting to capture the voles, they were observed to make flight movements appropriate to negotiating their way around objects that were once in their home environment but no longer were present.

Fentress' (1976) observations dovetail with those of others. No less a figure than the father of behaviourism, John Watson (see Gallistel, 1980), noted that when the arms of mazes in which rats were very familiar were changed in length, the rats still responded on the basis of their previous length. Thus they crashed head-on into the end wall of shortened arms and stopped short of the end in elongated arms. (Also, Gallistel (1990) and Oakley (1979) discuss examples showing that animals continue to make detour behaviour after the initial cause of the detour had been eliminated). There are two possible ways of interpreting such results. On the one hand, they might suggest the use of an inner representation of the form of a cognitive map of the way the world is expected to be. On the other hand, it might seem that under repetition, behaviour can assume some of the parameters of invariance that within classical ethology define a fixed action pattern (see Molt, 1965). How one might do a neat experiment to decide between these interpretations is not obvious.

Fentress (1976) found evidence that rapidly executed behavioural sequences can, under some conditions, acquire an autonomy not only from external stimuli but also from proprioceptive stimuli. Fentress reminds us of Karl Lashley's influential argument (Lashley, 1951) that rapidly executed sequences cannot rely upon sequential proprioceptive feedback. The Fentress model appears to dovetail with the conclusions drawn by Aldridge *et al.* (1993) concerning the role of the neostriatum: that at the beginning of a sequence 'neostriatal circuits temporarily switch motor control toward central pattern generators and away from sensory-guided systems'.

Not only does behaviour acquire a certain autonomy from external and proprioceptive inputs, there is also evidence (reviewed by Fentress) to show that it can develop an autonomy from the so-called higher brain regions: 'One might also tentatively postulate that in "higher" vertebrates subcortical (including brain stem) mechanisms are largely responsible for the articulation of stereotyped output sequences . . .'. With such a location of organization, the demands placed upon overall processing capacities would appear to be less. Fentress reviews evidence showing that stereotyped activities tend to appear during times of cortical deactivation by application of KCl or during recovery from surgical lesions (e.g. to hypothalamus). He argues: 'It is reasonable to postulate that behavioural situations that are variously defined in terms of "conflict", "thwarting", "stress", "overload", etc., reflect a processing capacity which is reduced with respect to any particular dimension of behaviour . . .'. It does indeed seem a reasonable claim, when there is some independent evidence to suppose that behaviour capacity is limited, as in depression of the cortex. However, there is a danger of circularity here in that overload and stress might simply come to be identified as those conditions that give rise to autonomy. In such terms, it is difficult to reconcile the model with the observation that stereotypies often appear in conditions where there would appear to be minimal processing demands placed upon the animal, described as boredom. One possible way of refining Fentress' model to account for such situations is suggested in Section 9.5.12.

In a further paper, Fentress (1977) suggests that 'reflexes may modulate mechanisms of intrinsic pattern generation without producing the details of that pattern generation *per se*' and that 'proprioceptive mechanisms may produce relatively "tonic" influences upon the detailed patterning of behavioural output, *even though* these patterning mechanisms are basically intrinsic to the inputs themselves'. Fentress also discusses the role of various factors (e.g. extrinsic disturbances) that seem to exert an indirect input to repetitive behaviour, either to suppress or enhance it. He also shows evidence of a rebound effect: removal of an inhibitory influence is followed by increased behaviour.

9.5.3.11   Fixated behaviour: the Feldman model

Feldman (1978) interprets stereotypies within a framework of theory and experimentation on what is termed fixated behaviour. As an example of this, Feldman notes that, if an animal is confronted with a difficult discrimination task, it sometimes tends to revert to a fixed way of responding by choosing one particular motor response or one particular stimulus towards which it responds. If stimuli that earlier were successfully discriminated are now reintroduced, the animal continues to respond in a fixated way. In other words, it fails to exploit the knowledge of the situation which it might be assumed still to possess. In the terms of the present analysis, it has moved to a mode of control dominated by a particular physically present stimulus. It fails to be controlled by the broader stimulus situation in which information might well be held in the form of knowledge of the world (e.g. (respond to A) → (access to food), (respond to B) → (no access)). Feldman notes that after such a stereotypy has been broken: '. . . the new response is acquired very rapidly suggesting the animals "knew" the correct solution but were prevented from responding on the basis of the acquired information'. This has some similarities to the situation described earlier (Section 9.5.3.6) wherein an animal will sometimes continue the stereotyped behaviour even after the original eliciting conditions have been changed.

Feldman (1978) relates such fixation to an apparently similar form exhibited in the learned helplessness paradigm (Section 5.8). Following uncontrollable aversive stimulation animals will sometimes fail to respond even when the situation changes such that active escape and/ or avoidance is now possible. It is possible that this might similarly be understood as a particularly prepotent response to the current stimulus dominating in the face of potential controls of behaviour that might require some kind of extrapolation, of the form that 'over there is safe'.

Compared with intact controls, Feldman (1978) sees animals with lesions in certain limbic structures as behaving similarly to that described as fixation. For example, cats with septal lesions learned a discrimination task as well as controls. However, when a reversal was called for, they simply carried on responding to the previously positive stimulus. In another study, monkeys were trained on a sequence: (1) respond to red stimulus followed by (2) respond to green stimulus and (3) reward given. Compared with controls, animals with hippocampal lesions tended to respond to the green stimulus first. Again the solution requires more than simply responding to physically present stimuli. Rather it might be argued that it requires a cognition involving a sequence of relationships not evident in the sensory information alone. Also one can speculate that something like a simple response reinforcement process would be likely to potentiate the power of the green stimulus (rather than the red), due to its closer proximity to food.

9.5.3.12 Behavioural hierarchies

A possible theoretical framework for understanding stereotypies is the notion of a behavioural hierarchy (Milner, 1961; Tinbergen, 1969; Shallice, 1972; Powers, 1973; Gallistel, 1980; Cools, 1985; Roitblat, 1991; Ridley, 1994; Toates, 1994a). Usually, in such a model of behaviour, the top level of the hierarchy is occupied by goals and cognitions. The lowest level corresponds to control loops that determine the state of individual motor neurons and thereby muscles. Intermediate levels correspond to the organization of particular behaviours (e.g. turn left). In such terms, Fentress' (1976) claim that behaviour develops autonomy might be seen as control shifting to a lower level in a hierarchy. Indeed, Dantzer (1986) suggested such a thing: 'Drawing upon classical hierarchical concepts of Jacksonian neurology, I propose that the occurrence of stereotypies reflects a cut-off of higher nervous functions coupled with a disinhibition of hypothalamic and brain-stem structures where the basic organization of most motor acts is hard-wired'.

According to the model proposed by Gallistel (1980), a low level of organization underlying, for example, reflexes is potentiated or depotentiated from a higher level. This means that individual building blocks of behaviour normally appear within a context that shows overall goal direction. A number of authors (discussed below) have, either explicitly or implicitly, been drawn to seeing stereotypies as an aberration of a control loop at a relatively low level in such a hierarchy. However, although this might indeed capture the essence of the determining process, we might still need to consider an initial goal-directed and top-down influence within the hierarchy.

Isaacson and Gispen (1990), in the context of stereotypies, note that a consequence of prefrontal brain abnormality can be a disruption of hierarchical control such that: '. . . behaviour becomes based on a less

well-differentiated world and actions are based more closely on acquired stimulus–response associations without regard to "higher-
order" contingencies'. Isaacson and Gispen note a similarity between
events seen in certain states of stress and human psychotic disorders.
In both cases the adaptiveness of behaviour is reduced by as they term
it 'restrictions of attentional, cognitive or performance characteristics',
associated with malfunction in the brain's prefrontal area. Also a
similarity between stereotypy and the behaviour of rats with damage
to the lateral hypothalamus can be recorded. Teitelbaum et al. (1990)
describe the lack of co-ordination shown by such a rat: '. . . it appears to
lack goal-directedness, responding reflexively to each configuration of
surfaces it encounters', and 'such an animal is merely a collection of
parts that are acting independently and may work at cross-purposes'.

Using a notion of hierarchy, Robbins and Sahakian (1983) relate
their data on AM-induced stereotypies (see Section 9.5.3.13) to the
action selection model of Norman and Shallice (see e.g. Shallice, 1972).
In this model, schemas represent various actions and also a certain
amount of specification of component responses and their spatio-
temporal sequence to accomplish the action. An established schema
can be selected on the basis of a combination of: (1) top-down influences
from motivational state among other things and (2) environmental
stimuli. However, established schemas are relatively easily triggered
by environmental stimuli even in the absence of top-down potentiation,
triggering and guidance being said to be automatic. In such terms,
according to Robbins and Sahakian: 'By increasing DA release,
amphetamine-like stimulants are assumed to bring schemas above the
activational threshold and facilitate their execution'. In a language
implying a top-down depotentiation (Gallistel, 1980) within a hierarchy, Robbins et al. (1990) write of the forebrain influences that 'normally antagonize the autonomous and stereotyped behaviour that can
result from overactivation'.

A model particularly relevant to the present discussion is that of
Milner (1961). He suggests that, at a level above that of the pools of
motor neurons which constitute the final effector stage, there exist
'innately organized nuclei for controlling such activities as walking,
reaching, grasping, chewing, sniffing, scratching, and so on'. These
were termed by him as 'actions', although this is a rather different use
of the term, as compared to, say, that of Dickinson (1985). They constitute the building blocks of more complex behaviour. According to
Milner, actions require a sequential activation of various groups of
muscles. Furthermore, they require repetition of the sequence until
they are switched off, presumably by a depotentiation signal from

higher in the hierarchy. Stimulation of the basal ganglia can reveal such motor organization.

Note that Milner's (1961) 'actions' represent precisely the level of organization that is most commonly seen as displacement activity and stereotypies. It is suggested here that stereotypies should be seen as a maladaptive sensitization at this level in the hierarchy. How this maladaptive sensitization arises might be explained by considering how the hierarchical control of behaviour normally is executed. It requires a balance between: (a) the intrinsic sensitivity within the control loops that organize the so-called actions, described by Milner, and (b) the signal of potentiation and depotentiation from higher in the hierarchy to the level of the actions. In the case of well-performed actions having a high probability of occurrence in any case, factor (a) will be high. Stereotypy might then exert a self-reinforcing effect within this local organization. Concerning factor (b), an abnormal descending influence could arise from either: (1) a monotonous environment in which there is not sufficient information to maintain a species-typical level of goal direction and associated descending potentiation and depotentiation or from (2) overstimulation as in a conflict situation.

It is tentatively proposed that a displacement activity is a transient switch in weighting in the hierarchy to a particular low-level control loop, at which point behavioural control will be exerted mainly by sensory input. It is transient as the normal context of goal-directed activity reasserts itself. Note that displacement activities commonly involve such things as grooming and scratching, preening, that represent species-typical organization at the level of Milner's 'actions'. In such terms, stereotypies would reflect a chronic state of maladaptive (de)potentiation. Also displacement activities occur commonly at times of ambivalence (Tinbergen, 1969), in other words, at times when no clear-cut goal strategy can be switched in. Possibly, ambivalent potentiation and depotentiation signals (or rapidly changing signals) might be sent downwards in the hierarchy. In other cases, the displacement activity is appropriate to the motivational state but inappropriate to the stimulus context (Tinbergen, 1969), suggesting hierarchical depotentiation in the terms expressed here, analogous to some kind of energy discharge in Tinbergen's terms.

In keeping with such a model is the observation that: (1) stereotypy is sometimes disrupted by very high levels of arousal and (2) stressors can sometimes actually lower the level of stereotypies induced by stimulant drugs (reviewed by Mason, 1992). There is, however, one potential problem with this line of thought: situations that trigger stereotypies, such as frustration and thwarting, are by definition those of failed expectations when, it might be reasoned, routines would be interrupted and emotion and cognitive control fully exerted (Simon, 1967; Toates, 1988, 1994b, 1995b; Oatley, 1992; Wiepkema and Koolhaas, 1993). Novelty and disturbance similarly imply a breaking of routine. Why high-level control should immediately switch out after being recruited remains to be explained. In a similar vein, Mason (1991) reviews evidence that arousal-reducing drugs lower stereotypies in isolation-reared chimpanzees as does familiarization with a novel environment. (Wiepkema and Koolhaas, 1992, developed an argument that raises a similar issue to the logic advanced here.)

Kennes et al. (1988) suggest a transition in the process underlying stereotypies. In the early stages, they are sensitive to endogenous opioids but 'thereafter only motoric automatisms remain, essentially under dopaminergic control'. This is claimed on the grounds that stereotypies are sensitive to reduction by opioid blockers only in the early stages whereas their sensitivity to DA blockers remains throughout. They also note that stereotypies can gain autonomy from their original eliciting conditions such that even if a source of conflict is removed the stereotypy can remain. In their early stages, stereotypies can be inhibited by tranquillizers whereas they are immune to this effect once well established (see Mason, 1991, and see also Cole and Koob, 1991, for analogous effects with CRF). Thus Mason suggests a transition from control by emotional factors to control exerted by emotionally neutral processes, in line with the kind of shift of control first introduced in Section 1.3.2 in which emotion is switched out as routines are switched in. Wemelsfelder (1993) also proposes such a distinction but one in which initially stereotypies are indicative of frustration whereas something with less active connotations, like depression, might characterize the mental state associated with their maintenance.

Milner (1961) suggests that once a course of goal-directed behaviour has been selected:

> . . . it facilitates various responses subliminally, and the sensory input again selects the one of these that leads most directly to the goal. The response requires that various actions be performed in the correct sequence; at this level most of the selecting sensory input is provided by the proprioceptors, and the organization is more and more dependent on the innate mechanisms . . ..

Stereotypies would seem to be a case of out-of-context behaviour that gets stuck at one stage of such a sequence. Such increased weighting being given to proprioception might correspond to what Mason and Turner (1993) refer to as increased centralization as opposed to external stimulus control in the determination of behaviour. However, as was noted in Section 9.5.3.10, with high repetition even proprioceptive information might come to play a less important part.

In terms of a hierarchy of control and based upon the language of Dickinson (1985), cognition can be seen as a high-level control over goal-directed behaviour, whereas lower-level controls are responsible for habits (Toates, 1994a,b, 1995a,b), although one should not assume that all well-practised behaviour has a subcortical locus of organization (Lashley, 1921). Some neuroanatomical pointers suggest that the habit system, defined as distinct from a cognitive system, is implicated in stereotyped behaviour. Thus DA depletion within the caudate nucleus reduces or eliminates stereotypy induced by d-AM (reviewed by Cooper and Dourish, 1990). Robbins et al. (1990) associate the striatum with the control of stereotyped behaviour. These brain regions associated with the control of stereotyped behaviour overlap with the regions associated by Petri and Mishkin (1994) with the habit system.

Such a model of stereotypies might enable them to be understood within a broader context as an exaggeration of a switch in behavioural control that would normally serve an adaptive function. In terms of a hierarchy of behavioural control, stereotypies might be seen as a switch from cognitive to procedural control that would under more normal conditions occur with repetition of a given response in a given context (Toates, 1994a,b, 1995a,b). Under more normal conditions, such a switch can be seen as an adaptive answer to problems for which a routine solution can suffice. The switch constitutes a move in weighting to lower hierarchical levels and can spare high level cognitive control for solving novel problems. This process has been described as one of moving from cognition to stimulus–response control (Toates, 1994a,b, 1995a,b) in line with assumptions of other writers (Hirsh, 1974; see earlier discussion in this section). It implies increased weighting being given to immediate stimulus input. However, as was noted in Section 9.5.3.10 there is evidence that autonomy goes even further than this and behaviour can gain autonomy even from stimulus input. Possibly we should view a two-stage autonomy process: (1) autonomy from (high-level) goal direction corresponding to increased weight being given to actual stimulus input and (2) autonomy from stimulus input corresponding to greater weighting being given to central (but low hierarchical level) programmes.

The present approach would place stereotypies in a context of other situations in which a shift to a habit is 'maladaptive', albeit under somewhat bizarre conditions. For instance, the phenomenon of 'the misbehaviour of organisms' (Breland and Breland, 1961) refers to a tendency for well-trained instrumental behaviour to degenerate into species-typical behaviour with a subsequent loss of reward. The suggestion was made (Toates, 1994a,b) that this should be understood as a shift from cognitive control to habit control, at which point well-formed species typical habits can intrude and compete. Interestingly, the kind of rooting behaviour that pigs show under such conditions is not unlike certain stereotypies (see Section 9.5.3.6). Something such as a somersaulting stereotypy in voles that seems to be susceptible to imitation (Cooper and Nicol, 1994) might start out under cognitive control and then with repetition switch to procedural control. The fact that with experience stereotypies become immune to disruption by naloxone, described as an emancipation from their original opioid basis (Wiepkema and Schouten, 1992), might give a clue to the process here. Opioids might serve in a sensitization rather than classical neurotransmitter role (cf. Watkins and Mayer, 1982). According to such a model, it is not obvious that stereotypies either result from stress, imply suffering or represent anything like coping, although the model is not necessarily incompatible with this being the case. Indeed, in the context of an hierarchical model, Dantzer (1986) goes so far as to argue: 'This view makes superfluous any speculation on the mental state of affected animals because they would be unable to feel any emotion while they are engaged in their stereotypies, but it provides no excuse for the design and use of facilities that result in such abnormal behaviour'.

In a hierarchical model, the hippocampus might be expected to correspond to behavioural control exerted at a high level (Toates, 1994a,b, 1995a,b). Its role is usually interpreted as the physical base *par excellence* of the cognitive mediation of behaviour (Hirsh, 1974; O'Keefe and Nadel, 1978; see also Chapter 7). As Blozovski (1986) notes, maturation of the hippocampus is associated with: (1) suppression of certain otherwise prepotent responses and (2) co-ordination of responses into an overall goal-directed strategy. In the terms developed here, in its role of cognitive control (Hirsh, 1974), the hippocampus would play a part in the sensitization and desensitization of responses (and not just to their inhibition) according to overall goals.

The hippocampally lesioned rat behaves much like a stimulus–response automaton (Hirsh, 1974). Similarly, Oakley (1983) noted that the rat with neocortex removed fits a stimulus–response model and seems impaired in its ability to exert cognitive control. One might expect then hippocampally lesioned rats and also rats with cortical damage to show an increased tendency to stereotypy. There is some evidence that the cortex and hippocampus do indeed exert a moderating influence on stereotypies (reviewed by Cabib, 1993; Robbins *et al.*,

1990; see also discussion in Section 9.5.3.10 on cortical depression). Decorticates and hippocampals tended to show an elevated stereotypy score compared with sham-operated controls. Robbins *et al.* (1990) review the evidence of Devenport that food-deprived rats with hippocampal lesions respond to the signalled presentation of food with stereotypy and locomotion that is similar to that of AM-injected rats. It can be blocked by injection of the DA antagonist haloperidol.

Apparently, dovetailing with a model of hierarchical control, Robbins *et al.* (1990) relate stereotypy to the notion of arousal (Sections 1.2.2.2 and 9.5.3.9); stereotypies typically involve behaviours that are described as automatic (i.e. behaviour can be organized at a low level in hierarchy) and require little in the way of planning (i.e. require little in the way of complex top-down potentiation and depotentiation). They can be performed even at high levels of arousal, whereas more difficult tasks require a lower level of arousal for their optimal performance.*

9.5.3.13 *Amphetamines, stereotypies and stress*

So far we have discussed mainly stereotypies induced by particular environmental contexts, although occasional reference has been made to AM-induced stereotypies. This section takes a brief digression from the main argument to look more closely at AM-induced stereotypies, in the hope of gaining insight into more 'normal' stereotypies. It compares stereotypies induced in undrugged animals with those induced by AMs, as there are some important similarities. Looking at the AM-induced effects might illuminate more 'naturally' evoked stereotypies.

Antelman and Chiodo (1983) claim that 'it is a virtual truism that drugs induce their effects by simulating the influence of naturally occurring environmental stimuli'. In this case, the acute effects of AM would presumably induce a similar state to that of the traditionally described stressors, the most obvious being stereotypy. AM-induced stereotypy can be antagonized by such neuroleptic drugs as haloperidol (Cooper and Dourish, 1990).

---

* Robbins and Sahakian (1983) note that some psychologists have suggested that stereotypies serve a function in regulating brain arousal level; the otherwise overaroused animal showing stereotypy is limiting sensory input to one or two channels. However, they go on to note the weakness of this idea in accounting for stimulant-induced stereotypies in that novelty serves to reduce the stereotypy. On the basis of such an explanation, one might have supposed that novelty would increase arousal and promote stereotypies. However, in terms of a hierarchy, introducing novelty could: (1) remove familiar cues that have got themselves locked into the low-level control as the stimulus input (Robbins and Sahakian emphasize the role of environmental determinants) and (2) introduce some new top-down information.

AM has a variety of effects on behaviour. In a discrimination situation, injected animals can show difficulty in withholding responding to the unreinforced stimulus (Lyon and Robbins,1975; Ridley *et al.*, 1981). Also, the differential reinforcement of low response rate (DRL) schedule, in which reinforcement is given provided the animal both (1) responds and then (2) *withholds* responding for a period of time, is disrupted. Increased perseveration of certain aspects of behaviour is one characteristic induced by AM (Robbins and Sahakian, 1983), e.g. increased persistence of behaviour in the absence of (apparent) reinforcement. In this sense there would appear to be some resemblance between the AM-injected animal and the hippocampally lesioned animal. Perseverative route tracing in rats and grooming in cats and monkeys have been observed. Spontaneous alternation in a T-maze is reduced (see Lyon and Robbins, 1975). Thus AMs alter the nature of what at some level might be described as whole-body, goal-directed behaviour. However, stereotypies, which are the best known AM-induced effect, are generally restricted to a simple act such as licking and are seen as lacking any obvious goal. For instance, Robbins and Sahakian note a type of *perseverative sequence*, as they term them, which appears to be out-of-context and therefore meaningless. They suggest that such sequences can be viewed as 'higher order stereotypies' which, with increasing AM doses, can break up into component stereotypies. Similarly, Lyon and Robbins (1975) suggest that: 'stereotypy cannot be regarded as the perseveration of a simple response, but that the syndrome involves complicated response chains'.

AM-induced 'stereotypies' sometimes take a form that is suggestive more of goal-directed behaviour rather than simply the repetition of an invariant mechanical act (cf. Mason and Turner, 1993). For example, Robbins *et al.* (1990) discuss the case of an AM-injected guinea-pig that would pursue a cage-mate apparently *in order to* gnaw at one location on its fur. Trained on an operant task, AM-injected rats can show (1) increased persistence apparently directed towards a goal and (2) a commensurate reduction in such activities as grooming and rearing. Trained on an operant shock escape/avoidance task, the lever-pressing of AM-injected rats was reported (Randrup and Munkvad, 1970) to be: '. . . increased and blended with the sniffing, licking and biting into a stereotyped activity, which was performed continuously to the exclusion of all other forms of behaviour'.

AM-induced stereotypies tend to be species-specific (Segal and Schuckit, 1983). For example, stereotyped pecking is seen in the pigeon (see Lyon and Robbins, 1975). In rats, AM tends to produce stereotypies that are commonly exaggerations of unlearned behaviours, e.g. those under some kind of rhythmic control (e.g. licking, sniffing) and particularly oral behaviours (e.g. gnawing, chewing and biting) (Segal and Schuckit, 1983). Lyon and Robbins (1975) noted that, although gnawing, biting and licking figure prominently in AM-induced stereotypies in rats, their co-ordination, which would normally lead to food ingestion, is soon lost. In some cases, behaviour that would normally occur at the beginning of a response chain can increase in frequency causing a loss of later components. Suggestive of a top-down potentiation, is the finding that, in particular, hungry animals have a tendency to develop feeding-related stereotypies in response to AM (reviewed by Mason, 1993).

In some respects, AM-induced stereotypy looks like an exaggeration of particular stimulus–response links, ones that have a high probability of occurrence in any case in the animal's normal commerce with a particular environment. For example, AM-induced drinking as a means of shock avoidance shows great perseverance (Teitelbaum and Derks, 1958). If the spout is removed the rat continues to direct licking through the empty aperture. However, this should not be viewed as a vacuum activity. Moving the rat back to its home cage terminates such licking, thus demonstrating the powerful environmental control over such behaviour (avoidance learning tells a similar story).

Robbins et al. (1990) discuss the issue of a possible reinforcing effect of AM-induced stereotypies. They raise the possibility that: (1) the reinforcing effect of AM is based upon the release of DA and (2) that whatever response happens to occur when AM exerts is effect will automatically be reinforced. In such terms, even the kinaesthetic feedback from operant behaviour might constitute a conditioned reinforcer whose effect becomes increased by the drug. In a similar vein, Hill (1970) speculates: '. . . that the proprioceptive and kinesthetic stimuli associated with locomotion, rearing and sniffing had their own CR properties conditioned in the extraexperimental history of the rats . . .'. Robbins and Sahakian (1983) develop the logic of Hill that AM might enhance the controlling influence of secondary reinforcing stimuli. They propose the possibility of an: '. . . association of enhanced reinforcing effect with the motor feedback of responding itself. Thus, the motor output may then acquire conditioned reinforcing properties of its own and become perseverative for that reason'. This would amount to positive feedback as described earlier (Section 9.5.3.7).

However, Robbins et al. (1990) go on to argue that the reinforcement hypothesis fails to explain the species-typical nature of stereotypies, i.e. that different individuals within a population tend to show similar stereotypies. According to the hypothesis advanced here, species-typical behaviours organized at a relatively low level in a behavioural hierarchy are the output of preformed control loops. These would be susceptible to strengthening by repetition. However, attractive as such an explanation might be, it is probably safer to agree with the possibility suggested by Robbins *et al.* that: 'reinforcement contingencies play some role in determining the form of amphetamine-induced stereotyped behaviour, but that stereotypies do not arise solely from an exaggeration of central reinforcement mechanisms'.*

The reason for their caution in proposing a monolithic (reinforcement) model is that, for the self-administration of AMs, there is some evidence of regulation of the plasma concentration of AM (this is also true of other self-administered drugs; Bozarth, 1987), such that the high levels which induce stereotypy are less favoured than lower doses. One might suggest both a high-level reward process and a lower-level reinforcement process.

As evidence for the relevance of AM to the effect of stressors, Antelman and Chiodo (1983) note, among other things, that both stressors and AM increase β-endorphin and corticosteroid levels. Similarly, both are followed by an increase in the turnover and/or release of DA and noradrenaline in the brain. Brain serotonin is affected in a similar way in response to both situations. However, if AM simulates the action of stressors, it is perhaps somewhat paradoxical that animals will opt to self-administer both AM and ACTH. Such a paradox is compounded by the observation, reviewed by Antelman and Chiado, that the neuroendocrine consequences of the profoundly positively reinforcing stimulus of electrical brain stimulation (e.g. depletion of brain noradrenaline levels) can be indistinguishable from that of applying stressors. Indeed, Antelman and Chiado employ such brain stimulation as a stressor.

So is AM a reinforcer in the conventional sense? Lyon and Robbins (1975) argue that: 'one of the effects of amphetamine is to strengthen the tendency to persevere or repeat responses previously learned in the given situation or which are present in that situation when the drug effect begins'; and further the implication of their hypothesis is that AM will 'act somewhat arbitrarily in conjunction with the reinforcing effects which are already present, by strengthening the tendency for

* From the discussion of Robbins and Sahakian concerning increased perseveration of lever-pressing in the absence of primary reinforcement, one can articulate two such possible factors: enhancement of either (1) a motor act *per se*, irrespective of the consequences derived from this act, or (2) the controlling influence of secondary reinforcers or a combination of the two. Support for the role of factor 2 comes from an experiment in which a neutral cue was paired with water reward. Rats injected with pipradol (which has both DA releasing and serotonin releasing effects) later preferentially opted to press a lever that delivered the previously neutral cue.

certain motor patterns, but *not others*, to be repeated. In this sense, according to our hypothesis, amphetamine is not in itself a reinforcing agent'.

9.5.4.14 Conclusions

Ideally, this section would present a theoretical framework to bring some order and synthesis to the results on stereotypies and fit them into a broader context of behavioural understanding. A number of factors that might play a part in stereotypies have been noted: emergence out of what is initially goal-directed behaviour, species-typical approach or avoidance behaviour, positive reinforcement and its apparent synonym in this case, positive feedback, a coping process based upon the HPA axis, opioids and DA. Although these have been discussed mainly in separate sections, a full understanding will doubtless require a contribution from each and additional factors as yet undiscussed. For instance, the fact that stereotypies commonly occur *after* a limited period of feeding might be understood in terms of an interaction between: (1) some kind of cognitive potentiation corresponding to the frustration of an excited motivational state (cues predictive of food excite feeding motivation and associated endocrine changes; Weingarten, 1984; Woods, 1991); (2) sensitization of rooting, chewing, licking and biting patterns (depending upon species and context) by their performance in feeding, involving opioid-mediated positive feedback; and (3) an excitation of HPA activity induced by presentation of cues predictive of food and then a suppression of this axis by motor acts normally associated with feeding (see Section 5.11). This is largely speculation but it is the kind of speculation involving interactions that might be needed to solve the riddle.

9.6 CONCLUSIONS

Considerations of animal husbandry and welfare raise a similar set of questions to those discussed elsewhere on stress, e.g. the role of corticosteroids, definitional problems on what is stress, individual differences in reaction to potential stressors and the role of coping strategies. In some cases, it is possible to draw a fairly unambiguous criterion of stress and welfare. For instance, chronically elevated corticosterone levels are indicative of stress that is likely to be associated with pathology.

One central topic that emerges throughout this chapter as well as in others concerns the *consequences* of performing behaviour, quite apart from changes in the external world that result. A consensus is emerging in applied ethology that allowing animals to perform certain of their repertoire of species-typical behaviours is conducive to good husbandry. For example, the consequences of chewing and swallowing movements for the transit of nutrients along the alimentary tract were noted. In a similar vein, Section 5.9 discussed the effects on physiological state of performing aggression. The message is the same throughout: behaviour *per se* has important consequences. However, we need care when considering the welfare implications of stereotypies. On the one hand, they are probably quite reasonably seen as indicative of a suboptimal environmental regime. On the other hand, given that the animal is in such an environment, stereotypy might provide some kind of beneficial feedback to the system.

Consideration of a hierarchy of behavioural control might offer some hope of a theoretical framework for understanding stereotypies. In such terms, stereotypy would represent a shift in weighting from top-down to bottom-up control over behaviour. Such a shift would represent both a loss of the ability to exert top-down control, arising from either an impossibly dull environment or one of overstimulation or failure of control, combined with a powerful habit forming input of behavioural repetition.

Chapter 10

Implications for Health and Pathology

10.1 INTRODUCTION

The relationship between stress and health is an enormous area of discourse that fires the popular imagination. However, trying to define the exact role of stress in human health and disease is problematic. Still more difficult is the attempt to tease apart the possible processes whereby stress could exert a role. One factor among so many to consider is that stressed individuals might pay more attention to otherwise unnoticed physiological states. Previously unlabelled sensations might assume the form of symptoms of disease (Cohen and Williamson, 1991).

One popular focus of attention at the moment is the possible effect of stress on the immune system which might render the stressed individual more vulnerable to both cancer and infectious illness (discussed later). However, any such effects of stress are likely to be exerted in combination with other changes that might affect disease risk. For example, stress could be accompanied by behavioural changes that might themselves affect immunity, e.g. increased smoking and drinking or eating poorer quality food (Cohen and Williamson, 1991). What is true of infectious illness might also be true to some extent of other 'stress effects', e.g. on circulatory system pathology. However, with this caution in mind this chapter will explore some of the possible processes linking stress with health and disease.

10.2 CIRCULATORY SYSTEM PATHOLOGY

There is a vast literature detailing the part of stress in the development of hypertension in humans, some animal models of which have been briefly mentioned (Chapter 6). The general conclusion is that stress interacts with such factors as diet in the generation of this condition (reviewed by Schneiderman and McCabe, 1985). The effect of stressors in inducing abnormal arterial blood pressure seems to be mediated principally by the sympathetic–adrenal–medullary (SAM) system. Schneiderman and McCabe conclude that there is little evidence to suggest that, in general, behavioural variables can, on their own, induce chronic hypertension. Rather they might more normally act synergistically with, for example, dietary factors or renal disorders. There can be a genetic bias towards hypertension.

As was noted in Chapter 2, at the time of exposure to a stressor, free fatty acids are released under the influence of adrenaline, noradrenaline and other hormones (Mason, 1968; Archer, 1979). Chronic exposure to stressors, with sympathetic nervous system (SNS) activation, is known to play a part in hardening of the arteries (arteriosclerosis), acting in interaction with other factors such as diet (reviewed by Schneiderman and McCabe, 1985). Fatty deposits are formed at the walls of blood vessels (see Figure 10.1).

There are differences between the physiological reactions to, on the one hand, exposure to stressors not accompanied by physical exertion and, on the other, aerobic exercise, even though both situations involve activation of the SNS (reviewed by Schneiderman and McCabe, 1985). Both involve the mobilization of lipid stores from adipose tissue. These are then hydrolysed to free fatty acids and can be utilized as an energy substrate for muscular exertion. In the case of hard exercise, the free fatty acids are therefore cleared from the circulation. By contrast, if

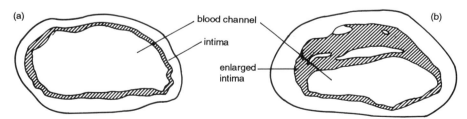

Figure 10.1. Cross-section of human artery (a) normal and (b) atherosclerotic. Note the fatty deposits on the inner layer (intima) of the vessel in (b). (Reproduced with permission from Archer, 1979, *Animals under Stress*, figure 6-1, p. 39. Copyright Williams & Wilkins)

the free fatty acids are not utilized, e.g. stress not accompanied by exertion, some of them are converted in the liver to triglycerides. Ultimately, following further conversion, lipids can reappear in the circulation and form atherosclerotic plaques. High blood pressure accelerates the formation of such deposits and catecholamines appear also to play a part, emphasizing the multicausality of such pathology.

Personality is much discussed in the context of coronary disease. In humans, the so-called Type A personality, characterized by hostility, impatience and excessive competition, is particularly associated with atherosclerosis (reviewed by Schneiderman and McCabe, 1985). However, according to some authors, the broad term 'Type A' seems now to cover too many personality traits to give a fine-grained description of exactly what is toxic. Some Type A traits might even be beneficial. Attempts to specify precisely what is toxic were made by Williams (1989) and Wright (1988). Although their conclusions differ slightly, there is every reason to believe that reconciliation can be achieved.

Williams' (1989, 1991) analysis suggested that one particular aspect of the Type A personality, hostility, was a good predictor of coronary heart disease (CHD). It might come as some comfort to the reader to know that, according to Williams, Type A personality traits such as excessive drive to achieve and time urgency are not good predictors except insofar as they are associated with hostility. On their own, high drive to achieve and rapid performance of tasks might even be beneficial to the coronary system. According to Williams, the biological basis of this phenomenon consists of a sympathetically mediated hyperreactivity of the cardiovascular system accompanied by a relatively weak parasympathetic antagonism. In its biological roots the autonomic nervous system (ANS) is of course 'designed' to be responsive to external threats. In the case of hostile personality types, then not only are the number of external stimuli capable of being interpreted as threatening larger than normal (e.g. that guy in front driving too slowly is there to annoy me; the old man fumbling in the check-out queue should shop somewhere else) but also presumably, by cognitive mediation, threats can be intrinsically generated simply by thinking processes. Eternal vigilance in the face of a hostile world is the price of such a personality type. Such behavioural and cognitive performance corresponds for the most part to a system being an open-loop (Section 1.3.9). In such terms, the parasympathetic inhibition might be seen as a negative feedback effect triggered by the changed circumstances when a threat has passed but in the hostile personality the threat passes more slowly. Elevated levels of catecholamines acting in synergy with elevated levels of cortisol and (at least in males) testosterone are implicated in the excessive coronary excitation (Williams, 1989, pp. 81 and 89). Williams (1991) mentions the possibility of abnormally low levels of CNS serotonin as being at the biological roots of this phenomenon.

A slightly different line of theoretical reasoning is that developed by Wright (1988). Examining a large number of patients with CHD, Wright was impressed by the presence of one particular component of the Type A personality, made up of a cluster of three behavioural traits, described as: (1) time urgency; (2) chronic activation; and (3) multiphasia. Time urgency was a term used to refer to an excessive concern over the optimal usage of each moment of time, e.g. frequently changing lanes to gain just a couple of car lengths' advantage. 'Chronic activation' refers to a tendency to remain aroused, active and 'in control' for most, if not all, of the day and for everyday. The term 'multiphasic' simply means trying to do many things at the same time.

Based upon the presence of such personality traits, Wright (1988) suggests that a person who takes an aggressive approach towards performing tasks might also be aggressive in interpersonal relations. Wright suggests that such situations whether social or non-social will be associated with the same neuroendocrine consequences (e.g. increased secretion of catecholamines, a release of metabolic fuels into the bloodstream, increased heart rate and increased blood flow to skeletal muscles), which might help to reconcile Wright's ideas with those of Williams.

Some of the behaviour traits observed by Wright (1988) in Type A personalities are suggestive of a negative feedback system having excessive gain (i.e. excessive sensitivity to error between actual and desired values; Toates, 1975) and being on open-loop. Wright notes:

> (a) a frequent straining type of facial grimace, even during minimal exertion; (b) dramatic or overly forceful movements while conducting minimal tasks such as opening and closing drawers or bottles and while inserting or extracting their contents (e.g. some wives of Type A men report that they cannot get caps off toothpaste tubes because their husbands close them so tightly); (c) overly forceful speech style, both in volume and content; (d) rapid eating; (e) frequent, breathy sighs; (h) repetitive (or fidgety) movements of the feet, fingers, or jaw; (i) an intense look with frequently inhibited smile or laugh; (j) a kind of wide-eyed look or protruding cornea.

Breathy sighs are, when performed by Type As, most usually a reaction to situations of minimal exertion which are, none the less, something like the signs of breathlessness that would be appropriate for hard physical work, indicative of inappropriately high arousal in Type As. According to Wright (1988) both the anticipatory response (high level of catecholamine secretion) and the concluding response (deep sigh) that would be appropriate for exertion are present but without the natural intervening response of exertion. Wright describes the Type A as in 'a kind of "suspended suspense", with a resulting emotional and hormonal surplus'. Offering possible reconciliation with Williams' approach, Wright suggests that anger might be secondary to time urgency:

How does such behaviour cause damage to the coronary arteries? Wright (1988) discusses two theories, which are not necessarily mutually exclusive. According to the mechanical theory, stress (including even such characteristic Type A stress as that involved in trying to overtake another motorist) causes a vasoconstriction in peripheral regions of the body associated with an acceleration of heart rate. According to the chemical theory, excessive levels of catecholamines are associated with arterial damage. These excessive levels arise from a very wide range of situations (many interpreted as quite innocuous by non-Type As) becoming associated with triggering the Type A's catecholamine response.

Why are excessive levels of catecholamines toxic when certain catecholamine provoking situations (e.g. jogging) are felt to be good for the cardiac system? Wright suggests two reasons. There might be a difference between acute elevation, as in a 1 hour jog, and chronic elevation everyday of the year. In addition, jogging might stimulate CNS processes that dampen catecholamine reactivity for the remainder of the day. Wright also suggests the possibility that adrenaline might be metabolized differently under the two conditions; in exercise, it might be broken down more quickly. Perhaps the most obvious factor is that in jogging a large fraction of the fatty acids circulating in the bloodstream will be metabolized.

The study of Type As raises a profound issue with important implications for therapy. In general, control is said to be a good thing (Section 5.7), with loss of control being detrimental to health. Certain therapies involve teaching the patient to exert more control. However, perhaps too much control (or *trying* to exert too much) can be a bad thing, as there is evidence to show that Type As attempt to exert inordinate degrees of (maladaptive) control over others. They take on to themselves excessive responsibility, something that is associated with increased output of adrenaline and noradrenaline.

It is interesting to consider what is reinforcing (Section 9.5.3.7) about Type A behaviour. Wright (1988) raises the question of whether Type As might become addicted to their own adrenaline. They report being uncomfortable when not doing anything and this might be a kind of withdrawal reaction. Wright asks whether Type As' activity immediately upon waking might be analogous to some individuals' first cigarette or cup of coffee. As an additional factor, Wright suggests that Type A behaviour might be seen as another instance of obsessive–compulsive neurosis (Toates, 1990). There are certainly some important similarities. Like the Type A, the obsessional sets impossibly high goals that can never be achieved, e.g. absolute certainty, cleanliness or perfection. Obsessionality, similarly, is a full-time occupation that demands eternal vigilance in the face of threats, real or imagined. As with the argument developed here for stress, there is the argument that obsessionality is characterized by a negative feedback loop going on to open-loop (see Toates, 1990). For both Type As and for obsessionals, Wright suggests that:

> . . . simply making a response may have more to do with increasing the probability that the response will reoccur in the future than it does with whether the response is reinforced. (This refers to the developmental or etiological phase of the problem. During the treatment phase, *not* making a response seems to affect the probability that a response will *not* be made in the future more than does whether the response is punished or simply not reinforced).

Applying Wright's logic in terms of the theoretical line developed here, it would be argued that behaviour might involve its own intrinsic reinforcement process and therefore Type A behaviour and obsessions might have something in common with stereotypies (see Section 9.5.3).

Something analogous to the human Type A behaviour pattern has been observed in baboons. As with comparable human studies, highest levels of serum cholesterol were associated with active strategies that were not too successful, i.e. the behaviour of subordinate and 'upwardly struggling' members of the group. Sapolsky (1988; see also Section 6.6) found that subordinate male olive baboons had relatively low plasma high-density lipoprotein (HDL) concentrations. He notes that, in both human and non-human primates, atherosclerosis and CHD bear a direct relationship to low-density lipoprotein (LDL) concentration and an *inverse* relation to HDL concentration. Sapolsky notes that, in association with LDL, cholesterol appears to promote atherosclerosis. HDL, by contrast, seem to act to counter this effect. (Ventricular fibrillation is a further example of stress-related coronary pathology, but its discussion goes beyond our scope here. The interested reader can consult Schneiderman and McCabe, 1985.)

In a study of male macaques (*Macaca fasicularis*), Manuck *et al*. (1986) found highest levels of atherosclerosis in dominant males whose dominance was being challenged by social instability. Introducing new animals into a formerly stable social group challenged the dominant male. It was suggested that the elevated heart rate associated with social instability could be an important causal factor in atherosclerosis. Manuck *et al.* also found that, in combination with social instability, a high cholesterol diet contributed to atherosclerosis.

Endogenous opioids seem to play a part in dampening the sympathetic reaction to stressors and there is the possibility that some individuals might be deficient in this pathway (McCubbin, 1993). This would be of obvious relevance in hypertension. Interesting individual differences might be evident in the levels of such opioid-mediated inhibition (McCubbin, 1991), which might map on to active versus passive tendencies to cope. In this context, one is reminded of the results discussed in Section 5.2 that grooming by another individual causes a rise in endogenous opioid levels in Talpoin monkeys. In pigtail macaques, such grooming is associated with a heart rate reduction (see Maestripieri *et al.*, 1992). The logic that stroking a pet might be good for the coronary health of the stroker quite apart from the pet might make sense in such terms.

10.3 TOUGHENING UP

Dienstbier (1989) develops an interesting argument regarding stress and stressors and their relation to physical and psychological health. He starts by questioning the common implicit assumption that arousal of physiological processes by a stressor is inevitably a negative thing. Some authors assume that such arousal is associated with psychosomatic disease. Dientsbier marshalls evidence from a number of sources, using human and non-human subjects, to qualify this negative view, as follows.

Suppose young rats were exposed to stressors such as handling or electric shock. When adult, such rats are found to have higher adrenal weights but to show less fearfulness than control subjects. (This result suggests that excessive sheltering of young children from exposure to any potential stressor might be counter-productive.) One effect of early handling might be to increase the number of steroid receptors in the brain (McEwen *et al.*, 1986). This could strengthen the corticosteroid feedback effect and restrain the basal level (see Chapter 2). Rats, exposed to stressors when young, were later found to have lower base rates of catecholamines and corticosteroids in spite of the larger adrenal glands. When exposed to stressors, relative to controls not stressed when young they showed: (1) a lower response of the corticosteroid system and (2) sharper 'catecholamine spikes', meaning a faster and higher rise from the baseline and a quicker return to the baseline. Frankenhaeuser (1976) discusses this phenomenon in the following terms: 'A rapid drop in catecholamine secretion as demands decrease— quick "unwinding"—implies an "economic" mode of response, whereas a slow drop indicates poor adjustment in the sense that the organism "overreacts" by mobilizing resources which are no longer needed'. In the case of humans, Frankenhaeuser interprets the slow decline in cognitive terms. She associates it with either, 'a slowness in the re-evaluation of environmental demands, or it may be part of a conscious effort to maintain a wide margin of safety'. Slow 'decreasers' tend to have a higher neuroticism score on the Eysenck Personality Inventory (Frankenhaeuser, 1976).

As was discussed in Chapter 5, exposure of rats to an acute stressor can lead to changes in metabolism of brain noradrenaline. However, daily exposure to a stressor can protect against such depletion, a procedure sometimes termed 'toughening up'. Dienstbier (1989) reviews evidence showing that such toughening can be of an active type in which the subject performs an appropriate response, e.g. swimming by rats placed in water or aerobic exercise in humans. However, (and perhaps more suprisingly) it might simply be of a passive kind, e.g. exposure to cold or (with suitable parameters) uncontrollable shock.

Dienstbier (1989) reviews a number of studies, carried out mainly in Scandinavia, showing that performance on tasks both intellectually demanding, such as examinations, and physically demanding, such as parachute jumping, correlates positively with the magnitude of increase in peripheral catecholamine secretion accompanying the task. There is also a positive correlation between the magnitude of the catecholamine spike and measures of emotional stability. Dienstbier concludes: '. . . although causality from catecholamine availability to both personality and performance is not proved, a reasonably strong case can be made'.

In developing his argument on the positive and negative connotations of stress, Dienstbier (1989) emphasizes the distinction between SAM and pituitary–adrenocortical arousal. Thus, whereas measures of catecholamines tend to correlate positively with success at intellectual and physical tasks, the association with corticosteroids tends to be a negative one. From animal studies, Dienstbier notes the high corticosteroid levels associated with situations of minimal predictability and control. He refers to these as 'situations of stress, rather than challenge'. Either actual, or at least perceived, coping (in Dienstbier's terms, making the situation 'challenging') serves to prevent both high levels of corticosteroids and catecholamine exhaustion. In the

Scandinavian research, humans experiencing high levels of control at a task showed elevations in catecholamine secretion but cortisol levels were below base levels.

Considering optimal performance, Dienstbier (1989) associates the acquisition of coping with the return of cortisol response to the baseline level, whereas: '. . . peak catecholamine responses should decline only to the level needed to sustain active coping'. In these terms, the time parameters of an emotionally stable individual showing competence in dealing with stressors is characterized as follows:

> In comparison with those of less fit individuals, SNS–adrenal–medullary and adrenal–cortical base rates for the fit individual are low, but in a challenge/threat situation, SNS–adrenal–medullary arousal onset is fast and strong, whereas cortisol remains relatively low; arousal decline is fast with stressor offset; and across repeated similar episodes, arousal levels for both kinds of peripheral arousal decline more quickly than in less fit controls (this is particularly apparent with cortisol). If stress is continuous, the fit individual will sustain SNS–adrenal–medullary arousal longer, and both catecholamine depletion and large pituitary–adrenal–cortical responses will be delayed.

The model has obvious implications for health. Normally, it has been assumed that the physiological consequences of SAM arousal, such as elevations of heart rate and blood pressure, release of free fatty acids and cholesterol, result in hypertension and cardiovascular disease. Dienstbier qualifies this assumption, arguing that health is compromised largely in those situations where the arousal is not associated with control. As an example of such lack of control, Henry (1976) discusses the development of hypertension in baboons placed in a situation where access to a mate was denied over long periods and repeated attempts to gain access were frustrated.

In support of the beneficial effects of 'tough responding', Dienstbier notes that corticosteroids generally depress immune system function, whereas some aspects of immune function are enhanced by catecholamines. Manipulations that lead to toughness, e.g. early exposure to stressors (particularly if they are controllable), can enhance later immune function.

Dienstbier (1989) acknowledges that the Type A personality is associated with CHD (see Section 10.2). This personality type is characterized by, among other things, the setting of high goals and showing hard work. Normally, it is assumed that the link between this personality and disease is mediated by overactivity of the SAM system. Potentially, this would appear to set a profound problem for a model that associates tough responding with good health. Dienstbier's answer is that for a person to show tough responding is not synonymous with having a Type A personality. Neither a tough response nor challenge seeking are associated with CHD. Dienstbier notes that a number of traits in addition to challenge seeking are associated with the Type A personality, e.g. tension, neuroticism, hostility and anger suppression. As was noted in Section 10.2, some argue that the hostility and anger suppression features of the Type A personality, rather than challenge seeking, are associated with CHD. Dienstbier reviews evidence suggesting that the risks of CHD for the Type A personality arise from arousal maintained over long periods, months rather than minutes. In contrast to the tough individual, characterized by a sharp elevation of catecholamine secretion in response to a stressor and fast return to baseline, the high risk percentage of Type As seem to have a relatively slow recovery to baseline. Dienstbier suggests that the major risk to health for the Type A personality might arise from pituitary–adrenocortical arousal. Although the Type A's catecholamine response to a challenge is elevated compared with control subjects, the corticosteroid response is even greater. Possibly the combination is the problem (see also Henry, 1976).

10.4 STRESS, THE IMMUNE SYSTEM AND DISEASE

The immune system is of interest in any study of stress, as it both affects, and is affected by, stress hormones (Chapter 4). For instance, in the studies of Sapolsky (1990) on free-living olive baboons, described in Chapter 6, it was found that subordinates, having a relatively high basal cortisol secretion rate exhibited fewer circulating lymphocytes, as compared with dominants.

Some evidence suggests that negative psychological states such as depression and bereavement increase a subject's vulnerability to infection (reviewed by Ballieux and Heijnen, 1987). The responses of both B cells and T cells are lowered under these conditions. However, although laboratory evidence shows that stress exerts an effect on the immune system, some have urged caution in assuming that this is necessarily reflected in any straightforward way in disease. In 1984, Cohen and Williamson (1984) were able to argue: 'There is sufficient evidence to convince us that stress influences the immune system. However, it is not clear that either the nature or the magnitude of change found in these studies alters disease susceptibility . . .'.

More recent reviews (e.g. Anderson *et al.*, 1994) have encouraged a less cautious view, that there is a real relationship between stressful events in life, immune suppression and disease susceptibility. On a more optimistic note, social support is seen as an influence to enhance the efficacy of the immune system and health. Examples reviewed include: (1) increased susceptibility to colds as a function of stress; (2) a stronger immune response to a vaccination and enhanced natural killer (NK) cell activity among those receiving social support; and (3) increased white blood cell counts among breast cancer patients receiving relaxation training.

Laboratory studies have shown that having a coping strategy can ameliorate the impact of stressors on the disruption of immune function. In an experiment by Laudenslager *et al.* (1983), rats were exposed to either escapable or inescapable shock. Shocks were matched for intensity and timing. Lymphocyte proliferation in response to mitogens was studied. In one case, escapable shock did not affect this and in another it enhanced it, whereas inescapable shock had a strongly suppressive effect. A difference in corticosteroid levels between the conditions of control and no control could play a crucial part in mediating these effects. However, it would be wrong to attribute all of the effect of stressors on the immune system to mediation via the corticosteroids. Other pathways might well also be implicated (Ader, 1987). Laudenslager *et al.* note: (1) the release of opioids in response to inescapable shock (see also Section 8.6) and (2) that injection of opioid antagonists can inhibit tumour growth and increase the life of tumour-bearing animals. Thus, comparing controllable and uncontrollable conditions, differences in opioid release might play a part in differences in immunosuppression.

Shavit and Martin (1987) note that a primary immune surveillance role against viral infection and tumour growth is mediated via cytotoxic T lymphocytes and NK cells. In their analysis, Shavit and Martin build upon the observation that the properties of stress-induced analgesia (SIA; see Chapter 8), specifically whether it is opioid- or non-opioid-mediated, depend upon the parameters of shock applied. Thus, rats were exposed to stressors corresponding to either an opioid- or non-opioid-based form of SIA and the effect upon NK cell activity noted. The opioid-based effect resulted in a reduction of NK cell activity to 74% of normal, an effect which was prevented by naloxone. In the absence of an opioid-based effect, naloxone had no effect. The non-opioid-based effect did not suppress NK cell activity. The effects of opioid- and non-opioid-based foot shock on tumour growth were also investigated. Rats subjected to the opioid, but not non-opioid, form had a reduced survival time compared with controls that were unstressed. The effect of the opioid-based stress was antagonized by naloxone and a similar effect to the stressor was obtained with morphine injection. Putting the result into a broader context, the authors note that such a difference in result deriving from a small difference in shock parameter casts doubt on the notion of one single intervening variable 'stress' (Chapter 1) that mediates between input and output.

How might opioids influence tumour growth? Shavit and Martin (1987) note that some tumour cells have opioid receptors, raising the possibility of a direct effect. Secondly, they might exert their effect via a hormonal link, most likely via adrenal corticosteroids. Finally, their effect could be mediated via a direct effect upon the immune system, because, as already noted, there are opioid effects on NK cell activity.

10.5 DEPRESSION

10.5.1 Introduction

A relationship between depression and stress has often been suspected. Is it possible to get any insight into the phenomenon of depression when viewed in the terms developed so far? There is more than one possible perspective that can be taken towards this topic, as discussed now.

10.5.2 An Ethological Perspective

One approach is to consider the possible adaptive significance of behaviours which then become grossly and maladaptively exaggerated in the case of full depression. Suppose, for the higher primates, separation of an infant from its caregiver occurs (introduced in Section 5.2) and an obstacle keeps them apart. Aggressive behaviour is likely to be shown by both parties as they struggle to regain contact (see review by Hamburg *et al.*, 1975). Should such an active strategy fail, something that appears similar to human depression is likely to be shown. Hamburg *et al.* argue that the depression reaction serves to warn the animal that something is wrong. This might be rephrased to state that the situation is *insoluble*; this is a situation to be avoided: '. . . something is wrong, attention must be paid, learning capacities utilized, resources mobilized to correct the situation'.

It also signals that something is wrong to other animals, presumably among other potential caregivers.

At its biological roots, for a number of species depression appears to be a response that is switched in when aggressive behaviour has failed to deliver a positive outcome (Hamburg *et al.*, 1975). In some primate species, mild depression might be seen to be adaptive in that it encourages change and solicits sympathy from others. The retardation of movement and the posture of despair minimize risk of attack from either conspecifics or predators, and possibly increase the chances of adoption (Thierry *et al.*, 1984). However, severe depression would seem to be maladaptive both behaviourally and in terms of increased susceptibility to disease. For both aggression and depression, excesses seem maladaptive whereas, in mild degrees, they might reasonably seem adaptive.

Thierry *et al.* (1984) propose an evolutionary model to explain features of depression, which they term a 'searching–waiting strategy model'. This model is based on the assumption that each situation of depression is associated with the subject facing '. . . a problem of survival which has no apparent solution'. By this, they mean that: '. . . the subject *estimates* on account of its information from the environment and its internal state, that it faces a problem without immediate solution and which jeopardizes its life'.

The authors do not commit themselves to any particular cognitive process by which the estimation might be made; it might or might not involve conscious processes. They argue that, placed in such a situation, there are two possible behavioural patterns, as follows: (1) the animal can perform searching behaviour, which might lead to a solution being found or (2) it might do nothing, simply waiting. The scientist can perform a cost–benefit analysis to determine the relative values of the two possibilities. Maybe, by analogy, the subject in this situation, at some level in the nervous system, also performs a kind of cost–benefit analysis. Depression is to be viewed as a pathological development of the adaptive behaviour described by this model.

These authors argue that the 'behavioural despair' test (described in Chapter 6) may be an animal model of some *features* of depression (they would not wish to overstate the similarities). This refers to the immobility that is sometimes displayed by rodents when placed in water. Such immobility is reduced by treatments that are sometimes effective in human depression, e.g. antidepressant drugs and electroconvulsive therapy. In this model, the floating rat and the depressed human are assumed to share the common feature of 'psychomotor inhibition in a solutionless aversive environment'. The phenomenon is further interpreted in terms of an alternation between 'searching for an exit' (the active swimming attempts) and waiting (floating). The authors suggest that such alternation might reflect an adaptive strategy in the wild. For example, after a subject falls into a fast-flowing river the best chances of escape might be to alternate between the two strategies depending upon the subject and the exact physical context. It is assumed that the subject's strategy is based upon an 'estimation of the situation'.

Koolhaas *et al*. (1990) propose an animal model of depression. It is based upon the assumption that 'loss of control is the crucial factor in the development of depression'. Koolhaas *et al*. note that, in the terms of such a model, a reduction in exploration and an increased tendency to passivity in the face of challenge are two of the criteria denoting depression. The model derives from exposure of rats to a relatively natural social stressor: a single session of encounter with, and defeat by, a dominant rat. It was found that, as a result of the encounter, rats were *sensitized* to the application of a mild stressor, the effect taking a few weeks to develop.

In the experiment of Koolhaas *et al*. (1990), there was background white noise in the animal's cage. When this is stopped, rats normally explore their environment. Placed in this situation, rats that had earlier been exposed to the social stress showed a tendency to immobility rather than exploration. The tendency to immobility was corrected by treatment with an antidepressant, the serotonin reuptake inhibitor clomipramine. In a forced swimming test, rats exposed to defeat showed a longer period of immobility and a lower latency to immobility compared with non-stressed controls. Thus, exposure to a social stressor increases the probability of a more passive reaction to two non-social stressors applied weeks later. The authors refer to an 'autonomous process' being induced by the social stressor to account for the changes occurring in the weeks between the application of social and non-social stresses. They suggest that, in studies of chronic stress, possibly the time elapsing since the first application of the stressor rather than continuous application of the stressor is crucial.

In terms of animal models, some aspects of depression might indeed involve a learning process but others might be seen as an unconditional reaction to aversive stimulation (Minor *et al*., 1994a,b). Minor *et al*. suggest that a disruption of the brain's energy metabolism might underlie the helplessness effect. This state can be induced artificially by mimicking the changes involved in disrupting energy homeostasis and is a state characterized by loss of interest in incentive objects (cf. Wise, 1994). Echoing earlier stress theorists, this state is suggested by Minor *et al*. to be one of conservation–withdrawal and loss of commerce with the environment.

10.5.3 Depression and the Hypothalamic–Pituitary–Adrenocortical Axis

There are relationships between events in the hypothalamic–pituitary–adrenocortical (HPA) axis and depression, although what is cause and what is effect is not always clear, if even a meaningful dichotomy to make. Also, as is not entirely surprising, the reports sometimes seem contradictory.

Depression is commonly characterized by hypersecretion of hormones in the HPA axis (Dubrovsky, 1993). More specifically, in humans, cortisol secretion rate is commonly abnormally high (reviewed by Carroll and Mendels, 1976; Depue and Kleiman, 1979). Both plasma and cerebrospinal fluid (CSF) cortisol levels are elevated in depressed patients (Carroll and Mendels, 1976). Several investigators (but not all) have reported elevated adrenocorticotrophic hormone (ACTH) secretion in depression (reviewed by Kronfol and Schlechte, 1986). In the context of HPA activation, some researchers have drawn a distinction between types of depression. Thus, on the evidence of patients examined, Sachar (1970) associates elevated cortisol levels with the anxiety that commonly accompanies some situations of depression, i.e. emotional arousal and disorganization. By contrast, based upon Sachar's sample, 'apathetic depression' is not associated with elevated cortisol levels.

There is evidence that corticosteroids and/or their metabolites can influence the CNS via receptors and thereby shift mood towards depression (discussed by McEwen, 1979; Schatzberg et al., 1985; Barnes, 1986). However, administration of cortisol has also been reported to be associated with euphoria, although this might reflect a more transient effect (Michael and Gibbons, 1963). There are occasional reports of patients suffering from Cushing's disorder, characterized by hypersecretion of corticosteroids, exhibiting euphoria whereas some Addison's syndrome patients, characterized by loss of corticosteroids, experience depression (Baxter and Rousseau, 1979; McEwen, 1979). However, the hyperactivity of corticosteroids that characterizes Cushing's disorder is more commonly associated with depression (Dubrovsky, 1993).

Carroll and Mendels conclude: '. . . the evidence points strongly to a significantly increased exposure of the tissues and CNS of depressed patients to active cortisol'. However, the brains of suicide victims have been found to have a *lower* than normal cortisol concentration, suggesting the possibility of a steroid binding deficiency (Carroll and Mendels, 1976). This might be related to a phenomenon that has been noted earlier (Section 2.3.2.5): exposure of the brain to excessive levels of corticosteroids can lead to loss of receptors. In this context, Panksepp (1990) speculates: 'When higher limbic aspects of this system begin to dysfunction, because of glucocorticoid receptor mediated metabolic "burnout" in the affected systems, the gateway to chronic despair, depression, and withdrawal from active confrontation with the world may be opened'.

So how do we explain the high secretion rate of corticosteroids in depression? It might reflect either increased input from corticotrophic-releasing factor (CRF)/ACTH or increased sensitivity of the adrenal cortex to ACTH. Depue and Kleiman (1979) suggest the possibility that it might arise from an alteration in central noradrenaline metabolism (given that there seems to exist a noradrenergic inhibition of the HPA axis, as discussed in Chapter 3). Reciprocally, abnormal ACTH and corticosterone levels might affect central catecholamine metabolism (Anisman 1978), giving rise to the possibility of positive feedback effects. One such hypothesis, to account for psychotic depression, is that elevated corticosteroid levels boost dopamine (DA) synthesis (via a metabolic pathway described in Section 3.4; Schatzberg *et al.*, 1985). As there also seem to be excitatory catecholaminergic inputs to CRF secretion, the possibility of positive feedback would arise if elevated corticosteroid levels boosted such excitation (Dubrovsky, 1993).

Results obtained from stimulating the adrenal cortex with exogenous ACTH and observing the cortisol response, led Carroll and Mendels (1976) to conclude that the elevated cortisol levels seen in depressed patients are the result of increased hypothalamic–pituitary activity rather than increased sensitivity of the adrenal cortex to normal ACTH levels. As noted in Chapter 2, release of cortisol is episodic and Carroll and Mendels argue that the endocrine disturbance in depression arises from a disinhibition of the hypothalamic–pituitary axis. It is a failure of the normal inhibition exerted on the ACTH–cortisol system throughout most of the day.

Somewhat at odds with Carroll and Mendel's conclusions are the findings of Gold *et al.* (1988). Their depressed patients showed normal basal levels of ACTH even though their cortisol levels were elevated. Gold *et al.* suggest that under these conditions the normal ACTH response is the outcome of a balance between two abnormal influences upon the pituitary: excessive excitation from an elevated secretion of CRF and excessive inhibition from abnormally high levels of corticosteroids. Gold *et al.* suppose that, in early stages of depression, the patients would have shown elevated ACTH levels. This would be in response to elevated drive from CRF but before the sensitivity of the adrenal cortex would have changed, i.e. the high cortisol/ACTH response characteristic, just described. Many patients suffering from anorexia nervosa also show excessive levels of cortisol and their CSF levels of CRF are also elevated.

What is the exact role of CRF in depression? CRF secretion is, commonly, unusually high in depression (reviewed by Kronfol and Schlechte, 1986). The role of CRF as a transmitter in the brain and its known integrating role in endocrine, behavioural and autonomic responses to stressors (Chapter 3) make it a candidate for examination in the context of psychiatric disorders. There is a suggestion that both in its role as CNS neurotransmitter in various brain regions and more specifically as part of the HPA axis, there is an over-activity in CRF-related neurons in depression (Ritchie and Nemeroff, 1991). Rats injected with CRF behave in some ways suggestive of human depression, e.g. anorexia, decreased motivation towards sex, disruption of sleep (reviewed by Bond *et al.*, 1989; Gold *et al.*, 1988; see also Chapter 3). Gold *et al.* note that large doses of CRF produce anxiety reactions, e.g. lowered levels of exploration and a tendency to freezing. This might model melancholic depression, a condition associated with high anxiety levels. Smith and Nemeroff (1988) suggest that one might expect a hypersecretion of CRF in depression to be associated with a decrease in brain CRF receptors. Suicide victims were indeed found to have a relatively low CRF receptor density in the frontal cortex. Gold *et al.* (1988) addressed the question of CRF's role. The high secretion rate of cortisol seen in many patients suffering from depression and anorexia nervosa points to the possible implication of CRF. Gold *et al.* describe a 'blunted ACTH response' to CRF in depressed subjects (see also Ritchie and Nemeroff, 1991). However, in spite of this blunted ACTH response, depressed patients showed a marked cortisol response to the CRF. This led them to suppose that in depression the adrenal cortex is hyperresponsive to ACTH.

Gold *et al.* (1988) note that, in rats, excessive levels of corticosteroids can impair corticosteroid feedback upon CRF secretion. Older rats show higher levels of corticosteroids than younger ones. This might model the fact that older depressed patients show higher cortisol levels and more severe forms of melancholic disorder than younger subjects.

Gold *et al.* (1988) then speculated as to how CRF-sensitive brain regions might, in combination with other brain regions, form part of the physical basis of depression. They note the candidacy of the locus coeruleus (LC) in such a role. (Chapter 5 associated depression with increased activity within the LC.) Its electrical stimulation causes anxiety, vigilance and inhibition of exploration in unanaesthetized primates. During threat, its activity increases, whereas it diminishes when the animal is either sleeping, grooming or feeding. Gold *et al.* interpret the experimental evidence to show that in melancholic depression there is an activation of the LC noradrenaline system. They suggest that there might be a mutually reinforcing effect between CRF and the LC noradrenergic system.

That the abnormalities of the HPA axis seen in depression might have some part to play in the *causation* of depression is suggested by the fact that similar abnormalities are seen in Cushing's disorder. This disorder is characterized by a primary excessive cortisol secretion (Michael and Gibbons, 1963; Carroll and Mendels, 1976). As far as motivational, affective and cognitive changes are concerned, depression and Cushing's disease share a striking number of symptoms (e.g. irritability, depressed mood, difficulty of concentration, disturbance of sleep, decreased libido; Dubrovsky, 1993). (However, a distinction between Cushing's disease and administration of cortisol has been discussed by Michael and Gibbons, 1963.) The evidence suggests that in Cushing's disorder the depression is the consequence of the elevated corticosteroid levels; correction of the excessive levels of corticosteroids usually cures the depression (Dubrovsky, 1993). A distinction between primary depression and Cushing's disorder has been noted (see Dubrovsky, 1993). Thus, whereas both are associated with high levels of corticosteroids the causation is different. In control theory terms, it might be argued that in primary depression the initial causation is represented by an elevated set-point whereas in Cushing's disorder the negative feedback effect of corticosteroids on the pituitary is deficient.

One of the characteristics of both depression and Cushing's disorder is a bias in memory retrieval and information processing (Dubrovsky, 1993). The patients' bias is in favour of the retrieval and processing of negative events, e.g. self-deprecating features of their lives. Dubrovsky reasons that, as the hippocampus: (1) forms a target for corticosteroid action (Chapter 7) and (2) is known to be closely involved with memory retrieval, abnormal corticosteroid activity at this site might play a part in biased memory retrieval and disturbed attentional processes in depression. There is also the possibility of a bias exerted upon the laying down of memories having negative associations. However, whatever the contribution of corticosteroids to depression, their role is not indispensable for all types of depression. As Dubrovsky notes, some patients with Addison's disease exhibit depression and in animal studies the formation of learned helplessness is actually strengthened by adrenalectomy.

10.5.4 Catecholamines and Depression

The idea that noradrenaline deficiency lies at the base of depression derived from the observation that reserpine, which depletes the CNS of noradrenaline, is associated with depression in some patients (reviewed by Veith, 1991). There are a number of similarities between the effects of uncontrollable aversive events on rats and certain features of clinical depression in humans (Weiss and Simson, 1985; Anisman and Zacharko, 1986; Weiss et al., 1989). These include anorexia, loss of weight, sleep disturbances, deficits in grooming and motor activity and disturbances in dominance hierarchies. In humans, depression is associated with feelings of being unable to cope or control events and being helpless (Weiss and Simson, 1985). Such observations led Anisman and Zacharko (1982) to propose a model whereby exposure to stress can predispose towards depression. As discussed in Chapter 5, exposure to a stressor can lead to depletion of noradrenaline in the brain. Anisman and Zacharko suggested that in some cases, on exposure to uncontrollable stressors, individuals are unable to synthesize noradrenaline sufficiently fast to keep pace with its utilization, resulting in depletion of noradrenaline at certain CNS sites. This depletion would exert a bias towards depression; although see also Stone (1982) for a possible counter-argument and Sapolsky (1994, p. 208) for a discussion of various possible abnormalities. Given that at some level in the CNS an antagonism might well occur between noradrenergic and cholinergic systems, depression might also usefully be viewed in terms of activation of a cholinergically mediated behavioural inhibition system (Laborit, 1982). Of course, no one would suppose that depression should be simply *reduced* to abnormalities at certain synapses, a point acknowledged by Anisman and Zacharko. As Leshner (1982) reminds us one might usefully see the human reaction of depression in terms of a vicious circle (positive feedback) between changes at central synapses and depressive cognitions.

Based upon the depression model proposed by Weiss and Simson (1988) and introduced in Chapter 5, Figure 10.2 summarizes some of the similarities between the effects of uncontrollable shock in rats and depression in humans. The similarities are striking, although the

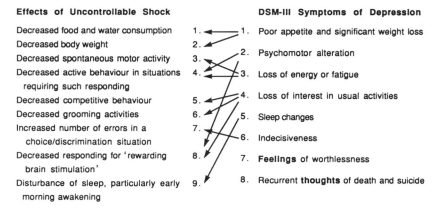

Figure 10.2. Comparisons of similarities between the effects of uncontrollable shock on a rat's behaviour and the symptoms of human depression. The arrows draw attention to points of similarity. (Source: Weiss and Simson, 1988)

effects of shock are short-lived relative to the course of human depression. At least some of the protracted course of human depression might be explicable in terms of the vicious circle just described.

Although over the last 10–20 years, the predominant view has been that depression is associated with catecholamine depletion in the brain, there is also some evidence to suggest quite the opposite—an association with elevated levels of noradrenaline secretion (reviewed by Dunn and Berridge, 1990a). This suggested the possibility of a positive feedback effect between elevated noradrenaline and CRF secretion levels at the biochemical basis of depression.

10.5.5 Depression and the Autonomic Nervous System

Other theorists approach depression from the perspective of ANS activity (Vingerhoets, 1985). A psychological state of helplessness and hopelessness following loss is associated with predominance of parasympathetic activity. Similarly, rats having no possibility of exerting control (the learned heplessness paradigm) show evidence of excessive parasympathetic nervous system (PNS) activity. Active strategies of fight and flight are associated with predominant sympathetic activity. In depression, there is some evidence of decreased sympathetic activity, as indexed by, for example, reduced activity of the sweat glands (reviewed by Vingerhoets, 1985). However, to complicate any neat summary that depression equals elevated PNS activity and decreased SNS activity, there is also evidence of increased SNS activity (at least as far as the cardiovascular system is concerned) in some depressed patients (Veith, 1991). As elevated SNS activity appears to correlate with elevated activity in the HPA axis (Veith, 1991), elevated CNS CRF might prove to be a common input to both. There are other (not mutually exclusive) possibilities. Reduced CNS somatostatin (SRIF) levels might be associated with SNS activation in depression mediated by a reduction in the inhibitory effect of SRIF on CRF (Veith, 1991). There is also the possibility that decreased levels of CNS noradrenaline (see Section 10.5.4) in depression cause a reduction in an inhibitory influence of noradrenaline on SNS outflow (Veith, 1991). Increased CNS acetylcholine activity might exert an excitatory effect upon SNS outflow, again possibly mediated via an excitatory influence on CRF release (see Section 3.3).

10.5.6 Conclusions

These various perspectives are not mutually exclusive explanations. Rather all of them could, and probably are, correct in part. The evidence suggests the value of looking at depression in terms of a failure of the kind of coping strategies that have been discussed throughout this book.

10.6   POST-TRAUMATIC STRESS DISORDER

Post-traumatic stress disorder (PTSD) has come into particular focus relatively recently. In Britain, this is especially in the aftermath of a series of disasters, e.g. the sinking of the ferry *Herald of Free Enterprise* and the Kings Cross fire in 1987. However, the disorder is not new; according to Burges Watson *et al.* (1988), Samuel Pepys showed signs of it following the Great Fire of London. A summary of some of the main criteria for PTSD is as follows, based upon Burges Watson *et al.* (1988) and Charney *et al.* (1993):

1. The subject has an experience that by universal consent would be described as highly distressing. Helplessness and terror are experienced. Although there is little or no option for action, it might be assumed that mechanisms of 'flight or fight' are activated.
2. Subsequently, over a long period, real or imagined reminders of the incident ('flashbacks') are suffered. Extinction of reactivity does not occur, rather sensitization can sometimes be seen. Sometimes the range of effective traumatic stimuli broadens.
3. Attempts are made to avoid reminders of the trauma.
4. Difficulties are experienced in sleep. Irritability and anger are shown. There is an exaggerated physiological response to stimuli that in some way approximate to, or symbolize, the traumatic event. Survivor guilt is sometimes shown.

Some authors (e.g. Michael and Gibbons, 1963) associate 'emotional arousal', whether characterized by anxiety, depression, fear or sadness, with elevated levels of cortisol. One might have supposed then that the PTSD patient would show a characteristic profile of helplessness involving high levels of cortisol. There is indeed some evidence that they have a reactive opioid response to stressors (McCubbin, 1993), normally associated with a passive, giving-up 'strategy'. However, although there is the occasional report of high levels of cortisol in PTSD, other reports show quite the opposite: a relatively low level (see Burges Watson *et al.*, 1988; Yehuda *et al.*, 1991). Mason *et al.* (1986) found low levels of urinary free cortisol and relatively high levels of urinary adrenaline and noradrenaline. There is some evidence of increased central noradrenergic activity (Charney *et al.*, 1993), suggestive of an active control system that has gone on to open-loop. An elevated activity of forebrain DA systems is also seen.

Mason *et al.* (1986) remark that the low level of activity of the HPA system is surprising in that one would suppose the disorder to share important features with anxiety and depression. However, the hormonal profile suggests an active coping strategy and raises interesting questions (discussed by Mason *et al.*) regarding the cognitive adjustments made by sufferers. Yehuda *et al.* (1991) suggest that because the hormonal profile is different in PTSD as compared to acute stress or depression, we should consider it to be a distinct disorder. In addition to differences in plasma cortisol and urinary cortisol excretion, they contrast a number of hormonal parameters of PTSD sufferers with those for sufferers of depression. For example, sufferers exhibited an elevation in number of glucocorticoid receptors (GRs) at lymphocytes, a number that had a positive correlation with the severity of PTSD symptoms. In contrast to sufferers from major depression, PTSD patients show suppression to dexamethasone (see discussion in depression section). There is evidence for exaggerated suppression in this disorder.

Learned helplessness would seem not to be a good model of PTSD as the former is something learned over many trials whereas PTSD arises often from a very brief exposure to a single powerful traumatic event (Foa *et al.*, 1992; Yehuda and Antelman, 1993). PTSD would seem to have more in common with a persistent but unsuccessful active avoidance situation (Chapter 7), with associated high sympathetic arousal (Foa *et al.*, 1992) and with a vigilance similar to that shown by phobics or obsessive–compulsives (Toates, 1990).

Thus, to summarize, major depressive disorder is commonly associated with decreased negative feedback (decreased 'gain') in the HPA axis, the altered components of the feedback system are an elevated level of production of cortisol and a reduction in the number of GRs. By contrast, in such terms PTSD would appear to be associated with an increased gain of the feedback pathway, involving a decreased basal cortisol level. Burges Watson *et al.* (1988) suggest that an imbalance in the noradrenaline and opioid release in the LC is implicated in PTSD.

Could there be a suitable animal model of PTSD or similar human conditions? Ottenweller *et al.* (1989) discuss a possible animal model of chronic stress. This would consist of the presence of both abnormal behaviour and visceral arousal at times when the stressor is not present. In their experiment, rats shocked in daily sessions exhibited decreases in food intake and exploration at times other than the shock sessions. A decrease in exploration of novel objects was noted in rats

2–3 days after exposure to a stressor (Rosellini and Widman, 1989). However, unlike PTSD patients, these rats showed increased glucocorticoid levels. Yehuda *et al.* (1991) review experiments with rats showing that, under some conditions of chronic repeated exposure to a given stressor, the HPA system can become underreactive. This cannot be attributed to atrophy of the adrenals, as a normal corticosterone response is shown to a novel situation. Such underreactivity seems to apply only to certain types of stressor, others consistently provoking an elevated HPA response. By analogy, in humans, evidence from soldiers exposed to combat and from the parents of chronically and fatally sick children reveals a low cortisol secretion. This seems to be due to a relatively strong negative feedback effect exerted by corticosteroids at both the brain and pituitary gland.

10.7   GASTROINTESTINAL FUNCTION AND ULCERATION

10.7.1   Introduction

Stress-related damage to the gastrointestinal system has been discussed at various places and in various contexts already in this book (Section 3.4 in the context of DA; Section 5.4.2, predictability; Section 5.4.3, control; Section 5.4.5, performing species-typical behaviour; Section 6.2.3, strain differences and susceptibility; Section 6.9.1, the ANS). Since at least Seyle's writings of 1936, ulcers of the stomach have traditionally played an important part in defining what constitutes stress (reviewed by Glavin *et al.*, 1991).

The motor activity of the alimentary tract is determined by the enteric nervous system (ENS), which consists of a network of local reflexes (Burks, 1991). However, the patterning of activation within these reflexes can be modulated by inputs from the CNS via the ANS, a process described as 'the ability to select ENS programmes that provide particular desired patterns of motility' (Burks, 1991). (In this sense, one can see a parallel with the role of the CNS in modulating behavioural reactions in a hierarchical mode of control; Section 9.5.3.12.) This gives the CNS the facility for differential activation or inhibition of different segments of the alimentary tract (stomach, small intestine and colon). Stressors commonly decrease gastric emptying rate but increase the intensity of colonic contractions (Burks, 1991).

Digestion, governed normally by parasympathetic activation, is inhibited at times of sympathetic activation (Sapolsky, 1994, p. 70). There is a reduction in saliva secretion and a dry mouth. Stomach contractions are inhibited as is peristalsis of the intestine. Blood flow to the alimentary tract is reduced in the interests of glucose and oxygen being made available elsewhere. At the termination of the stressor provoking sympathetic activation, the digestive process is normally resumed.

An ulcer is a lesion in the wall of an organ and the term *peptic ulcer* is employed to describe ulcers in the stomach and the immediately adjacent organs (Sapolsky, 1994, p. 71). Gastric ulcer is used to refer to those in the stomach whereas those at the border of the stomach and intestine are termed *duodenal ulcers*. Just how much responsibility can be attributed to stress as a causal factor in peptic ulcer formation is a matter of some debate but a role of sorts seems certain; Sapolsky identifies six possible (and not mutually exclusive) processes that could mediate the effect, as follows.

1. *Acid rebound.* Cells that line the stomach wall secrete hydrochloric acid that aids the breakdown of food. Confronted with such acid, protective processes occur within the stomach wall. At a time of sympathetic activation characterized as stress, the protective maintenance on the walls is inhibited. When the stressful period ends, feeding triggers a parasympathetically mediated secretion of acid which enters a stomach ill-equipped to defend itself. Thus it is the end of stressor application rather than the time of stressor application that is associated with ulcer formation.

2. *Acid overproduction.* Some individuals might have a tendency to produce abnormally high levels of acid secretion. Stress might have a role in impairing feedback that would otherwise switch off this high rate.

3. *Decrease in blood flow.* At the time of stressor exposure, the diversion of blood away from the gut to the muscles might be such as to starve the gut of oxygen.

4. *Bacteria.* There are bacteria in the stomach that can attack the walls. At a time when the immune system might be inhibited the bacteria can be more effective.

5. *Prostaglandins.* Suppose for whatever reason micro-ulcers are formed in the stomach. Normally, prostaglandins would aid the process of repair by means of increasing blood flow to the stomach wall. However, prostaglandin production is inhibited by corticosteroids.

6. *Stomach contractions.* Stress is associated with slow rhythmic contractions of the stomach, which, for some reason, seem to increase the risk of ulceration, possibly by transiently reducing blood flow to the stomach walls or by causing mechanical damage.

According to Weiner (1992, p. 189), three principal factors involved in duodenal ulcer formation are: (1) normal level of gastric acid secretion; (2) an increase in gastric contractions; and (3) a reduction in duodenal bicarbonate secretion. These constitute necessary but not sufficient conditions for lesion formation.

In the experimental literature on rats, restraint has been one of the most reliable stressors employed, as defined by its tendency to provoke ulcers (Glavin *et al.*, 1991). As this stressor can be associated with activation of both sympathetic and parasympathetic branches of the nervous system (Henry *et al.*, 1986), for reasons given in this section, it might be expected to be particularly ulcerogenic. Running wheel activity (Section 6.2.3) is another stressor that is associated with ulceration.

Weiner (1991b) reviews the multiple factors (e.g. genetically determined differences in susceptibility) involved in the causation of peptic ulceration in humans. Of particular interest here is the suggested link between, on the one hand, certain psychological/behavioural factors and, on the other, a vagally mediated excessive secretion of gastric acid and excessive motility that lead to duodenal ulceration. However, Weiner (1991a, 1992) concludes that gastric acid in the stomach plays a permissive part in the formation of ulcers, i.e. it has to be present for ulcer formation but increases in secretion cannot explain the origin of ulceration. (Indeed, as Taché, 1991, notes, most stressors cause a decrease in acid secretion.) Weiner presents evidence that changes in the pattern of gastric contractions (appearance of a slow, regular rhythm of contractions) with exposure to a stressor are an important causal factor.

Similarly, Taché (1991) argues for a multiple causality of gastric ulceration, with the possibility that the weighting of the different component factors might vary according to the nature of the stressor. She continues:

All or part of such alterations as peripheral sympathetic and parasympathetic activation, stimulation of the pituitary–adrenal axis leading to the discharge of catecholamine and corticosterone, increased gastric acid, histamine and serotonin secretion, and high-amplitude gastric contractions, decreased gastric mucus or bicarbonate secretion and blood flow, disturbance of gastric mucosal microcirculation, inhibition of prostaglandin biosynthesis, formation of oxygen-derived free radicals, and deficit in mucosal energy metabolism, may contribute to ulcer formation.

Taché suggests that centrally injected substances (e.g. CRF) that exert a protective effect against stress-induced ulcers might do so by the *combination* of effects that they induce: inhibition of the secretion of gastric acid and pepsin, inhibition of high amplitude gastric contractions and a stimulation of gastric bicarbonate and mucus secretion.

10.7.2 A Theory on the Process Underlying Ulceration

Sapolsky (1992) reviews one possible account of the origin of stress-related ulcers. At a time of sympathetically mediated stress, blood flow to the gastrointestinal tract is reduced since blood is diverted elsewhere. Thus the flow of oxygen and certain crucial nutrients to the gastrointestinal tract is severely slowed. Normally, there would be processes of reconstruction going on in the stomach walls, associated with mucus secretion. Such reconstruction and secretion protects the stomach from gastric acids, which might otherwise produce lesions in the wall. In a situation of chronic activation there will be a chronic inhibition of acid secretion. In this state, the process of reconstruction and mucus secretion is suspended. When the sympathetically mediated state of stress ends, acid secretion resumes at a normal rate. In this state, the stomach wall is vulnerable. In terms of this model, it is not so much the period of exposure to the stressor but its aftermath that is immediately associated with ulcer formation.

10.7.3 Stress Hormones and Ulcers

Weiner (1991a, 1992) discusses the much debated question of a possible link between corticosteroids and gastric ulceration. He notes that simply because restraint in rats is associated with increased corticosteroid secretion and gastric ulceration, should not lead us to conclude that, necessarily, the elevated corticosteroids cause the ulceration. Ulceration occurs even in adrenalectomized rats subject to restraint, leading Weiner to conclude that, 'the original idea that corticosterone plays a primary pathogenic role in erosion formation is likely to be incorrect'.

As noted already, Paré and Redei (1993) found an increased susceptibility of Wistar Kyoto (WKY) rats as compared with other strains. Both Wistar and WKY rats were subjected to restraint stress. The WKY but not the Wistars showed ulcers. Whereas the WKY rats had elevated plasma ACTH levels relative to the Wistars, there was no difference in corticosterone levels.

Somewhat surprisingly in the light of traditional assumptions, there are reports that, on exposure to a stressor, adrenalectomy is associated with an *increase* in gastric ulceration (Hernandez *et al.*, 1984). This suggested that an intact sympathetic adrenal system plays a part in maintaining integrity of the stomach wall. Which axis, the SAM or HPA, is implicated in the protective role of adrenal hormones? The results of Hernandez et al. would suggest that both are. Injection of either a synthetic corticosteroid or a β-adrenergic agonist caused a dose-related decrease in the magnitude of gastric ulceration.

Sapolsky (1992) notes that prostaglandins play a powerful part in repair of ulcers. As prostaglandin synthesis is inhibited by corticosteroids, a damaging effect of the latter might be seen not so much in causation but in prevention of self-repair.

10.7.4 Neurotransmitters and Gastric Ulceration

Glavin et al. (1991) discuss the notion of a 'brain–gut axis' and the possibility that 'stress ulcerogenesis may be a "brain-driven" event'. In a study reported by Glavin (1985), rats were depleted of brain noradrenaline prior to being exposed to the stressor of being restrained. Glavin reports that the frequency and severity of gastrointestinal ulceration were greater in the noradrenaline-depleted rats than in controls.

There is evidence that the PNS plays an active part in the development of stress ulcers. Antacids and anticholinergic drugs tend to counter the effects of restraint upon ulceration (see Glavin et al., 1984; Hernandez et al., 1984). Gastric lesions can be induced by injections of thyrotrophin-releasing factor (TRH) into the CSF whereas the intravenous route of injection does not have this effect (Taché, 1991). TRH increases parasympathetic outflow. Centrally injected CRF counters the development of ulcers (Taché, 1991), which might be accounted for by its action in biasing towards sympathetic and against parasympathetic outflow (Section 3.3). In rats, lesions of the central nucleus of the amygdala cause a reduction in parasympathetic activity and attenuate stress-induced gastric ulceration (see Wiersma et al., 1993).

In rats, a protective effect against gastric damage can be obtained from DA and its agonists (Taché, 1991; Glavin, 1993). This is particularly so when they are injected centrally, specifically into the mesolimbic DA tract. Rats showing high anxiety, relative to low anxiety rats: (1) were particularly prone to develop gastric ulcers; (2) had lower basal DA in the amygdala; (3) had higher basal levels of DA metabolites in the amygdala and striatum, suggestive of a higher DA turnover; and (4) a faster decline of amygdala DA in response to the stressor of cold restraint. Protection against gastric ulceration was afforded by injection of the DA agonist SKF 75670C, both in the case of damage induced by stress and by gastric loading with ethanol (described by Glavin as a non-stressor). The latter effect would tend to argue against an otherwise tempting and all-embracing explanation (see Section 3.4): that the role of maintaining DA is to help the animal show an active coping strategy in the face of a stressor. Glavin concludes that differences in central DA levels are associated with differences in susceptibility to gastric injury irrespective of whether this arises from a stressor or a so-called non-stressor, ethanol loading. Of course, one might want to include ethanol loading under the rubric of being a stressor. However, if it is a stressor then it presumably is not one about which it is meaningful to speak of reactions in terms of a choice between active goal-directed strategies or passivity. Thus Glavin argues that: 'increased ulcer susceptibility is a characteristic of the animal and not the method used to induce the gastric injury'. The characteristic is embodied in different DA states in the brain, specifically 'high anxious rats appear to have a more labile or reactive mesolimbic DA tract, particularly when challenged by exposure to a stressor'.

As noted in Section 6.2.3 and discussed further by Glavin *et al.*, WKY rats tend to show signs of a high proneness to ulceration, depression in the open field test, a strong tendency to float in a Porsolt forced-swimming task and a high tendency to learned helplessness. WKY rats also exhibit a particularly high ACTH response to the stressor of restraint. The evidence from WKY rats is suggestive of a possible association between depression and stress ulcer, which would fit with clinical reports of such an association in humans (reviewed by Glavin *et al.*, 1991). Hernandez *et al.* (1993), after surveying patients with peptic ulcer disease, reported that 'the distinct lack of social interactions and low level of leisure activities would suggest that these patients were basically depressed'. Similarly, Paré and Redei (1993) suggested, on the basis of their comparisons between WKY and other rat strains, that manipulations that reduce depression might reduce stress ulceration. They report some evidence that imipramine, an antidepressant, did have just this effect, although they caution on the assumption of its route of action on the basis of the different routes by which it might exert its effect. Paré and Redei note that WKY rats do not enter a session of inescapable exposure to a stressor with a depression reaction. Rather, they start the session with a high degree of anxiety. At first they are active and only show a 'behavioural inhibition' phase when apparently they find a solution impossible. Looking at individual differences, Glavin (1993) reported that rats that showed high anxiety, as measured in an open-field test, also exhibited a high proneness to gastric pathology.

In rats, injection of CRF, either intracerebrovascularly or in the lateral hypothalamus, reduces the extent of gastric ulceration that is caused by cold restraint (reviewed by Weiner, 1991a). CRF inhibits gastric acid secretion. Centrally administered CRF reduces gastric contractions via inhibition of vagal activity. Taché et al. (1989) examined the role of neurotransmitters, particularly central CRF and TRH, in the generation of gastric ulcers. They start their analysis with the observation that stressors tend to elicit a reduction in gastric acid secretion. In rats, CRF infused either into the CSF or into parts of the hypothalamus inhibits gastric acid secretion. Similarly, in dogs, the gastric acid secretion that would normally follow a meal is inhibited by an injection of CRF into the CSF. The action of CRF is mediated via the ANS.

Restraining an animal in a cold environment has the opposite effect to other stressors in that it stimulates the secretion of gastric acid (Taché et al., 1989). It appears to arise from increased parasympathetic activity. Cold is a stimulus to the release of thyrotrophin-releasing factor in the brain and TRH injections into the CSF stimulate secretion of gastric acid.

Taché et al. (1989) then discussed the neurochemistry of gastric motility and emptying. They noted that stressors tend to inhibit both activities. Injection of CRF into the CSF delays gastric emptying, acting through a CNS and vagally mediated route. On the basis that exogenous CRF can mimic the effect of stressors, they suggested that the effect of stressors is mediated via CRF. However, cold stress has the effect of increasing gastric motility and emptying, this being mediated by vagal cholinergic activity. Therefore, as with its effect on gastric secretion, cold exerts the opposite effect to other stressors. Taché et al. suggest that TRH release is implicated in the effect of cold stressors. Experiments have shown that injection of TRH into the brain results in a vagally mediated increase in gastric emptying.

Stress stimulates activity of the colon, while CRF, acting in the brain, appears to play a crucial part in mediating this effect (Taché et al., 1989). So how does this information assist in the understanding of gastric ulcers? Restraint in the cold is a powerful stimulus to ulcer formation and the cold-restraint 'model' could give a broader insight into the transmitters implicated in the process. Data cited by Taché et al. suggest that, under these conditions, endogenous TRH activity plays a part in ulcer formation and that injection of CRF, if anything, tends to reduce their formation. The role of TRH is vagally mediated and associated with parasympathetic activation. Taché et al. suggest that the role of TRH in promoting ulceration arises from a combination of increased secretion of gastric acid and increased motility. However, Taché et al. unfortunately leave unexplained the means by which stressors other than cold restraint exert their effects on ulcer formation.

10.7.5 The Rest-period Hypothesis

It is known that ulceration increases during a 'rest period' immediately following exposure to a stressor (Desiderato et al., 1974). Section 8.5 briefly mentioned the result that shock followed by a period in the same apparatus was more ulcerogenic than shock at the end of a period of confinement (Murison and Overmier, 1993). In rats, Desiderato et al. compared 6 h of exposure to a stressor followed by 2 h rest in the home cage with 8 h exposure to the stressor. They obtained the perhaps somewhat counterintuitive result that the former procedure produced more gastric ulceration than the latter. From this, they concluded that a transition from a stressful to a stress-free environment is what produces ulceration. As was noted in Section 6.9.3, some authors argue that, on exposure to certain stressors, a period of sympathetic activation is followed by a rebound effect. The rebound would, it is argued, be associated with vagal innervation and hydrochloric acid secretion into a stomach already damaged by sympathetic activity during exposure to the stressor itself (see Overmier and Murison, 1989). Such parasympathetic rebound (and associated slowing of heart rate) might also explain some cases of sudden death (Richter, 1957; Barry and Buckley, 1966).

However, experiments by Overmier et al. (1987) and Overmier and Murison (1989) seemed to question this interpretation. During the putative rebound period, conditional stimuli (CS) earlier associated with shock were presented. This actually increased ulceration, rather than decreasing it as might be supposed on the basis of a sympathetic–parasympathetic antagonism. This does seem to be evidence against the rebound hypothesis. However, the assumption that, in their experiments, parasympathetic rebound after exposure to shock was inhibited by cues to shock might, for at least two reasons, not be true (see discussion in Section 6.9.3). First, the CSs might not have elicited sympathetic arousal, although Overmier et al. argue that they did. Shock-associated CS presented in a context in which escape is impossible might elicit parasympathetic arousal (see Section 6.9.3). Shocks were administered and recovery experienced in chambers too small to allow much movement. There were two sources of evidence that Overmier et al. used to support the claim that such CSs elicit sympathetic activation. One of them (Black, 1971) in fact makes the point that, for autonomic conditioning the conditional response (CR) can be opposite in direction to the unconditional response. Thus, for example, a shock might elicit sympathetically mediated acceleration of the heart beat but a cue paired with shock might yield a parasympathetically mediated slowing. The other source of evidence that Overmier *et al.* cited (Jaworska and Soltysik, 1962) was based upon dogs rather than rats as in the Overmier *et al.* study, and species differences might be crucial. Secondly, even if the CSs elicit sympathetic arousal, this is not necessarily incompatible with parasympathetic arousal coexisting (see Sections 2.2 and 6.9.3). Indeed, in an experiment reported by Iwata and Le Doux (1988), a cue predictive of shock elicited *both* sympathetic and parasympathetic activation.

10.8 ALCOHOL

In studies of human health, there are some well-known harmful effects of alcohol on the heart. However, as far as CHD is concerned there is some evidence that small amounts of alcohol can have beneficial effects (Levenson, 1987). Moderate drinkers seem to be in a better position regarding a healthy heart than either heavy drinkers or abstainers. There are various possible routes for such an effect. One possible explanation lies in the observation that alcohol can reduce the magnitude of the increase in both heart rate and cardiac contractility shown in response to a stressor (Levenson, 1987). In rats, Pohorecky and Brick (1987) examined the plasma corticosterone level and non-esterified fatty acid level as a measure of stress, in rats treated with ethanol as compared with controls. On these two measures of stress, using a variety of stressors, it was found that low doses of ethanol had a stress-lowering effect. Pohorecky and Brick suggest that the site of action of alcohol evident in these studies is on the CNS. They suggest a further route by which low doses of alcohol could exert a protective effect on human health: by decreasing plasma levels of non-esterified fatty acids, the chances of lipid deposits in the heart are reduced.

10.9 CONCLUSIONS

Although not wishing to oversimplify, the model of stress developed in earlier chapters, in terms of (1) a failure of coping strategies to restore equilibrium and (2) overactivity on the part of either the SAM, parasympathetic and/or pituitary–adrenocortical axes has been shown to have considerable relevance to a number of behavioural phenomena. Circulatory disorders are usually associated with over-activity of the SAM system, although there may well be an interactive effect with the HPA system. The notion of toughening-up causes us to take care in our definitions of stress; not all activity on the part of the systems implicated in the stress response is a bad thing. Rather, optimal performance was seen in terms of a fast response by the SAM system and a quick return to baseline. A useful model of depression might be in terms of a failure of the passive coping strategy accompanied by over-activity of the HPA system. Disturbances of immune function can be associated with over-activity of the HPA system.

Chapter 11

Conclusions

11.1 A THEORETICAL MODEL OF STRESS

Evidence was presented to show that activation of the so-called stress hormones occurs in anticipation of bodily activity. Where the future demands are uncertain there is a particularly strong activation of the hypothalamic–pituitary–adrenocortical (HPA) system (e.g. allocation to one of several possible experiments as described in Section 5.6 or in a situation of novelty as described in Section 5.3). Where a potential signal turns out to have benign consequences (Section 5.4) or where the event signalled poses little demand (Section 5.10.1) there can be a diminution of the HPA response over trials. Even during the course of an agonistic encounter there can be a suppression of HPA activity when the consequences seem to be predictable and a coping strategy is available (Section 1.3.9). Chapter 1 proposed a tentative model of stress in terms of unresolved and prolonged disparity between reference values and the actual state of the world. In the subsequent chapters, the evidence was presented that such disparity is associated with inappropriately high activation of a hormonal axis.

The definition developed in this book might well be as open to the charge of circularity as the definition in terms of coping, but I feel that it has some conceptual value. It might not account unambiguously for every situation that we would term 'stress' but it can form a useful criterion. Other indices, which give pointers to stress but which cannot stand alone as criteria, such as hormonal profiles, can be interpreted in the context of the model. The definition starts with the assumption that there are potential stressors in an animal's environment, e.g. predators, electric shocks, excessive heat and cold. The animal is equipped with a number of strategies for dealing with such potential stressors. In some cases, one might accurately term these 'species-specific defense reactions', such as fleeing from a predator or freezing. If such strategies are successful, then the potential stressor does not impinge upon the animal or its contact is terminated. Fleeing places a distance between the subject and a predator. Successful attack drives away an intruder. In such cases, one can view the interaction between animal and its surroundings as a negative feedback system: disparity is introduced and the animal takes action such as to correct the disparity. Even freezing can be viewed in these terms. By freezing, the animal effects a change in the environment that would not otherwise have happened: a predator overlooks the subject or a superior conspecific does not attack. In cognitive terms, one might argue that the animal that freezes has cognitions (1) (move) → (harm) and (2) (freeze) → (avoid harm), and each successful freezing confirms the second cognition.

In the terms developed here, so long as the animal is working in this negative feedback mode, then it is not stressed. Stress is the situation that prevails over extended periods when *the negative feedback loop is opened*. That is to say, the animal takes behavioural and hormonal action appropriate to the stressor but the action fails to correct the state. In these terms, either active or passive coping strategies might go on open-loop. For an example of an active strategy going on open-loop, consider the case of a monkey which was prevented from gaining access to its partner. Aggressive gestures were fruitless over extended periods. Such situations are associated with an elevation in heart rate and blood pressure and a mobilization of energy reserves from fat deposits. However, as the animal cannot make an energetic response, the heart is pumping in excess of tissue needs and the mobilization is, in the terms of Obrist (1976), 'metabolically unjustified', meaning that the heart is pumping in excess of tissue metabolic needs. The subdominant tree shrew whose heart rate was shown in Figure 6.3 would be another example of this. Even an active avoidance task, although it might successfully avoid shocks, can sometimes still produce a metabolically unjustified level of mobilization of energy (Obrist, 1976). Obrist suggests that the increased heart rate and blood pressure seen under such conditions might be a model of the aetiology of certain cardiovascular disease states (e.g. hypertension).

For an example of a passive strategy failing, consider an animal whose freezing fails to deflect aggression of a more dominant animal. The submissive tree shrews described in Chapter 6 could be said to be stressed because of the metabolic inappropriateness of massive elevations in cortisol level in a situation of inactivity.

In these terms, stress is not an appropriate term to refer to the situation of application of, say, a single shock to an animal. We already have some good words and expressions to describe this situation, e.g. pain, punishment, aversive or noxious stimulation. As was noted (Chapter 2), some situations of pain (or assumed pain) are not associated with high corticosterone levels relative to the condition prior to the experience. As Arthur (1987) notes, if we associate stress with corticosterone levels: 'Physiological stress seems to be more closely related to the intention of the organism to be vigilant and to be ready to take corrective action than to distress and suffering'.

It is doubtful whether we really need the stress concept to refer to anticipation of pain either, as we already have the less ambiguous term 'fear' to describe this state. In this context, stress could be employed to refer to when the animal is subjected to shocks over extended periods, and neither active nor passive strategies can avoid them. It is a property of the whole system going on open-loop and is associated with certain pathological states.

The recent ideas of Minor *et al.* (1994a,b) in suggesting that stress can be defined in terms of a disruption of the metabolic homeostasis of the CNS was briefly noted in Chapters 1 and 5. This seemed to offer some promise of defining the states described here as passive stress but it is not clear whether it can be adapted to apply to states described here as active stress.

11.2   HORMONAL INDICES OF STRESS

The possibility of tying stress simply to a particular hormonal response was considered and the necessity for important qualifications made. Some authors implicitly assume that stress is virtually identical with a particular hormonal response, such as the level of corticosteroid hormones. Others refer to a particular hormone as one index or measure of stress. To identify stress with a certain level of hormone might seem to obviate much of the need for a stress concept—why bother with the problematic word 'stress' if a less ambiguous word such as 'corticosteroid level' or 'elevated catecholamine response' would suffice? However, corticosteroids can rise and fall for a variety of reasons that we would not wish to label as primarily stressor induced. For example, they show a powerful circadian rhythm. In certain disease syndromes whose organic basis is well understood, corticosteroids can rise abnormally. Hard physical exercise, which is not necessarily perceived as being stressful by human participants, is associated with a relatively high secretion of catecholamines. Hypoglycaemia is a powerful trigger for catecholamine secretion (Ganong, 1975).

The corticosteroid response to placing an animal in a hot environment can be an initial activation followed by a decline (see Lefcourt, 1986). The stressor and the metabolic consequences of the new environment interact to determine hormonal response, and logically one might argue that, in trying to use the HPA response as an index of stress, the latter can mask the former (Lefcourt, 1986).

Using the corticosteroid response as an index, we would find that electric shock (Natelson *et al.*, 1981) is no more stressful to a rat than simply moving its cage from one location to another (Ursin and Murison, 1986). But by the index of catecholamine secretion, it surely would be more stressful (cf. Natelson *et al.*, 1981). Maybe we would like to employ the term stress as a short-hand for 'a high level of either corticosteroids or catecholamines, or both'. But, suppose an animal were adrenalectomized and maintained on salt solution. Would we suppose that such an animal could not be stressed? I would argue that it would be if it were executing active or passive strategies that were unsuccessful. I suspect that common sense and empathy will continue to influence our interpretation of stress, much as some researchers would like to rely upon objective measures (Ursin and Murison, 1986).

By using corticosteroid responses as an index of stress we would have to say that a human subject is most stressed in the hours prior to rising, which sounds absurd. Corticosteroids play a vital role in various aspects of day-to-day living where it would not be considered appropriate to refer to stress. As Arthur (1987) notes: 'Vigilance and readiness for action are necessary in everyday living as well as in unusual stressful situations and the existence of the circadian cortisol rhythm suggests that human beings are primed for living and survival every morning'.

To say that a hormone such as adrenaline is 'an index of stress' or 'barometer of stress' (Natelson *et al.*, 1981) or is reliably released 'in response to stress', is rather different to claiming that the hormone is synonymous with stress. It implies that there is a state somewhere in the animal (presumably in its CNS) that *is* stress. Shortly following the appearance of this state, a hormone is reliably released. A problem with this definition comes in trying to obtain any independent evidence for the existence of such a state that does not simply depend upon the hormone in question. A further problem is the differentiation between possible corticosteroid and catecholamine indexes; some situations provoke predominantly one or other response and some animals show a bias to one or the other.

To attach stress to hormone levels whether as a definition or as a measure in the absence of other indices is fraught with several problems. We need to see the hormonal response in the context of the animal's situation and behaviour to gain a useful impression of stress. Is the hormonal response behaviourally and metabolically appropriate? Is the state short-lived or chronic? For example, anticipation of food is associated with an elevated corticosteroid level (Chapter 5) but in the terms developed here it is not necessarily a stressful situation. The appearance and ingestion of food is rapidly followed by a return of corticosteroids to baseline. The evidence is that corticosteroids are released in anticipation of action (Chapter 5). Hunger *per se* does not reliably provoke their release but hunger *and* the anticipation of food does, so their release is appropriate. In these terms, by contrast, the massive release of corticosteroids over a long period of time in, say, the submissive tree shrew (Chapter 6) would be an index of stress, as the animal remains immobile, it fails to resolve the underlying problem and the corticosteroid level is metabolically inappropriate.

If any candidate has emerged in the present study as a 'stress-substance' then perhaps it is corticotrophin-releasing factor (CRF). It plays a crucial role in endocrine, behavioural and autonomic responses to stressors (De Souza and Battaglia, 1988). Behaviourally, its intracerebrovascular (i.c.v.) administration causes increased locomotion in a familiar environment, increased grooming and rearing, as well as decreases in feeding (Ritchie and Nemeroff, 1991). It has effects on raising plasma adrenaline and noradrenaline via its action in the brain mediated by the sympathetic nervous system (SNS; Chapter 2). It also plays a crucial part in the HPA axis (Chapter 2) and affects such brain processes as attention and arousal. Dunn and Berridge (1990) suggest that '. . . it is possible that the secretion of brain CRF may be both necessary and sufficient to define stress'. The parallel release of CRF, arginine vasopressin and oxytocin (Sawchenko, 1991) by, say, haemorrhage, with effects on both the HPA and autonomic nervous systems might also seem a candidate in defining stress. Given its role in both SNS and HPA systems, CRF might be a candidate for a crucial role in Selye's hypothesis of non-specificity in stress (Dunn and Berridge, 1990). As Koob *et al.* (1988) note, in these various actions, CRF could be seen as providing a basis for the much discussed association between stress and arousal (Chapter 1). Whether the system's behaviour is biased towards either sympathetic–adrenal–medullary (SAM) or pituitary–adrenocortical responding, CRF would play a role (a more specific aspect of stress). However, restraint is still needed as the i.c.v. administration of CRF does not produce all of the effects of stressors (Ritchie and Nemeroff, 1991). For example, it fails to induce analgesia.

Looking at the HPA axis gives a broader significance to the term 'stress hormones' in that various levels of this axis exert inhibition upon reproductive function. Thereby, the hormones of the axis could be described as acting in an integrated fashion. Thus we have seen the inhibitory roles of CRF on luteinizing hormone (LH) and sexual behaviour (Section 3.3). In olive baboons, stressor-induced opiates exert inhibition on LH secretion (Sapolsky, 1988; Chapter 5).

11.3 COPING

A possible approach that is explicit or implicit in much of the literature is to try to use the notion of coping strategy as a central theme for a definition. Coping is generally defined in terms of hormonal consequences. The model proposed here is rather similar, although the emphasis is upon the index of closing a feedback loop, i.e. a measure involving an effect upon the world. For instance, in terms of coping, one might argue that an animal is in a state of stress if it is unable to terminate the impact of a potential stressor. Another animal having the capacity to terminate the potential stressor is not stressed, or is at least less stressed, than that lacking the capacity for such coping. In some cases, one can objectively define a coping strategy both in terms of consequences and hormonal profile. For example, a rat that can terminate an electric shock by turning a wheel could unambiguously be said to have a coping strategy compared to its passive yoked control: the external world is changed as a result of its behaviour. In other cases, the notion of coping is employed in situations in which it does not escape from circularity. The inclination is to define any strategy, even doing nothing, that results in a restraint of the rise in corticosteroid levels as a coping strategy. For instance, Henry (1976) argues that the progressive recruitment of the SAM system over repeated sessions of immobilization is a reflection of the animal's gaining some control: the perception of a predictable outcome.

11.4 A MODEL OF STRESS, THE HORMONE REACTION AND PATHOLOGY

Confronted by a novel potential stressor, both the SAM and pituitary–adrenocortical systems will tend to be activated. The animal will follow some strategy, either active or passive, which might succeed in correcting the disturbance. In future, it will tend to repeat this strategy when confronted by the same potential stressor. If an active strategy worked in the past, the stressor will tend to provoke activation of the SAM system, accompanied by an increase in activity of the pituitary–adrenocortical system. After the strategy is successful, there will be a tendency for the hormonal systems to return to their basal levels. If the strategy is not successful, then one of several things might happen. The subject might persist with the same strategy, which might be associated with activation of the SAM and the HPA systems beyond their optimal range. This is an open-loop situation: stress. The animal might try fleeing, which might (closed-loop) or might not (open-loop: stress) be successful. The animal might switch to a passive strategy, which again might be successful at deflecting attack or unsuccessful (open-loop). An animal which persists with either an active or passive strategy in the face of repeated failure over extended periods of time might be described as chronically stressed. These open-loop states would each be characterized by an abnormal hormonal profile and a risk of associated pathology. In the case of tree shrews (Chapter 6), even though the strategy largely worked in the sense of deflecting attack, the animal would be stressed by the criteria of: (1) that it is in an environment not of its choosing and (2) of inappropriate hormonal secretion and pathology.

Defined in this way, one would not include in the definition of stress physical challenges that can activate the HPA in the absence of a psychological component and an attempt at corrective behaviour, e.g. a surreptitious insulin-induced hypoglycaemia. However, the way in which stress is defined will to a considerable extent depend upon the *purpose* behind the explanation. The explanation developed here is based upon the need to sharpen the vocabulary of behavioural science and to scrutinize the need for a particular word 'stress' in this context. In other contexts, it might be more useful to group together all of those situations, whether behavioural or not, that can exert a common effect upon the HPA axis. I cannot argue that the proposed model is the only logical one.

11.5 THE ROLE OF CORTICOSTEROIDS

The role of corticosteroids has emerged as essentially twofold. First, they prepare the body for activity. Times of uncertainty, such as entering a novel environment or being handled by the experimenter, are associated with activation of the HPA axis. In an adaptive sense, such situations might well be followed by the need to fight or flee. Times of *anticipation of a significant event*, e.g. arrival of food or an aversive event, cause an elevation of corticosteroid levels (Chapter 5). Experiencing the anticipated event (e.g. unavoidable shock), in some cases accompanied by engaging in an appropriate activity (e.g. consuming food), is often associated with a reduction in corticosterone level or even a full return to baseline (e.g. feeding, Chapter 5). It might be useful to view the extreme rise of corticosterone activity that is associated with, for example, the submissive tree shrews described in Chapter 6 as an example of a protracted anticipation of a state that would permit activity but which, in practice, the constraints of the context never permit to be realized.

The second role attributed to corticosteroids is one of restraining or switching off some of the body's defence functions, such as inflammation and immune function (Chapters 4 and 10). Considering the acute application of a natural stressor (e.g. wounding by a predator that had earlier been sighted and which had evoked anticipatory action), the two roles would be played at different times. The first would occur in anticipation of an escape attempt, whereas the second would occur some time after injury had been sustained. For example, tissue damage would be associated with inflammation and an immune response which would later be terminated by corticosteroid action.

11.6   APPLIED ETHOLOGY

Since the theoretical context within which the present model arose was one of applied ethology it is appropriate to ask whether there are implications of it for the future development of this discipline. The model is based upon the notion of disparity correction and it was suggested that frustration might arise by animals being thwarted in their goals (Section 9.4.1). The model incorporates the assumption that in such correction, the performance of species-typical behaviour can have consequences for physiological states (Section 9.4.2). In the terms of the model, elevated HPA activation might arise from over- or under-stimulation (Section 9.2.2).

The situation in which stereotypies are exhibited often seems to involve a negative feedback loop going on to open-loop and the animal performing behaviour in a fruitless attempt to close the loop (Chapter 9). Whether some intrinsic loop involving a hormone or neurotransmitter is closed by such behaviour remains to be seen.

Some see the value of the stress concept as being a state that is prepathological (Dawkins, 1980; Moberg, 1985). Identifying the existence of this state is of clear practical significance; it can provide an early warning of possible pathology, such as gastric ulceration or impaired immune function (Chapters 9 and 10). However, the definition is only useful for some pathological states and does not escape from the circularity. It specifically refers to those pathologies generally associated with inappropriately high activity by the SAM and pituitary–adrenocortical systems.

11.7   FUTURE DIRECTIONS

One clear implication of the theoretical development presented here is a belief in the value of a purposive model of behaviour in which animals set goals, are motivated to meet them and monitor the efficacy of their achievement (Powers, 1973; Wiepkema, 1985, 1987, 1990; Toates, 1986, 1994c). A number of authors have mentioned in passing the validity of such an explanatory principle (Tinbergen, 1969; Laborit, 1986) but most stop short of its full acceptance. Such a model would also involve central states described as affective or hedonic.

A theme that has emerged in several places is that of a hierarchy of control (Section 9.5.3.12) possibly with the hippocampus playing a pivotal part in exerting full cognitive control over behaviour. In such terms, one might make sense of the rich density of corticosteroid receptors in the hippocampus (Chapter 7) as a factor in the maintenance of vigilance and cognitive control over behaviour in the face of a possibility of switching into more automatic routines. However, the contradictions in applying such ideas to stereotypies were acknowledged (Chapter 9).

The capacity to form predictions about the future involves the use of information that might in reality prove to be 'wrong'. If so, stress reactions can be activated. To return to the theme of Chapter 1, stress is a possibility in cases where there is flexibility of behaviour and information might turn out to be wrong or unreliable. Flexibility is a bonus but the possibility of stress is the inevitable price to be paid for this.

Extending the theoretical ideas developed here to a broader context of behavioural control might provide some insights into the emergence of states of affect and consciousness. Chapter 1 developed a particular argument concerning the part that affective states play in the control of behaviour, i.e. as a monitor of the efficacy of flexible behaviour. Can the model say anything about the emergence of consciousness? In terms of the hierarchical control of behaviour discussed in Section 9.5.3.12, consciousness might be seen within the hierarchy as a specialized adaptation in a high-level cognitive control of behaviour. In such terms, consciousness would be seen as setting high-level goals that are put into effect by lower levels in the hierarchy. At such a high level, consciousness might normally be rather remote from a *direct and immediate* involvement in response production. In keeping with Gray's (1993) observation, consciousness could not directly mediate between stimuli and responses. So is consciousness merely a monitor of the efficacy of action? This would contradict intuition which suggests an active role of consciousness in behaviour. A possible resolution is to see consciousness as a monitor but, in conjunction with affect, also setting overall directions to behaviour. Given such overall direction, the lower levels would actually select appropriate behaviour based upon stimulus input. In such terms, the role of consciousness would be that of the potentiation and depotentiation (Gallistel, 1980) of lower hierarchical levels. This means that consciousness is not merely some passive epiphenomenon (which raises problems concerning how it emerged in evolution) but an overall goal setter and monitor of efficacy. As such it would form an integral part of a negative feedback system whose goals might or might not be realized.

References

Abbott, B.B., Schoen, L.S. and Badia, P. (1984) Predictable and unpredictable shock: Behavioural measures of aversion and physiological measures of stress. *Psychological Bulletin,* **96**, 45–71.

Ader, R. (1987) Conditioned immune responses: adrenocortical influences. In *Progress in Brain Research*, Vol. 72 (eds E.R. de Kloet, V.M. Wiegant and D. de Wied), Elsevier, Amsterdam, pp. 79–90.

Aldridge, J.W., Berridge, K.C., Herman, M. and Zimmer, L. (1993) Neuronal coding of serial order: Syntax of grooming in the neostriatum. *Psychological Science,* **4**, 391–395.

Allen, J.P., Allen, C.F., Greer, M.A. and Jacobs, J.J. (1973) Stress-induced secretion of ACTH. In *Brain–Pituitary–Adrenal Interrelationships* (eds A. Brodish and E.S. Redgate), Karger, Basel, pp. 99–127.

Amir, S., Brown, Z.W. and Amit, Z. (1980) The role of endorphins in stress: Evidence and speculations. *Neuroscience and Biobehavioural Reviews,* **4**, 77–86.

Amit, Z. and Galina, Z.H. (1986) Stress-induced analgesia: Adaptive pain suppression. *Physiological Reviews,* **66**, 1091–1120.

Amit, Z. and Galina, Z.H. (1988) Stress induced analgesia plays an adaptive role in the organization of behavioural responding. *Brain Research Bulletin,* **21**, 955–958.

Andersen, B.L., Kiecolt-Glaser, J.K. and Glaser, R. (1994) A biobehavioural model of cancer stress and disease course. *American Psychologist,* **49**, 389–404.

Anderson, D.C. (1993) Does ACTH mediate the punishment-intensification effect of prolonged, fixed-duration treatment shocks? *Psychobiology,* **21**, 43–49.

Anisman, H. (1975) Time-dependent variations in aversively motivated behaviours: Nonassociative effects of cholinergic and catecholaminergic activity. *Psychological Review,* **82**, 359–385.

Anisman, H. (1978) Neurochemical changes elicited by stress. In *Psychopharmacology of Aversively Motivated Behaviour* (eds H. Anisman and G. Bignami), New York, Plenum Press, pp. 119–172.

Anisman, H. and Zacharko, R.M. (1982) Depression: The predisposing influence of stress. *Behavioural and Brain Sciences,* **5**, 89–137.

Anisman, H. and Zacharko, R.M. (1986) Behavioural and neurochemical consequences associated with stressors. *Annals of the New York Academy of Sciences,* **467**, 205–225.

Anisman, H., Pizzino, A. and Sklar, L.S. (1980) Coping with stress, norepinephrine depletion and escape performance. *Brain Research,* **191**, 583–588.

Antelman, S.M. and Brown, T.S. (1972) Hippocampal lesions and shuttlebox avoidance behaviour: A fear hypothesis. *Physiology and Behaviour,* **9**, 15–20.

Antelman, S.M. and Chiodo, L.A. (1983) Amphetamine as a stressor. In *Stimulants: Neurochemical, Behavioural and Clinical Perspectives* (ed. I. Creese), Raven Press, New York, pp. 269–299.

Archer, J. (1976) The organization of aggression and fear in vertebrates. In *Perspectives in Ethology 2* (eds P.P.G. Bateson and P. Klopfer), Plenum, New York, pp. 231–298.

Archer, J. (1979) *Animals under Stress.* Edward Arnold, London.

Archer, J. (1988) *The Behavioural Biology of Aggression.* Cambridge University Press, Cambridge.

Arthur, A.Z. (1987) Stress as a state of anticipatory vigilance. *Perceptual and Motor Skills,* **64**, 75–85.

Ashmore, J. and Morgan, D. (1967) Metabolic effects of adrenal glucocorticoid hormones. Carbohydrate, protein, lipid and nucleic acid metabolism. In *The Adrenal Cortex* (ed A.B. Eisenstein), Little, Brown and Company, Boston, pp. 249–267.

Atrens, D.M. (1984) Self-stimulation and psychotropic drugs: A methodological and conceptual critique. In *Animal Models in Psychopathology* (ed. N.W. Bond), Academic Press, Sydney, pp. 227–256.

Auerbach, P. and Carlton, P.L. (1971) Retention deficit correlated with a deficit in the corticosteroid response to stress. *Science,* **173**, 1148–1149.

Ax, A.F. (1953) The physiological differentiation between fear and anger in humans. *Psychosomatic Medicine,* **15**, 433–442.

Axelrod, J. and Reisine, T.D. (1984) Stress hormones: their interaction and regulation. *Science,* **224**, 452–459.

Ballieux, R.E. and Heijnen, C.J. (1987) Brain and immune system: a one-way conversation or a genuine dialogue? In *Progress in Brain Research,* Vol. 72 (eds E.R. de Kloet, V.M. Wiegant and D. de Wied), Elsevier, Amsterdam, pp. 71–77.

Ballieux, R.E. and Heijnen, C.J. (1989) Stress and immune response. In *Frontiers of Stress Research* (eds H. Weiner, I. Florin, R. Murison and D. Hellhammer), Hans Huber, Toronto, pp. 51–55.

Bandura, A., Taylor, C.B., Williams, S.L., Mefford, I.N. and Barchas, J.D. (1985) Catecholamine secretion as a function of perceived coping self-efficacy. *Journal of Consulting and Clinical Psychology,* **53**, 406–414.

Bandura, A., Cioffi, D., Taylor, C.B. and Brouillard, M.E. (1988) Perceived self-efficacy in coping with cognitive stressors and opioid activation. *Journal of Personality and Social Psychology,* **55**, 479–488.

Barnes, D.M. (1986) Steroids may influence changes in mood. *Science,* **232**, 1344–1345.

Barnett, J.L. (1987) The physiological concept of stress is useful for assessing welfare. *Australian Veterinary Journal,* **64**, 195–196.

Barnett, J.L., Winfield, C.G., Cronin, G.M., Hemsworth, P.H. and Dewar, A.M. (1985) The effect of individual and group housing on behavioural and physiological responses related to the welfare of pregnant pigs. *Applied Animal Behaviour Science,* **14**, 149–161.

Barry, H. and Buckley, J.P. (1966) Drug effects on animal performance and the stress syndrome. *Journal of Pharmaceutical Sciences,* **55**, 1159–1183.

Bateson, P. (1991) Assessment of pain in animals. *Animal Behaviour,* **42**, 827–839.

Baxter, J.D. and Rousseau, G.G. (1979) Glucocorticoid hormone action: An overview. In *Glucocorticoid Hormone Action* (eds J.D. Baxter and G.G. Rousseau), Springer-verlag, Berlin, pp. 1–24.

Baxter, M.R. (1983) Ethology in environmental design. *Applied Animal Ethology*, **9**, 207–220.

Becker, J.B. (1992) Hormonal influences on extrapyramidal sensorimotor function and hippocampal plasticity. In *Behavioural Endocrinology* (eds J.B. Becker, S.M. Breedlove and D. Crews), The MIT Press, Cambridge, pp. 325–356.

Bélanger, D. and Feldman, S.M. (1962) Effects of water deprivation upon heart rate and instrumental activity in the rat. *Journal of Comparative and Physiological Psychology*, **55**, 220–225.

Beninger, R.J. (1989) Methods for determining the effects of drugs on learning. In *Neuromethods*, Vol. 13, *Psychopharmacology* (eds A.A. Boulton, G.B. Baker and A.J. Greenshaw), Humana Press, Clifton, pp. 623–685.

Benus, I. (1988) Aggression and coping. Doctoral dissertation. Rijksuniversiteit, Groningen.

Benus, R.F., Bohus, B., Koolhaas, J.M. and van Oortmerssen, G.A. (1989) Behavioural strategies of aggressive and non-aggressive male mice in active shock avoidance. *Behavioural Processes*, **20**, 1–12.

Bernardi, M., Genedani, S., Tagliavini, S. and Bertolini, A. (1989) Effect of castration and testosterone in experimental models of depression in mice. *Behavioural Neuroscience*, **103**, 1148–1150.

Berntson, G.G., Cacioppo, J.T. and Quigley, K.S. (1991) Autonomic determinism: The modes of autonomic control, the doctrine of autonomic space and the laws of autonomic constraint. *Psychological Review*, **98**, 459–487.

Berridge, K.C. and Fentress, J.C. (1985) Trigeminal–taste interaction in palatability processing. *Science*, **228**, 747–750.

Berridge, K.C. and Grill, H.J. (1984) Isohedonic tastes support a two-dimensional hypothesis of palatability. *Appetite*, **5**, 221–231.

Berridge, K.C. and Valenstein, E.S. (1991) What psychological process mediates feeding evoked by electrical stimulation of the lateral hypothalamus? *Behavioural Neuroscience*, **105**, 3–14.

Berridge, K.C., Venier, I.L. and Robinson, T.E. (1989) Taste reactivity analysis of 6-hydroxydopamine-induced aphagia: Implications for arousal and anhedonia hypotheses of dopamine function. *Behavioural Neuroscience*, **103**, 36–45.

Besedovsky, H., Del Rey, A., Sorkin, E., Da Prada, M., Burri, R. and Honegger, C. (1983) The immune response evokes changes in brain noradrenergic neurons. *Science*, **221**, 564–566.

Bignami, G. and Michalek, H. (1978) Cholinergic mechanisms and aversively motivated behaviours. In *Psychopharmacology of Aversively Motivated Behaviour* (eds H. Anisman and G. Bignami), Plenum, New York, pp. 173–255.

Bindra, D. (1978) How adaptive behaviour is produced: a perceptual–motivational alternative to response-reinforcement. *Behavioural and Brain Sciences*, **1**, 41–91.

Black, A.H. (1971) Autonomic aversive conditioning in infrahuman subjects. In *Aversive Conditioning and Learning* (ed. F.R. Brush), Academic Press, New York, pp. 3–104.

Blackburn, J.R., Phillips, A.G., Jakubovic, A. and Fibiger, H.C. (1989) Dopamine and preparatory behaviour: II. A neurochemical analysis. *Behavioural Neuroscience*, **103**, 15–23.

Blalock, J.E. (1987) Virus-induced increases in plasma corticosterone. *Science,* **238**, 1424–1425.

Blalock, J.E. (1988) Immunologically-mediated pituitary–adrenal activation. In *Mechanisms of Physical and Emotional Stress* (eds G.P. Chrousos, D.L. Loriaux and P.W. Gold), Plenum, New York, pp. 217–223.

Blokhuis, H.J. and van der Haar, J.W. (1992) Effects of pecking incentives during rearing on feather pecking of laying hens. *British Poultry Science,* **33**, 17–24.

Blozovski, D. (1986) L'hippocampe et le comportement. *La Recherche,* **17**, 330–337.

Bohus, B. (1970) Central nervous structures and the effect of ACTH and corticosteroids on avoidance behaviour: A study with intracerebral implantation of corticosteroids in the rat. In *Pituitary, Adrenal and the Brain—Progress in Brain Research,* Vol. 32 (eds D. de Wied and J.A.W.M. Weijnen), Elsevier, Amsterdam, pp. 171–184.

Bohus, B. and de Kloet, E.R. (1981) Adrenal steroids and extinction behaviour: Antagonism by progesterone, deoxycorticosterone and dexamethasone of a specific effect of corticosterone. *Life Sciences,* **28**, 433–440.

Bohus, B. and De Wied, D. (1980) Pituitary–adrenal system hormones and adaptive behaviour. In *General, Comparative and Clinical Endocrinology of the Adrenal Cortex* (eds I. Chester Jones and I.W. Henderson), Academic Press, London, pp. 265–347.

Bohus, B. and Lissak, K. (1968) Adrenocortical hormones and avoidance behaviour of rats. *International Journal of Neuropharmacology,* **7**, 301–306.

Bohus, B., De Kloet, E.R. and Veldhuis, H.D. (1982) Adrenal steroids and behavioural adaptation: Relationship to brain corticoid receptors. In *Adrenal Actions on Brain* (eds D. Ganten and D. Pfaff), Springer-Verlag, Berlin, pp. 107–148.

Bohus, B., Benus, R.F., Fokkema, D.S., Koolhaas, J.M., Nyakas, C., van Oortmerssen, G.A., Prins, A.J.A., de Ruiter, A.J.H., Scheurink, A.J.W. and Steffens, A.B. (1987a) Neuroendocrine states and behavioural and physiological stress responses. In *Progress in Behaviour Research,* Vol. 72 (eds E.R. de Kloet, V.M. Wiegant and D. de Wied), Elsevier, Amsterdam, pp. 57–70.

Bohus, B., Koolhaas, J.M., Nyakas, C., Steffens, A.B., Fokkema, D.S. and Scheurink, A.J.W. (1987b) Physiology of stress: A behavioural view. In *Biology of Stress in Farm Animals: An Integrative Approach* (eds P.R. Wiepkema and P.W.M. van Adrichem), Martinus Nijhoff, Dordrecht, pp. 57–70.

Bolles, R.C. (1970) Species-specific defense reactions and avoidance learning. *Psychological Review,* **77**, 32–48.

Bolles, R.C. (1972) Reinforcement, expectancy and learning. *Psychological Review,* **79**, 394–409.

Bolles, R.C. (1979) *Learning Theory.* Holt, Rinehart and Winston, New York.

Bolles, R.C. (1988) The bathwater and everything. *Behavioural and Brain Sciences,* **11**, 449–450.

Bolles, R.C. and Fanselow, M.S. (1980) A perceptual–defensive–recuperative model of fear and pain. *Behavioural and Brain Sciences,* **3**, 291–323.

Bolles, R.C. and Moot, S.A. (1973) The rat's anticipation of two meals a day. *Journal of Comparative and Physiological Psychology,* **83**, 510–514.

Bond, P.E., Owens, M.J., Butler, P.D., Bissette, G. and Nemeroff, C.B. (1989) Corticotrophin-releasing factor: Possible involvement in the pathogenesis of affective disorders. In *Molecular Biology of Stress* (eds S. Breznitz and O. Zinder), Alan R. Liss, New York, pp. 67–76.

Borrell, J., de Kloet, E.R., Versteeg, D.H.G. and Bohus, B. (1983) Inhibitory avoidance deficit following short-term adrenalectomy in the rat: The role of adrenal catecholamines. *Behavioural and Neural Biology*, **39**, 241–258.

Bozarth, M.A. (1987) *Methods of Assessing the Reinforcing Properties of Abused Drugs*. Springer-Verlag, New York.

Bradbury, M.W.B., Burden, J., Hillhouse, E.W. and Jones, M.T. (1974) Stimulation electrically and by acetylcholine of the rat hypothalamus *in vitro*. *Journal of Physiology*, **239**, 269–283.

Brain, P.F. (1971) Possible role of the pituitary/adrenocortical axis in aggressive behaviour. *Nature*, **233**, 489.

Brain, P.F. (1980) Adaptive aspects of hormonal correlates of attack and defense in laboratory mice: A study in ethobiology. In *Progress in Brain Research*, Vol. 53, *Adaptive Capabilities of the Nervous System* (eds P.S. McConnell, G.J. Boer, H.J. Romijn, N.E. Van de Poll and M.A. Corner), Elsevier/North-Holland Biomedical Press, Amsterdam, pp. 391–413.

Breland, K. and Breland, M. (1961) The misbehaviour of organisms. *American Psychologist*, **16**, 681–684.

Brett, L.P. and Levine, S. (1981) The pituitary–adrenal response to 'minimized' schedule-induced drinking. *Physiology and Behaviour*, **26**, 153–158.

Brick, J. and Pohorecky, L.A. (1987) The limbic system and ethanol-induced changes in plasma corticosterone and nonesterified fatty acids. In *Stress and Addiction* (eds E. Gottheil, K.A. Druley, S. Pashko and S.P. Weinstein), Brunner/Mazel Publishers, New York, pp. 101–121.

Broom, D.M. (1991) Assessing welfare and suffering. *Behavioural Processes*, **25**, 117–123.

Brown, M.R. (1991) Brain peptide regulation of autonomic nervous and neuroendocrine functions. In *Stress—Neurobiology and Neuroendocrinology* (eds M.R. Brown, G.F. Koob and C. Rivier), Marcel Dekker, New York, pp. 193–215.

Brown, M.R. and Fisher, L.A. (1985) Corticotropin-releasing factor: effect on the autonomic nervous system and visceral systems. *Federation Proceedings*, **44**, 243–248.

Bruner, A. (1969) Reinforcement strength in classical conditioning of leg flexion, freezing and heart rate in cats. *Conditioned Reflex*, **4**, 24–31.

Brush, F.R. and Shain, C.N. (1989) Endogenous opioids and behaviour. In *Psychoendocrinology* (eds F.R. Brush and S. Levine), Academic Press, San Diego, pp. 379–435.

Buckingham, J.C. and Hodges, J.R. (1979) Hypothalamic receptors influencing the secretion of corticotrophin releasing hormone in the rat. *Journal of Physiology*, **290**, 421–431.

Burchfield, S.R. (1979) The stress response: A new perspective. *Psychosomatic Medicine*, **41**, 661–672.

Burchfield, S.R., Woods, S.C. and Elich, M.S. (1980) Pituitary adrenocortical response to chronic intermittent stress. *Physiology and Behaviour*, **24**, 297–302.

Burges Watson, I.P., Hoffman, L. and Wilson, G.V. (1988) The neuropsychiatry of post-traumatic stress disorder. *British Journal of Psychiatry*, **152**, 164–173.

Burks, T.F. (1991) Role of stress in the development of disorders of gastrointestinal motility. In *Stress—Neurobiology and Neuroendocrinology* (eds M.R. Brown, G.F. Koob and C. Rivier), Marcel Dekker, New York, pp. 565–583.

Cabanac, M. (1992) Pleasure: the common currency. *Journal of Theoretical Biology*, **155**, 173–200.

Cabanac, M. and Gosselin, F. (1993) Emotional fever in the lizard *Callopistes maculatus* (Teiidae). *Animal Behaviour*, **46**, 200–202.

Cabanac, M. and Johnson, K.G. (1983) Analysis of conflict between palatability and cold exposure in rats. *Physiology and Behaviour*, **31**, 249–253.

Cabanac, M. and Russek, M. (1982) *Régulation et Controle en Biologie*. Les Presses de l'Université Laval, Quebec.

Cabib, S. (1993) Neurobiological basis of stereotypies. In *Stereotypic Animal Behaviour—Fundamentals and Applications to Welfare* (eds A.B. Lawrence and J. Rushen), CAB International, Wallingford, pp. 119–145.

Cabib, S. and Puglisi-Allegra, S. (1990) Social behaviour of the house mouse: A potential model for preclinical studies on stress. In *Psychobiology of Stress* (eds S. Puglisi and A. Oliverio), Kluwer, Dordrecht, pp. 31–40.

Cabib, S., Puglisi-Allegra, S. and Oliverio, A. (1984) Chronic stress enhances apomorphine-induced stereotyped behaviour in mice: involvement of endogenous opioids. *Brain Research* **298**, 138–140.

Candland, D.K. and Leshner, A.I. (1974) A model of agonistic behaviour: Endocrine and autonomic correlates. In *Limbic and Autonomic Nervous Systems Research* (ed. L.V. DiCara), Plenum Press, New York, pp. 137–163.

Carli, G., Farabollini, F. and Lupo di Prisco, C. (1979) Plasma corticosterone and its relation to susceptibility to animal hypnosis in rabbits. *Neuroscience Letters*, **11**, 271–274.

Carlton, P.L. (1969) Brain acetylcholine and inhibition. In *Reinforcement and Behaviour* (ed. J.T. Tapp), Academic Press, New York, pp. 286–327.

Carroll, B.J. and Mendels, J. (1976) Neuroendocrine regulation in affective disorders. In *Hormones, Behaviour and Psychopathology* (ed. E.J. Sachar), Raven Press, New York, pp. 193–224.

Charlton, B.G. and Ferrier, I.N. (1989) Hypothalamo–pituitary–adrenal axis abnormalities in depression: a review and a model. *Psychological Medicine*, **19**, 331–336.

Charney, D.S., Deutch, A.Y., Krystal, J.H., Southwick, S.M. and Davis, M. (1993) Psychobiologic mechanisms of posttraumatic stress disorder. *Archives of General Psychiatry*, **50**, 294–305.

Cherek, D.R., Thompson, T. and Heistad, G.T. (1973) Responding maintained by the opportunity to attack during an interval food reinforcement schedule. *Journal of the Experimental Analysis of Behaviour*, **19**, 113–123.

Cherkin, A. and Meinecke, R.O. (1971) Suppression of fighting behaviour in rabbits by paired emergence from anaesthesia. *Nature*, **231**, 195–196.

Chrousos, G.P., Loriaux, D.L. and Gold, P.W. (1988) The concept of stress and its historical development. In *Mechanisms of Physical and Emotional Stress* (eds G.P. Chrousos, D.L. Loriaux and P.W. Gold), Plenum Press, New York, pp. 3–7.

Coe, C.L., Stanton, M.E. and Levine, S. (1983) Adrenal responses to reinforcement and extinction: Role of expectancy versus instrumental responding. *Behavioural Neuroscience*, **97**, 654–657.

Cohen, D.H. (1974) Analysis of the final common path for heart rate conditioning. In *Cardiovascular Psychophysiology* (eds P.A. Obrist, A.H. Black, J. Brener and L.V. DiCara), Aldine Publishing Company, Chicago, pp. 117–135.

Cohen, D.H. and Obrist, P.A. (1975) Interactions between behaviour and the cardiovascular system. *Circulation Research*, **37**, 693–706.

Cohen, D.H. and Pitts, L.H. (1968) Vagal and sympathetic components of conditioned cardioacceleration in the pigeon. *Brain Research*, **9**, 15–31.

Cohen, P.S., Looney, T.A., Campagnoni, F.R. and Lawler, C.P. (1985) A two-state model of reinforcer-induced motivation. In *Affect, Conditioning and Cognition: Essays on the Determinants of Behaviour* (eds F.R. Brush and J.B. Overmier), Lawrence Erlbaum, Hillsdale, pp. 281–297.

Cohen, S. and Williamson, G.M. (1991) Stress and infectious disease in humans. *Psychological Bulletin*, **109**, 5–24.

Cole, B.J. and Koob, G.F. (1991) Corticotropin-releasing factor, stress, and animal behaviour. In *Stress, Neuropeptides and Systemic Disease* (eds J.A. McCubbin, P.G. Kaufmann and C.B. Nemeroff), Academic Press, San Diego, pp. 119–148.

Colpaert, F.C., De Witte, P., Maoli, A.N., Awouters, F., Niemegeers, C.J.E. and Janssen, P.A.J. (1980) Self-administration of the analgesic suprofin in arthritic rats: evidence of *Mycobacterium butyricum*-induced arthritis as an experimental model of chronic pain. *Life Sciences*, **27**, 921–928.

Cools, A.R. (1985) Brain and behaviour: Hierarchy of feedback systems and control of input. In *Perspectives in Ethology* Vol. 6 (eds P.P.G. Bateson and P.H. Klopfer), Plenum, New York, pp. 109–168.

Conner, R.L., Vernikos-Danellis, J. and Levine, S. (1971) Stress, fighting and neuroendocrine function. *Nature*, **234**, 564–566.

Cooper, J.J. and Nicol, C.J. (1993) The 'coping' hypothesis of stereotypic behaviour: a reply to Rushen. *Animal Behaviour*, **45**, 616–618.

Cooper, J.J. and Nicol, C.J. (1994) Neighbour effects on the development of locomotor stereotypies in bank voles, *Clethrionomys glareolus*. *Animal Behaviour*, **47**, 214–216.

Cooper, S.J. and Dourish, C.T. (1990) An introduction to the concept of stereotypy and a historical perspective on the role of brain dopamine. In *Neurobiology of Stereotyped Behaviour* (eds S.J. Cooper and C.T. Dourish), Clarendon Press, Oxford, pp. 1–24.

Coover, G.D., Goldman, L. and Levine, S. (1971) Plasma corticosterone levels during extinction of a lever-press response in hippocampectomized rats. *Physiology and Behaviour*, **7**, 727–732.

Coover, G.D., Sutton, B.R. and Heybach, J.P. (1977) Conditioning decreases in plasma corticosterone level in rats by pairing stimuli with daily feedings. *Journal of Comparative and Physiological Psychology*, **91**, 716–726.

Coover, G.D., Murison, R., Sundberg, H., Jellestad, F. and Ursin, H. (1984) Plasma corticosterone and meal expectancy in rats: Effects of low probability cues. *Physiology and Behaviour*, **33**, 179–184.

Corley, K.C., Mauck, H.P. and Shiel, F.O. (1975) Cardiac responses associated with 'yoked-chair' shock avoidance in squirrel monkeys. *Psychophysiology*, **12**, 439–444.

Craddock, C.G. (1978) Corticosteroid-induced lymphopenia, immunosuppression and body defense. *Annals of Internal Medicine*, **88**, 564–566.

Cronin, G.J., Wiepkema, P.R. and Van Ree, J.M. (1985) Endogenous opioids are involved in abnormal stereotyped behaviours of tethered sows. *Neuropeptides*, **6**, 527–530.

Crow, T.J. and Deakin, J.F.W. (1985) Neurohumoral transmission, behaviour and mental disorder. In *Handbook of Psychiatry*, Vol. 5, *The Scientific Foundations of Psychiatry*, (ed. M. Shepherd), Cambridge University Press, Cambridge, pp. 137–182.

Dallman, M.F. (1991) Regulation of adrenocortical function following stress. In *Stress—Neurobiology and Neuroendocrinology* (eds M.R. Brown, G.F. Koob and C. Rivier), Marcel Dekker, New York, pp. 173–192.

Dallman, M.F., Akana, S.F., Cascio, C.S., Darlington, D.N., Jacobsen, L. and Levin, N. (1987) Regulation of ACTH secretion: Variations on a theme of B. In *Recent Progress in Hormone Research*, Vol. 43, (ed. J.H. Clark), Academic Press, Orlando, pp. 113–173.

Dantzer, R. (1986) Behavioural, physiological and functional aspects of stereotyped behaviour: A review and a reinterpretation. *Journal of Animal Science*, **62**, 1776–1786.

Dantzer, R. (1991) Stress, stereotypies and welfare. *Behavioural Processes*, **25**, 95–102.

Dantzer, R. and Mittelman, G. (1993) Functional consequences of behavioural stereotypy. In *Stereotypic Animal Behaviour—Fundamentals and Applications to Welfare* (eds A.B. Lawrence and J. Rushen), CAB International, Wallingford, pp. 147–172.

Dantzer, R. and Mormède, P. (1981) Pituitary–adrenal consequences of adjunctive activities in pigs. *Hormones and Behaviour*, **15**, 386–395.

Dantzer, R. and Mormède, P. (1983a) Stress in farm animals: A need for re-evaluation. *Journal of Animal Science*, **57**, 6–18.

Dantzer, R. and Mormède, P. (1983b) De-arousal properties of stereotyped behaviour: Evidence from pituitary–adrenal correlates in pigs. *Applied Animal Ethology*, **10**, 233–244.

Dantzer, R., Terlouw, C., Mormède, P. and Le Moal, M. (1988a) Schedule-induced polydipsia experience decreases plasma corticosterone levels but increases plasma prolactin levels. *Physiology and Behaviour*, **43**, 275–279.

Dantzer, R., Terlouw, C., Tazi, A., Koolhaas, J.M., Bohus, B., Koob, G.F. and LeMoal, M. (1988b) The propensity for schedule-induced polydipsia is related to differences in conditioned avoidance behaviour and defense reactions in a defeat test. *Physiology and Behaviour*, **43**, 269–273.

Daughaday, W.H. (1967) The binding of corticosteroids by plasma protein. In *The Adrenal Cortex* (ed. A.B. Eisenstein), Little, Brown and Company, Boston, pp. 385–403.

Davis, H., Memmott, J. Macfadden, L. and Levine, S. (1976) Pituitary–adrenal activity under different appetitive extinction procedures. *Physiology and Behaviour*, **17**, 687–690.

Dawkins, M.S. (1980) *Animal Suffering*. Chapman and Hall, London.

De Boer, S.F., Slangen, J.L. and Van der Gugten, J. (1988) Adaptation of plasma catecholamine and corticosterone responses to short-term repeated noise stress in rats. *Physiology and Behaviour*, **44**, 273–280.

De Boer, S.F., De Beun, R., Slangen, J.L. and Van der Gugten, J. (1990) Dynamics of plasma catecholamine and corticosterone concentrations during reinforced and extinguished operant behaviour in rats. *Physiology and Behaviour*, **47**, 691–698.

De Kloet, E.R. and Veldhuis, H.D. (1985) Adrenocortical hormone action. In *Handbook of Neurochemistry*, Vol. 8, *Neurochemical System* (ed. A. Lajtha), Plenum, New York, pp. 47–91.

Delft, A.M.L. van (1970) The relation between pretraining plasma corticosterone levels and the acquisition of an avoidance response in the rat. In *Pituitary, Adrenal and the Brain* (Vol. 32, Progress in Brain Research), (eds. D. de Wied and J.A.W.M. Weijnen), Elsevier, Amsterdam. pp. 192–199.

Delius, J.D., Craig, B. and Chaudoir, C. (1976) Adrenocorticotropic hormone, glucose and displacement activities in pigeons. *Zeitschrift für Tierpsychologie*, **40**, 183–193.

De Passillé, A.M.B., Christopherson, R.J. and Rushen, J. (1991) Sucking behaviour affects the post-prandial secretion of digestive juices in the calf. In *Applied Animal Behaviour: Past, Present and Future* (eds M.C. Appleby, R.I. Horrell, J.C. Petherick, and S.M. Rutter), Universities Federation for Animal Welfare, Potters Bar, pp. 130–131.

Depue, R.A. and Kleiman, R.M. (1979) Free cortisol as a peripheral index of central vulnerability to major forms of polar depressive disorders: Examining stress-biology interactions in subsyndromal high-risk persons. In *The Psychobiology of the Depressive Disorders: Implications for the Effects of Stress* (ed. R.A. Depue), Academic Press, New York, pp. 177–204.

Deroche, V., Piazza, P.V., Deminere, J-M., Le Moal, M. and Simon, H. (1993) Rats orally self-administer corticosterone. *Brain Research*, **622**, 315–320.

Deshmukh, V.D. and Deshmukh, S.V. (1990) Stress-adaptation failure hypothesis of Alzheimer's disease. *Medical Hypotheses*, **32**, 293–295.

Desiderato, O., MacKinnon, J.R. and Hissom, H. (1974) Development of gastric ulcers in rats following stress termination. *Journal of Comparative and Physiological Psychology*, **87**, 208–214.

De Souza, E.B. and Appel, N.M. (1991) Distribution of brain and pituitary receptors involved in mediating stress responses. In *Stress—Neurobiology and Neuroendocrinology* (eds M.R. Brown, G.F. Koob and C. Rivier), Marcel Dekker, New York, pp. 91–117.

De Souza, E.B. and Battaglia, G. (1988) Corticotropin-releasing hormone (CRH) receptors in brain. In *Mechanisms of Physical and Emotional Stress* (eds G.P. Chrousos, D.L. Loriaux and P.W. Gold), Plenum Press, New York, pp. 123–136.

De Souza, E.B., Grigoriadis, D.E. and Webster, E.L. (1991) Role of brain, pituitary and spleen corticotropin-releasing factor receptors in the stress response. In *Stress Revisited 1. Neuroendocrinology of Stress* (eds G. Jasmin and M. Cantin), Karger, Basel, pp. 23–44.

Deutsch, J.A. (1979) Intragastric infusion and pressure. *Behavioural and Brain Sciences*, **1**, 105.

De Wied, D. (1969) Effects of peptide hormones on behaviour. In *Frontiers in Neuroendocrinology 1969* (eds W.F. Ganong and L. Martini), Oxford University Press, New York, pp. 97–140.

De Wied, D. (1977) Pituitary adrenal system hormones and behaviour. *Acta Endocrinologica* (Suppl.), **214**, 9–18.

De Wied, D., Bohus, B., Gispen, W.H., Urban, I. and van Wimersma Greidanus, T.B. (1976) Hormonal influences on motivational, learning and memory processes. In *Hormones, Behaviour and Psychopathology* (ed. E.J. Sachar), Raven Press, New York, pp. 1–14.

Dickinson, A. (1980) *Contemporary Animal Learning Theory*. Cambridge University Press.

Dickinson, A. (1985) Actions and habits: the development of behavioural autonomy. *Philosophical Transactions of the Royal Society of London B*, **308**, 67–78.

Dickinson, A. and Balleine, B. (1992) Actions and responses: the dual psychology of behaviour. In *Problems in the Philosophy and Psychology of Spatial Representation* (eds N. Eilan, R.A. McCarthy and M.W. Brewer), Blackwell, Oxford, pp. 277–293.

Dickinson, A. and Dearing, M.F. (1979) Appetitive-aversive interaction and inhibitory processes. In *Mechanisms of Learning and Motivation* (eds A. Dickinson and R.A. Boakes), Lawrence Erlbaum, Hillsdale, pp. 203–231.

Dienstbier, R.A.. (1989) Arousal and physiological toughness: Implications for mental and physical health. *Psychological Review*, **96**, 84–100.

Di Gusto, E.L., Cairncross, K. and King, M.G. (1971) Hormonal influences on fear-motivated responses. *Psychological Bulletin*, **75**, 432–444.

Dimsdale, J.E. and Moss, J. (1980) Plasma catecholamines in stress and exercise. *Journal of the American Medical Association*, **243**, 340–342.

Doerr, H.O. and Hokanson, J.E. (1968) Food deprivation, performance and heart rate in the rat. *Journal of Comparative and Physiological Psychology*, **65**, 227–231.

Dubrovsky, B. (1993) Effects of adrenal cortex hormones on limbic structures: Some experimental and clinical correlations related to depression. *Journal of Psychiatry and Neuroscience*, **18**, 4–16.

Duncan, I.J.H. and Poole, T.B. (1990) Promoting the welfare of farm and captive animals. In *Managing the Behaviour of Animals* (eds P. Monaghan and D. Wood-Gush), Chapman and Hall, London, pp. 193–232.

Duncan, I.J.H., Rushen, J. and Lawrence, A.B. (1993) Conclusions and implications for animal welfare. In *Stereotypic Animal Behaviour— Fundamentals and Applications to Welfare* (eds A.B. Lawrence and J. Rushen), CAB International, Wallingford, pp. 193–206.

Dunn, A.J. (1988) Systemic interleukin-1 administration stimulates hypothalamic norepinephrine metabolism paralleling the increased plasma corticosterone. *Life Sciences*, **43**, 429–435.

Dunn, A.J. (1989) Psychoneuroimmunology for the psychoneuroendocrinologist: A review of animal studies of nervous system–immune system interactions. *Psychoneuroendocrinology*, **14**, 251–274.

Dunn, A.J. and Berridge, C.W. (1990a) Physiological and behavioural responses to corticotropin-releasing factor administration: is CRF a mediator of anxiety or stress responses? *Brain Research Reviews*, **15**, 71–100.

Dunn, A.J. and Berridge, C.W. (1990b) Corticotrophin-releasing factor as the mediator of stress responses. In *Psychobiology of Stress* (eds S. Puglisi and A. Oliverio), Kluwer, Dordrecht, pp. 81–93.

Dunn, A.J. and Kramarcy, N.R. (1984) Neurochemical responses in stress: Relationships between the hypothalamic–pituitary–adrenal and catecholamine systems. In *Handbook of Psychopharmacology*, Vol. 18, *Drugs, Neurotransmitters and Behaviour* (eds L.L. Iversen, S.D. Iversen and S.H. Snyder), Plenum, New York, pp. 455–515.

Dunn, A.J., Antoon, M. and Chapman, Y. (1991) Reduction of exploratory behaviour by intraperitoneal injection of interleukin-1 involves brain corticotrophin-releasing factor. *Brain Research Bulletin*, **26**, 539–542.

Dupont, A., Endröczi, E. and Fortier, C. (1971) Relationship of pituitary–thyroid and pituitary–adrenocortical activities to conditioned behaviour in the rat. In *Influence of Hormones on the Nervous System* (ed. D.H. Ford), Karger, Basel, pp. 451–462.

Eichenbaum, H., Otto, T. and Cohen, N.J. (1994) Two functional components of the hippocampal memory system. *Behavioural and Brain Sciences*, **17**, 449–518.

Eikelboom, R. and Stewart, J. (1982) Conditioning of drug-induced physiological responses. *Psychological Review*, **89**, 507–528.

Eisemann, C.H., Jorgensen, W.K., Merritt, D.J., Rice, M.J., Cribb, B.W., Webb, P.D. and Zalucki, M.P. (1984) Do insects feel pain?—A biological view. *Experientia*, **40**, 164–167.

Elliott, R. (1969) Tonic heart rate: Experiments on the effects of collative variables lead to a hypothesis about its motivational significance. *Journal of Personality and Social Psychology*, **12**, 211–228.

Ely, D.L. and Henry J.P. (1978) Neuroendocrine response patterns in dominant and subordinate mice. *Hormones and Behaviour*, **10**, 156–169.

Endröczi, E. (1972) *Limbic System Learning and Pituitary–Adrenal Function*. Akademiai Kiado, Budapest.

Endröczi, E. and Nyakas, C. (1976) Brain catecholamines and homeostatic behaviour. In *Catecholamines and Stress* (eds Usdin, E., Kvetnansky, R. and Kopin, I.J.), Pergamon Press, Oxford, pp. 9–16.

Engel, B.T. (1985) Stress is a noun! No, a verb! No, an adjective! In *Stress and Coping* (eds T.M. Field, P.M. McCabe and N. Schneiderman), Lawrence Erlbaum, Hillsdale, pp. 3–12.

Epstein, A.N. (1982) Instinct and motivation as explanations for complex behaviour. In *The Physiological Mechanisms of Motivation* (ed. D.W. Pfaff), Springer, New York, pp. 25–58.

Espmark, Y. and Langvatn, R. (1985) Development and habituation of cardiac and behavioral response in young red deer calves (*Cervus elaphus*) exposed to alarm stimuli. *Journal of Mammalogy*, **66**, 702–711.

Exton, J.H. (1979) Regulation of gluconeogenesis by glucocorticoids. In *Glucocorticoid Hormone Action* (eds J.D. Baxter and G.G. Rousseau), Springer-Verlag, Berlin, pp. 535–546.

Fain, J.N. (1979) Inhibition of glucose transport in fat cells and activation of lipolysis by glucocorticoids. In *Glucocorticoid Hormone Action* (eds J.D. Baxter and G.G. Rousseau), Springer-Verlag, Berlin, pp. 547–560.

Fanselow, M.S. (1980) Conditional and unconditional components of post-shock freezing. *Pavlovian Journal of Biological Sciences*, **15**, 177–182.

Fanselow, M.S. (1991) Analgesia as a response to aversive Pavlovian conditional stimuli: Cognitive and emotional mediators. In *Fear, Avoidance and Phobias—A Fundamental Analysis* (ed. M.R. Denny), Lawrence Erlbaum, Hillsdale, pp. 61–86.

Fanselow, M.S. and Lester, L.S. (1988) A functional behaviouristic approach to aversively motivated behaviour: Predatory imminence as a determinant of the topography of defensive behaviour. In *Evolution and Learning* (eds R.C. Bolles and M.D. Beecher), Lawrence Erlbaum, Hillsdale, pp. 185–212.

Fanselow, M.S. and Sigmundi, R.A. (1986) Species-specific danger signals, endogenous opioid analgesia and defensive behaviour. *Journal of Experimental Psychology: Animal Behaviour Processes*, **12**, 301–309.

Fantino, M., Hosotte, J. and Apfelbaum, M. (1986) An opioid antagonist, naltrexone, reduces preference for sucrose in humans. *American Journal of Physiology*, **251**, R91–96.

Fehm, H-L. and Born, J. (1989) In *Frontiers of Stress Research* (eds H. Weiner, I. Florin, R. Murison and D. Hellhammer), Hans Huber, Toronto, pp. 250–261.

Feldman, R.S. (1978) Environmental and physiological determinants of fixated behaviour in mammals. In *1st World Congress on Ethology Applied to Zootechnics*, Editorial Garsi, Madrid, pp. 486–492.

Feldman, S. (1989) Afferent neural pathways and hypothalamic neurotransmitters regulating adrenocortical secretion. In *Frontiers of Stress Re-*

search (eds H. Weiner, I. Florin, R. Murison and D. Hellhammer), Hans Huber, Toronto, pp. 201–208.

Feldman, S. and Dafny, N. (1970) Effects of adrenocortical hormones on the electrical activity of the brain. In *Pituitary, Adrenal and the Brain*, Vol. 32, Progress in Brain Research (eds D. de Wied and J.A.W.M. Weijnen), Elsevier, Amsterdam, pp. 90–101.

Fentress, J.C. (1976) Dynamic boundaries of patterned behaviour: interaction and self-organization. In *Growing Points in Ethology* (eds P.P.G. Bateson and R.A. Hinde), Cambridge University Press, Cambridge, pp. 135–169.

Fentress, J.C. (1977) The tonic hypothesis and the patterning of behaviour. *Annals of the New York Academy of Sciences*, **290**, 370–395.

Fibiger, H.C., Zis, A.P. and Phillips, A.G. (1975) Haloperidol-induced disruption of conditioned avoidance responding: Attenuation by prior training or by anticholinergic drugs. *European Journal of Pharmacology*, **30**, 309–314.

File, S.E. and Peet, L.A. (1980) The sensitivity of the rat corticosterone response to environmental manipulations and to chronic chlordiazepoxide treatment. *Physiology and Behaviour, 25*, 753–758.

Fiorito, G. and Scotto, P. (1992) Observational learning in *Octopus vulgaris. Science, 256*, 545–547.

Fitzgerald, R.D. and Teyler, T.J. (1970) Trace and delayed heart-rate conditioning in rats as a function of US intensity. *Journal of Comparative and Physiological Psychology*, **70**, 242–253.

Foa, E.B., Zinbarg, R. and Rothbaum, B.O. (1992) Uncontrollability and unpredictability in post-traumatic stress disorder: An animal model. *Psychological Bulletin*, **112**, 218–238.

Fokkema, D.S., Smit, K., Van Der Gugten, J. and Koolhaas, J.M. (1988) A coherent pattern among social behaviour, blood pressure, corticosterone and catecholamine measures in individual male rats. *Physiology and Behaviour,* **42**, 485–489.

Foo, H. and Westbrook, R.F. (1994) The form of the conditioned hypoalgesic response resulting from preexposure to a heat stressor depends on the pain test used. *Psychobiology, 22*, 173–179.

Forsyth, R.P. (1974) Mechanisms of the cardiovascular responses to environmental stressors. In *Cardiovascular Psychophysiology* (eds P.A. Obrist, A.H. Black, J. Brener and L.V. DiCara), Aldine Publishing Company, Chicago, pp. 5–32.

Fortier, C. (1966) Nervous control of ACTH secretion. In *The Pituitary Gland* (eds G.W. Harris and B.T. Donovan), Butterworths, London, pp. 195–234.

Fowler, H. and Miller, N.E. (1963) Facilitation and inhibition of runway performance by hind- and forepaw shock of various intensities. *Journal of Comparative and Physiological Psychology, 56*, 801–805.

Fowles, D.C. (1982) Heart rate as an index of anxiety: Failure of a hypothesis. In *Perspectives in Cardiovascular Psychophysiology* (eds J.T. Cacioppo and R.E. Petty), The Guilford Press, New York, pp. 93–123.

Frankenhaeuser, M. (1976) The role of peripheral catecholamines in adaptation to understimulation and overstimulation. In *Psychopathology of Human Adaptation* (ed. G. Serban), Plenum, New York, pp. 173–191.

Fraser, A.F. and Broom, D.M. (1990) *Farm Animal Behaviour and Welfare.* Baillière Tindall, London.

Fraser, D., Ritchie, J.S.D. and Fraser, A.F. (1975) The term 'stress' in a veterinary context. *British Veterinary Journal*, **131**, 653–662.

Freeman, B.M. (1971) Stress and the domestic fowl: a physiological appraisal. *World's Poultry Science Journal*, **27**, 263–275.

Freeman, B.M. (1975) Physiological basis of stress. *Proceedings of the Royal Society of Medicine*, **68**, 427–429.

Freeman, B.M. (1985) Stress and the domestic fowl: Physiological fact or fantasy? *World Poultry Science Journal*, **41**, 45–51.

Freeman, B.M., Manning, A.C.C. and Flack, I.H. (1983) Adrenal cortical activity in the domestic fowl *Gallus domesticus*, following withdrawal of food or water. *Comparative Biochemistry and Physiology*, **79A**, 639–641.

Freeman, B.M., Manning, A.C.C. and Flack, I.H. (1984) Changes in plasma corticosterone concentrations in the water-deprived fowl, *Gallus domesticus*. *Comparative Biochemistry and Physiology*, **79A**, 457–458.

Frith, C.D. and Done, D.J. (1990) Stereotyped behaviour in madness and in health. In *Neurobiology of Stereotyped Behaviour* (eds S.J. Cooper and C.T. Dourish), Clarendon Press, Oxford, pp. 232–259.

Furedy, J.J. and Riley, D.M. (1987) Human Pavlovian autonomic conditioning and the cognitive paradigm. In *Cognitive Processes and Pavlovian Conditioning in Humans* (ed. G. Davey), John Wiley, Chichester, pp. 1–25.

Gabrielsen, G., Kanwisher, J. and Steen, J.B. (1977) 'Emotional' bradycardia: A telemetry study on incubating willow grouse (*Lagopus lagopus*), *Acta Physiologica Scandinavica*, **100**, 255–257.

Gallistel, C.R. (1980) *The Organization of Action—A New Synthesis*. Lawrence Erlbaum, Hillsdale.

Gallistel, C.R. (1990) *The Organization of Learning*. The MIT Press, Cambridge.

Gallup, G.G., Boren, J.L., Suarez, S.D. and Wallnau, L.B. (1983) The psychopharmacology of tonic immobility in chickens. In *The Brain and Behaviour of the Fowl* (ed. T. Ookawa), Japan Scientific Societies Press, Tokyo, pp. 43–59.

Ganong, W.F. (1975) *Review of Medical Physiology*. Lange Medical Publications, Los Altos.

Ganong, W.F., Kramer, N., Reid, I.A., Boryczka, A.T. and Shackelford, R. (1976) Inhibition of stress-induced ACTH secretion by norepinephrine in the dog: Mechanism of action. In *Catecholamines and Stress* (eds E. Usdin, R. Kvetnansky and I.J. Kopin), Pergamon Press, Oxford, pp. 139–143.

Garcia, J. (1989) Food for Tolman: Cognition and cathexis in concert. In *Aversion, Avoidance and Anxiety—Perspectives on Aversively Motivated Behaviour* (eds T. Archer and L-G. Nilsson), Lawrence Erlbaum, Hillsdale, pp. 45–85.

Garrud, P., Gray, J.A. and De Wied, D. (1974) Pituitary–adrenal hormones and extinction of rewarded behaviour in the rat. *Physiology and Behaviour*, **12**, 109–119.

Gilad, G.M., Mahon, B.D., Finkelstein, Y., Koffler, B. and Gilad, V.H. (1985) Stress-induced activation of the hippocampal cholinergic system and the pituitary–adrenocortical axis. *Brain Research*, **347**, 404–408.

Glavin, G.B. (1985) Stress and brain noradrenaline: A review. *Neuroscience and Biobehavioural Reviews*, **9**, 233–243.

Glavin, G.B. (1993) Vulnerability to stress ulcerogenesis in rats differing in anxiety: A dopaminergic correlate. *Journal of Physiology (Paris)*, **87**, 239–243.

Glavin, G.B., Murison, R., Overmier, J.B., Pare, W.P., Bakke, H.K., Henke, P.G. and Hernandez, D.E. (1991) The neurobiology of stress ulcers. *Brain Research Reviews*, **16**, 301–343.

Glickman, S.E. and Schiff, B.B. (1967) A biological theory of reinforcement. *Psychological Review,* **74**, 81–109.

Goesling, W.J., Buchholz, A.R. and Carreira, C.J. (1974) Conditioned immobility and ulcer development in rats. *Journal of General Psychology,* **91**, 231–236.

Gold, P.W., Kling, M.A., Whitfield, H.J., Rabin, D., Margioris, A., Kalogeras, K., Demitrack, M., Loriaux, D.L. and Chrousos, G.P. (1988) The clinical implications of corticotropin-releasing hormone. In *Mechanisms of Physical and Emotional Stress* (eds G.P. Chrousos, D.L. Loriaux and P.W. Gold), Plenum, New York, pp. 507–519.

Goldman, L., Coover, G.D. and Levine, S. (1973) Bidirectional effects of reinforcement shifts on pituitary adrenal activity. *Physiology and Behaviour,* **10**, 209–214.

Goldstein, R., Beideman, L.R. and Stern, J.A. (1970) Effect of water deprivation and saline-induced thirst on the conditioned heart rate response of the rat. *Physiology and Behaviour,* **5**, 583–587.

Granner, D.K. (1979) The role of glucocorticoid hormones as biological amplifiers. In *Glucocorticoid Hormone Action* (eds J.D. Baxter and G.G. Rousseau), Springer-Verlag, Berlin, pp. 593–611.

Grau, J.W. (1987) The central representation of an aversive event maintains the opioid and nonopioid forms of analgesia. *Behavioural Neuroscience,* **101**, 272–288.

Gray, G.D., Bergfors, A.M., Levin, R. and Levine, S. (1978) Comparison of the effects of restricted morning or evening water intake on adrenocortical activity in female rats. *Neuroendocrinology,* **25**, 236–246.

Gray, J.A. (1982) Multiple book review of *The Neuropsychology of anxiety: An enquiry into the Functions of the Septohippocampal System. Behavioural and Brain Sciences,* **5**, 469–534.

Gray, J.A. (1987) *The Psychology of Fear and Stress.* Cambridge University Press.

Gray, J.A. (1991) Neural systems, emotion and personality. In *Neurobiology of Learning, Emotion and Affect* (ed. J. Madden IV), Raven Press, New York, pp. 273–306.

Gray, J.A. (1993) Discussion in *Experimental and Theoretical Studies of Consciousness* (Ciba Foundation Symposium 174) (eds R. Bock and J. Marsh), John Wiley, Chichester, pp. 165–166.

Gray, T.S. (1991) Limbic pathways and neurotransmitters as mediators of autonomic and neuroendocrine response to stress. The amygdala. In *Stress—Neurobiology and Neuroendocrinology* (eds M.R. Brown, G.F. Koob and C. Rivier), Marcel Dekker, New York, pp. 73–89.

Grossman, A.B. (1991) Regulation of human pituitary responses to stress. In *Stress—Neurobiology and Neuroendocrinology* (eds M.R. Brown, G.F. Koob and C. Rivier), Marcel Dekker, New York, pp. 151–171.

Groves, P.M. and Thompson, R.F. (1970) Habituation: A dual process theory. *Psychological Review,* **77**, 419–450.

Guile, M.N. and McCutcheon, N.B. (1980) Prepared responses and gastric lesions in rats. *Physiological Psychology,* **8**, 480–482.

Guile, M.N. and McCutcheon, N.B. (1984) Effects of naltrexone and signaling inescapable electric shock on nociception and gastric lesions in rats. *Behavioural Neuroscience,* **98**, 695–702.

Guth, S., Seward, J.P. and Levine, S. (1971) Differential manipulation of passive avoidance by exogenous ACTH. *Hormones and Behaviour,* **2**, 127–138.

Guyton, A.C. (1971) *Basic Human Physiology: Normal Function and Mechanisms of Disease*. W.B. Saunders, Philadelphia.

Guyton, A.C. (1991) *Textbook of Medical Physiology*. W.B. Saunders, Philadelphia.

Hall, G. and Honey, R.C. (1990) Context-specific conditioning in the conditioned-emotional-response procedure. *Journal of Experimental Psychology: Animal Behaviour Processes*, **16**, 271–278.

Haller, J. (1993) Adrenomedullar catecholamine liberation and carbohydrate metabolism during the first 30 min of an aggressive encounter in rats. *Physiology and Behaviour*, **54**, 195–197.

Hamburg, D.A., Hamburg, B.A. and Barchas, J.D. (1975) Anger and depression in the perspective of behavioural biology. In *Emotions—Their Parameters and Measurements*. Raven Press, New York, pp. 235–278.

Hanson, J.D., Larson, M.E. and Snowdon, C.T. (1976) The effects of control over high intensity noise on plasma cortisol levels in rhesus monkeys. *Behavioural Biology*, **16**, 333–340.

Harris-Warrick, R.M. and Flamm, R.E. (1986) Chemical modulation of a small central pattern generator circuit. *Trends in Neural Sciences*, **9**, 432–437.

Hart, B.L. (1988) Biological basis of the behaviour of sick animals. *Neuroscience and Biobehavioural Reviews*, **12**, 123–137.

Harvey, S., Phillips, J.G., Rees, A. and Hall, T.R. (1984) Stress and adrenal function. *The Journal of Experimental Zoology*, **232**, 633–645.

Hawkins, R.D. and Advokat, C. (1977) Effects of behavioural state on the gill-withdrawal reflex in *Aplysia Californica*. In *Aspects of Behavioural Neurobiology*, Vol. III, (Society for Neuroscience Symposia) (ed. J.A. Ferrendelli), Society for Neuroscience, Bethesda, pp. 16–32.

Hayes, R.L., Bennett, G.J., Newlon, P.G. and Mayer, D.J. (1978) Behavioural and physiological studies of non-narcotic analgesia in the rat elicited by certain environmental stimuli. *Brain Research*, **155**, 69–90.

Hedge, G.A. and Smelik, P.G. (1968) Corticotropin release: Inhibition by intrahypothalamic implantation of atropine. *Science*, **159**, 891–892.

Hemsworth, P.H. and Barnett, J.L. (1987) Human–animal interactions. In *The Veterinary Clinics of North America*, Vol. 3, No. 2 (ed. E.O. Price), W.B. Saunders, Philadelphia, pp. 339–356.

Henkin, R.I. (1970) The effects of corticosteroids and ACTH on sensory systems. In *Pituitary, Adrenal and the Brain*, Vol. 32, Progress in Brain Research (eds D. de Wied and J.A.W.M. Weijnen), Elsevier, Amsterdam, pp. 270–294.

Hennessy, J.W. and Levine, S. (1979) Stress, arousal and the pituitary–adrenal system: A psychoendocrine hypothesis. In: *Progress in Psychobiology and Physiological Psychology*, Vol. 8 (eds J.M. Sprague and A.N. Epstein), Academic Press, New York, pp. 133–178.

Hennessy, J.W., Smotherman, W.P. and Levine, S. (1976) Conditioned taste aversion and the pituitary–adrenal system. *Behavioural Biology*, **16**, 413–424.

Hennessy, M.B. and Levine, S. (1978) Sensitive pituitary-adrenal responsiveness to varying intensities of psychological stimulation. *Physiology and Behaviour*, **21**, 295–297.

Hennessy, M.B., Becker, L.A. and O'Neil, D.R. (1991) Peripherally administered CRH suppresses the vocalizations of isolated guinea pig pups. *Physiology and Behaviour*, **50**, 17–22.

Henry, J.P. (1976) Mechanisms of psychosomatic disease in animals. *Advances in Veterinary Science and Comparative Medicine*, **20**, 115–145.

Henry, J.P. (1980) Present concept of stress theory. In *Catecholamines and Stress: Recent Advances* (eds E. Usdin, R. Kvetnansky and I.J. Kopin), Elsevier/North-Holland, New York, pp. 557–571.

Henry, J.P. (1982) The relation of social to biological processes in disease. *Social Science and Medicine*, **16**, 369–380.

Henry, JP., Kross, M.E., Stephens, P.M. and Watson, F.M.C. (1976) Evidence that differing psychological stimuli lead to adrenal cortical stimulation by autonomic pathways. In *Catecholamines and Stress* (eds E. Usdin, R. Kvetnansky and I.J. Kopin), Pergamon Press, Oxford, pp. 457–468.

Henry, J.P., Stephen, P.M. and Ely, D.L. (1986) Psychosocial hypertension and the defence and defeat reactions. *Journal of Hypertension*, **4**, 687–697.

Herman, B.H. and Panksepp, J. (1978) Effects of morphine and naloxone on separation distress and approach attachment: Evidence for opiate mediation of social affect. *Pharmacology Biochemistry and Behaviour*, **9**, 213–220.

Herman, J.P., Schafer, M.K.-H., Young, E.A., Thompson, R., Douglass, J., Akil, H. and Watson, S.J. (1989) Evidence for hippocampal regulation of neuroendocrine neurons of the hypothalamo–pituitary–adrenocortical axis. *Journal of Neuroscience*, **9**, 3072–3082.

Hernandez, D.E., Arandia, D. and Dehasa, M. (1993) Role of psychosomatic factors in peptic ulcer disease. *Journal of Physiology (Paris)*, **87**, 223–227.

Hernandez, D.E., Adcock, J.W., Nemeroff, C.B. and Prange, A.J. (1984) The role of the adrenal gland in cytoprotection against stress-induced gastric ulcers in rats. *Journal of Neuroscience Research*, **11**, 193–201.

Heybach, J.P. and Vernikos-Danellis, J. (1979a) Inhibition of the pituitary–adrenal response to stress during deprivation-induced feeding. *Endocrinology*, **104**, 967–973.

Heybach, J.P. and Vernikos-Danellis, J. (1979b) Inhibition of adrenocorticotrophin secretion during deprivation-induced eating and drinking in rats. *Neuroendocrinology*, **28**, 329–338.

Heyes, C.M. and Dawson, G.R. (1990) A demonstration of observational learning in rats using a biodirectional control. *Quarterly Journal of Experimental Psychology*, **42B**, 59–71.

Hill, R.T. (1970) Facilitation of conditioned reinforcement as a mechanism of psychomotor stimulation. In *Amphetamines and Related Compounds* (eds E. Costa and S. Garanttini), Raven Press, New York, pp. 781–795.

Hillhouse, E.W., Burden, J. and Jones, M.T. (1975) The effect of various putative neurotransmitters on the release of corticotrophin releasing hormone from the hypothalamus of the rat *in vitro*. I. The effect of acetylcholine and noradrenaline. *Neuroendocrinology*, **17**, 1–11.

Hirsh, R. (1974) The hippocampus and contextual retrieval of information from memory: A theory. *Behavioural Biology*, **12**, 421–444.

Hogan, J.A. and Roper, T.J. (1978) A comparison of the properties of different reinforcers. In *Advances in the Study of Behaviour*, Vol. 8 (eds J.S. Rosenblatt, R.A. Hinde, C. Beer and M-C. Busnel), Academic Press, New York, pp. 155–255.

Hollis, K.L. (1984) The biological function of Pavlovian conditioning: the best defense is a good offense. *Journal of Experimental Psychology: Animal Behaviour Processes*, **10**, 413–425.

Holst, D. von (1986) Vegetative and somatic components of tree shrews' behaviour. *Journal of the Autonomic Nervous System*, (Suppl.) 657–670.

Houston, A. and Sumida, B. (1985) A positive feedback model for switching between two activities. *Animal Behaviour,* **33**, 315–325.

Hucklebridge, F.H., Gamal-el-Din, L. and Brain, P.F. (1981) Social status and the adrenal medulla in the house mouse (*Mus musculus* L.). *Behavioural and Neural Biology,* **33**, 345–363.

Hughes, B.O. (1980) The assessment of behavioural needs. In *The Laying Hen and its Environment* (ed. R. Moss), The Hague, Martinus Nijhoff, pp. 149–159.

Hughes, B.O. (1988) Discussion 2 (in Proceedings from Workshop in Behavioural Needs). *Applied Animal Behaviour Science,* **19**, 356–367.

Hughes, B.O. and Duncan, I.J.H. (1988a) The notion of ethological 'need', models of motivation and animal welfare. *Animal Behaviour,* **36**, 1696–1707.

Hughes, B.O. and Duncan, I.J.H. (1988b). Behavioural needs: Can they be explained in terms of motivational models? *Applied Animal Behaviour Science,* **19**, 352–355.

Imperato, A., Angelucci, L., Casolini, P., Zocchi, A. and Puglisi-Allegra, S. (1992) Repeated stressful experiences differently affect limbic dopamine release during and following stress. *Brain Research,* **577**, 194–199.

Ingram, D.L., Dauncey, M.J., Barrand, M.A. and Callingham, B.A. (1980) Variations in plasma catecholamines in the young pig in response to extremes of ambient temperature compared with exercise and feeding. In *Catecholamines and Stress: Recent Advances* (eds E. Usdin, R. Kvetnansky and I.J. Kopin), Elsevier/North-Holland, Amsterdam, pp. 273–278.

Isaacson, R.L. and Gispen, W.H. (1990) Neuropeptides and the issue of stereotypy in behaviour. In *Neurobiology of Stereotyped Behaviour* (eds S.J. Cooper and C.T. Dourish), Clarendon Press, Oxford, pp. 117–141.

Iwata, J. and LeDoux, J.E. (1988) Dissociation of associative and nonassociative concomitants of classical fear conditioning in the freely behaving rat. *Behavioural Neuroscience,* **102**, 66–76.

Jacquet, Y.F. (1978) Opiate effects after adrenocorticotropin or B-endorphin injection in the periaqueductal gray matter of rats. *Science,* **201**, 1032–1034.

Jacquet, Y.F. (1980) B-endorphin and ACTH: inhibitory and excitatory neurohormones of pain and fear. *Behavioural and Brain Sciences,* **3**, 312–313.

Jaworska, K. and Soltysik, S. (1962) Studies on the aversive classical conditioning 3. Cardiac responses to conditioned and unconditioned defensive (aversive) stimuli. *Acta Biologiae Experimentalis,* **22**, 193–214.

Jefferys, D. and Funder, J.W. (1987) Glucocorticoids, adrenal medullary opioids and the retention of a behavioural response after stress. *Endocrinology,* 121, 1006–1009.

Jensen, P. (1995) Stress as a motivational state. *Acta Agriculturae Scandinavica,* in press.

Jensen, P. and Toates, F.M. (1993) Who needs 'behavioural needs'? Motivational aspects of the needs of animals. *Applied Animal Behaviour Science,* **37**, 161–181.

Jewell, D.S. and Mylander, M. (1988) The psychology of stress: Run silent, run deep. In *Mechanisms of Physical and Emotional Stress* (eds G.P. Chrousos, D.L. Loriaux and P.W. Gold), Plenum, New York, pp. 489–505.

Johnson, J.T. and Levine, S. (1973) Influence of water deprivation on adrenocortical rhythms. *Neuroendocrinology,* **11**, 268–273.

Jones, G.H., Mittleman, G. and Robbins, T.W. (1989) Attenuation of amphetamine-stereotypy by mesostriatal dopamine depletion enhances plasma corticosterone: Implications for stereotypy as a coping response. *Behavioural and Neural Biology,* **51**, 80–91.

Jurcovicova, J., Jezova, D. and Vigas, M. (1980) The role of central catecholamines in rat growth hormone response during stress. In *Catecholamines and Stress: Recent Advances* (eds E. Usdin, R. Kvetnansky and I.J. Kopin), Elsevier/North-Holland, New York, pp. 167–170.

Kavaliers, M. (1987) Evidence for opioid and non-opioid forms of stress-induced analgesia in the snail *Cepaea nemoralis. Brain Research,* **410**, 111–115.

Kavaliers, M. (1988) Evolutionary and comparative aspects of nociception. *Brain Research Bulletin,* **21**, 923–931.

Kavaliers, M. (1989) Evolutionary aspects of the neuromodulation of nociceptive behaviours. *American Zoologist,* **29**, 1345–1353.

Kehoe, P. (1989) The neuropharmacology of neonatal rat's separation vocalizations. In *Molecular Biology of Stress* (eds S. Breznitz and O. Zinder), Alan R. Liss, New York, pp. 307–317.

Keiper, R.R. (1969) Causal factors of stereotypies in caged birds. *Animal Behaviour,* **17**, 114–119.

Keller-Wood, M.E. and Dallman, M.F. (1984) Corticosteroid inhibition of ACTH secretion. *Endocrine Reviews,* **5**, 1–24.

Kennedy, J. (1992) *The New Anthropomorphism.* Cambridge University Press.

Kennes, D., Ödberg, F.O., Bouquet, Y. and De Rycke, P.H. (1988) Changes in naloxone and haloperidol effects during the development of captivity-induced jumping stereotypy in bank voles. *European Journal of Pharmacology,* **153**, 19–24.

Keverne, E.B., Martensz, N.D. and Tuite, B. (1989) Beta-endorphin concentrations in cerebrospinal fluid of monkeys are influenced by grooming relationships. *Psychoneuroendocrinology,* **14**, 155–161.

Keyes, J.B. (1974) Effect of ACTH on ECS-produced amnesia of a passive avoidance task. *Physiological Psychology,* **2**, 307–309.

Kimble, G.A. and Perlmuter, L.C. (1970) The problem of volition. *Psychological Review,* **77**, 361–384.

Komisaruk, B.R. and Whipple, B. (1986) Vaginal stimulation-produced analgesia in rats and women. *Annals of the New York Academy of Sciences,* **467**, 30–39.

Koob, G.F. (1985) Stress, corticotrophin-releasing factor and behaviour. *Perspectives on Behavioural Medicine,* **2**, 39–52.

Koob, G.F. (1991) Behavioural responses to stress. Focus on corticotropin-releasing factor. In *Stress—Neurobiology and Neuroendocrinology* (eds M.R. Brown, G.F. Koob and C. Rivier), Marcel Dekker, New York, pp. 255–271.

Koob, G.F., Thatcher-Briton, K., Tazi, A. and Le Moal, M. (1988) Behavioural pharmacology of stress: Focus on CNS corticotropin-releasing factor. In *Mechanisms of Physical and Emotional Stress* (eds G.P. Chrousos, D.L. Loriaux and P.W. Gold), Plenum, New York, pp. 25–34.

Koolhaas, J.M., Hermann, P.M., Kemperman, C., Bohus, B., Van den Hoofdakker, R.H. and Beersma, D.G.M. (1990) Single social defeat in male rats induces a gradual but long lasting behavioural change: A model of depression? *Neuroscience Research Communications,* **7**, 35–41.

Kovacs, G.L., Telegdy, G. and Lissak, K. (1976) 5-hydroxytryptamine and the mediation of pituitary–adrenocortical hormones in the extinction of active avoidance behaviour. *Psychoneuroendocrinology,* **1**, 219–230.

Krebs, C.J., Gaines, M.S., Keller, B.L., Myers, J.H. and Tamarin, R.H. (1973) Population cycles in small rodents. *Science,* **179**, 35–41.

Krieger, D.T. (1974) Food and water restriction shifts corticosterone, temperature, activity and brain amine periodicity. *Endocrinology*, **95**, 1195–1201.

Krieger, H.P. and Krieger, D.T. (1970) Chemical stimulation of the brain: Effect on adrenal corticoid release. *American Journal of Physiology*, **218**, 1632–1641.

Krishnan, K.R.R., Doraiswamy, P.M., Venkataraman, S. and Reed, D.A. (1991) Current concepts in hypothalamo–pituitary–adrenal axis regulation. In *Stress, Neuropeptides and Systemic Disease* (eds J.A. McCubbin, P.G. Kaufmann and C.B. Nemeroff), Academic Press, San Diego, pp. 19–35.

Kronfol, Z. and Schlechte, J. (1986) Depression, hormones and immunity. In *Enkephalins and Endorphins—Stress and the Immune System* (eds N.P. Plotnikoff, R.E. Faith, A.J. Murgo and R.A. Good), Plenum, New York, pp. 69–80.

Kuchel, O. (1991) Stress and catecholamines. In *Stress Revisited 1. Neuroendocrinology of Stress* (eds G. Jasmin and M. Cantin), Karger, Basel, pp. 80–103.

Kvetnansky, R. (1980) Recent progress in catecholamines under stress. In *Catecholamines and Stress: Recent Advances.* (eds E. Usdin, R. Kvetnansky and I. Kopin), Elsevier, North Holland, Amsterdam, pp. 7–18.

Kvetnansky, R., Mitro, A., Palkovits, M., Brownstein, M., Torda, T., Vigas, M. and Mikulaj, L. (1976) Catecholamines in individual hypothalamic nuclei in stressed rats. In *Catecholamines and Stress* (eds E. Usdin, R. Kvetnansky, and I.J. Kopin), Pergamon Press, Oxford, pp. 39–50.

Laborit, H. (1982) Depression and the action inhibitory system (AIS) *Behavioural and Brain Sciences, 5,* 111.

Laborit, H. (1986) *L'inhibition de l'action.* Masson, Paris.

Ladewig, J., de Passillé, A.M., Rushen, J., Schouten, W., Terlouw, E.M.C. and von Borell, E. (1993) Stress and the physiological correlates of stereotypic behaviour. In *Stereotypic Animal Behaviour—Fundamentals and Applications to Welfare* (eds A.B. Lawrence and J. Rushen), CAB International, Wallingford, pp. 97–118.

Lashley, K.S. (1951) The problem of serial order in behaviour. In *Cerebral Mechanisms in Behaviour* (ed. L.A. Jeffress), Wiley, New York, pp. 112–136.

Lashley, K.S. (1921) Studies of cerebral function in learning. II. The effects of long continued practice upon cerebral localization. *Journal of Comparative Psychology,* **1**, 453–468.

Laudenslager, M.L., Ryan, S.M., Drugan, R.C., Hyson, R.L. and Maier, S.F. (1983) Coping and immunosuppression: Inescapable but not escapable shock suppresses lymphocyte proliferation. *Science,* **221**, 568–570.

Lefcourt, A.M. (1986) Usage of the term 'stress' as it applies to cattle. *Vlaams Diergeneeskundig Tijdschrift*, **55**, 258–265.

Le Moal, M. and Simon, H. (1991) Mesocorticolimbic dopaminergic network: Functional and regulatory roles. *Physiological Reviews, 71,* 155–234.

Lenz, H.J. (1990) Mediation of gastrointestinal stress responses by corticotropin-releasing factor. *Annals of the New York Academy of Sciences,* **597**, 81–91.

Lenz, H.J., Raedler, A., Greten, H. and Brown, M.R. (1987) CRF initiates biological actions within the brain that are observed in response to stress. *American Journal of Physiology,* **252**, R34–39.

Leshner, A.I. (1980) The interaction of experience and neuroendocrine factors in determining behavioural adaptations to aggression. *Progress in Brain Research,* **53**, 427–438.

Leshner, A.I. (1982) An alternative hypothesis of depression. *Behavioural and Brain Sciences*, **5**, 111–112.

Leshner, A.I. and Politch, J.A. (1979) Hormonal control of submissiveness in mice: Irrelevance of the androgens and relevance of the pituitary–adrenal hormones. *Physiology and Behaviour*, **22**, 531–534.

Lester, L.S. and Fanselow, M.S. (1985) Exposure to a cat produces opioid analgesia in rats. *Behavioural Neuroscience*, **99**, 756–759.

Levenson, R.W. (1987) Alcohol, affect, and physiology: Positive effects in the early stages of drinking. In *Stress and Addiction* (eds E. Gottheil, K.A. Druley, S. Pashko and S.P. Weinstein), Brunner/Mazel Publishers, New York, pp. 173–196.

Levine, A.S. and Billington, C.J. (1991) Stress, peptides and regulation of ingestive behaviour. In *Stress, Neuropeptides and Systemic Disease* (eds J.A. McCubbin, P.G. Kaufmann and C.B. Nemeroff), Academic Press, San Diego, pp. 327–339.

Levine, S. (1971) Stress and behaviour. *Scientific American*, **224** (1), 26–31.

Levine, S. and Brush, F.R. (1967) Adrenocortical activity and avoidance learning as a function of time after avoidance training. *Physiology and Behaviour*, **2**, 385–388.

Levine, S. and Coe, C.L. (1985) The use and abuse of cortisol as a measure of stress. In *Stress and Coping* (eds T.M. Field, P.M. McCabe and N. Schneiderman), Lawrence Erlbaum, Hillsdale, pp. 149–159.

Levine, S. and Coover, G.D. (1976) Environmental control of suppression of the pituitary–adrenal system. *Physiology and Behaviour*, **17**, 35–37.

Levine, S. and Jones, L.E. (1965) Adrenocorticotropic hormone (ACTH) and passive avoidance learning. *Journal of Comparative and Physiological Psychology*, **59**, 357–360.

Levine, S., Weinberg, J. and Brett, L.P. (1979) Inhibition of pituitary–adrenal activity as a consequence of consummatory behaviour. *Psychoneuroendocrinology*, **4**, 275–286.

Lewis, D.J. (1979) Psychobiology of active and inactive memory. *Psychological Bulletin*, **86**, 1054–1083.

Lewis, J.W., Cannon, J.T. and Liebeskind, J.C. (1980) Opioid and nonopioid mechanisms of stress analgesia. *Science*, **208**, 623–625.

Lewis, J.W., Tordoff, M.G., Sherman, J.E. and Liebeskind, J.C. (1982) Adrenal medullary enkephalin-like peptides may mediate opioid stress analgesia. *Science*, **217**, 557–559.

Lewis, J.W., Cannon, J.T. and Liebeskind, J.C. (1983) Involvement of central muscarinic cholinergic mechanisms in opioid stress analgesia. *Brain Research*, **270**, 289–293.

Lewis, J.W., Morgan, M.M. and Marek, P. (1989) Stress-induced analgesia. In *Frontiers of Stress Research* (eds H. Weiner, I. Florin, R. Murison and D. Hellhammer), Hans Huber, Toronto, pp. 21–36.

Liddle, G.W. (1967) Cushing's syndrome. In *The Adrenal Cortex* (ed. A.B. Eisenstein), Little, Brown and Company, Boston, pp. 523–551.

Lieblich, I., Yirmiya, R. and Liebeskind, J.C. (1991) Intake of and preference for sweet solutions are attenuated in morphine-withdrawn rats. *Behavioural Neuroscience*, **105**, 965–970.

Ludlow, A.R. (1980) The evolution and simulation of a decision maker. In *Analysis of Motivational Processes* (eds F.M. Toates and T.R. Halliday), Academic Press, London, pp. 273–296.

Lundberg, U. and Frankenhaeuser, M. (1980) Pituitary–adrenal and sympathetic–adrenal correlates of distress and effort. *Journal of Psychosomatic Research*, **24**, 125–130.

Lyon, M. and Robbins, T. (1975) The action of central nervous system stimulant drugs: A general theory concerning amphetamine effects. In *Current Developments in Psychopharmacology*, Vol. 2 (eds W.B. Essman and L. Valzelli), Spectrum Publications, New York, pp. 79–163.

McCarty, R. (1983) Stress, behaviour and the sympathetic–adrenal medullary system. In *Stress and Alcohol Use* (eds L.A. Pohorecky and J. Brick), Elsevier, New York, pp. 7–22.

McKearney, J.W. (1968) Maintenance of responding under a fixed-interval schedule of electric shock presentation. *Science*, **160**, 1249–1251.

MacLennan, A.J., Drugan, R.C., Hyson, R.L., Maier, S.F., Madden, J. and Barchas, J.D. (1982) Corticosterone: A critical factor in an opioid form of stress-induced analgesia. *Science*, **215**, 1530–1532.

McCubbin, J.A. (1991) Diminished opioid inhibition of blood pressure and pituitary function in hypertension development. In *Stress, Neuropeptides and Systemic Disease* (eds J.A. McCubbin, P.G. Kaufmann and C.B. Nemeroff), Academic Press, San Diego, pp. 445–466.

McCubbin, J.A. (1993) Stress and endogenous opioids: Behavioural and circulatory interactions. *Biological Psychology*, **35**, 91–122.

McCubbin, J.A., Kizer, J.S. and Lipton, M.A. (1984) Naltrexone prevents footshock-induced performance deficit in rats. *Life Sciences*, **34**, 2057–2066.

McCullough, L.D., Sokolowski, J.D. and Salamone, J.D. (1993) A neurochemical and behavioural investigation of the involvement of nucleus accumbens dopamine in instrumental avoidance. *Neuroscience*, **52**, 919–925.

McEwen, B.S. (1970) Discussion comment. In *Pituitary, Adrenal and the Brain*, Vol. 32, Progress in Brain Research, (eds D. de Wied and J.A.W.M. Weijnen), Elsevier, Amsterdam, pp. 233–234.

McEwen, B.S. (1979) Influences of adrenocortical hormones on pituitary and brain function. In *Glucocorticoid Hormone Action* (eds J.D. Baxter and G.G. Rousseau), Springer-Verlag, Berlin, pp. 467–492.

McEwen, B.S. and Brinton, R.E. (1987) Neuroendocrine aspects of adaptation. In *Progress in Behaviour Research*, Vol. 72 (eds E.R. de Kloet, V.M. Wiegant and D. de Wied), Elsevier, Amsterdam, pp. 11–26.

McEwen, B.S. and Weiss, J.M. (1970) The uptake and action of corticosterone: Regional and subcellular studies on rat brain. In *Pituitary, Adrenal and the Brain*, Vol. 32, Progress in Brain Research (eds D. de Wied and J.A.W.M. Weijnen), Elsevier, Amsterdam, pp. 200–212.

McEwen, B.S., De Kloet, E.R. and Rostene, W. (1986) Adrenal steroid receptors and actions in the nervous system. *Physiological Reviews*, **66**, 1121–1188.

McEwen, B.S., Brinton, R.E. and Sapolsky, R.M. (1988) Glucocorticoid receptors and behaviour. In *Mechanisms of Physical and Emotional Stress* (eds G.P. Chrousos, D.L. Loriaux and P.W. Gold), Plenum, New York, pp. 35–45.

McEwen, B.S., Chao, H.M., Gannon, M.N. and Spencer, R.L. (1991) Characterization of brain adrenal steroid receptors and their involvement in the stress response. In *Stress—Neurobiology and Neuroendocrinology* (eds M.R. Brown, G.F. Koob and C. Rivier), Marcel Dekker, New York, pp. 275–292.

McFarland, D.J. and McFarland, F.J. (1968) Dynamic analysis of an avian drinking response. *Medical and Biological Engineering*, **6**, 659–668.

McNaughton, N. (1994) The hippocampus: relational processor or antiprocessor? *Behavioural and Brain Sciences*, **17**, 487–488.

Maestripieri, D., Schino, G., Aureli, F. and Troisi, A. (1992) A modest proposal: displacement activities as an indicator of emotions in primates. *Animal Behaviour,* **44**, 967–979.

Maickel, R.P., Matussek, N., Stern, D.N. and Brodie, B.B. (1967) The sympathetic nervous system as a homeostatic mechanism. I. Absolute need for sympathetic nervous function in body temperature maintenance of cold-exposed rats. *Journal of Pharmacology and Experimental Therapeutics,* **157**, 103–110.

Maier, S.F. (1989) Determinants of the nature of environmentally induced hypoalgesia. *Behavioural Neuroscience,* **1093**, 131–143.

Maier, S.F., Drugan, R.C. and Grau, J.W. (1982) Controllability, coping behaviour and stress-induced analgesia in the rat. *Pain,* **12**, 47–56.

Maier, S.F., Ryan, S.M., Barksdale, C.M. and Kalin, N.H. (1986) Stressor controllability and the pituitary–adrenal system. *Behavioural Neuroscience,* **100**, 669–674.

Maier, S.F., Watkins, L.R. and Fleshner, M. (1994) Psychoneuroimmunology. *American Psychologist,* **49**, 1004–1017.

Malmo, R.B. and Bélanger, D. (1967) Related physiological and behavioural changes: What are their determinants. *Research Publications of the Association for Research in Nervous and Mental Diseases,* **45**, 288–318.

Manuck, S.B., Kaplan, J.R. and Clarkson, T.B. (1986) Atherosclerosis, social dominance and cardiovascular reactivity. In *Biological and Psychological Factors in Cardiovascular Disease* (eds T.H. Schmidt, T.M. Dembroski and G. Blumchen), Springer-Verlag, Berlin, pp. 459–475.

Marx, M.H. (1972) Unconditioned chewing response in the rat as a measure of reaction to frustration. *Psychological Reports,* **30**, 613–614.

Mason, G.J. (1991) Sterotypies: a critical review. *Animal Behaviour,* **41**, 1015–1037.

Mason, G.J. (1993) Forms of stereotypic behaviour. In *Stereotypic Animal Behaviour—Fundamentals and Applications to Welfare* (eds A.B. Lawrence and J. Rushen), CAB International, Wallingford, pp. 7–40.

Mason, G.J. and Turner, M.A. (1993) Mechanisms involved in the development and control of stereotypies. In *Perspectives in Ethology,* Vol. 10 (eds P.P.G. Bateson, P.H. Klopfer and N.S. Thompson), Plenum, New York, pp. 53–85.

Mason, J.W. (1968) Organization of the multiple endocrine responses to avoidance in the monkey. *Psychosomatic Medicine,* **30**, 774–790.

Mason, J.W. (1971) A re-evaluation of the concept of 'non-specificity' in stress theory. *Journal of Psychiatric Research,* **8**, 323–333.

Mason, J.W. (1972) Organization of psychoendocrine mechanisms. In *Handbook of Psychophysiology* (eds N.S. Greenfield and R.A. Sternbach), Holt, Rinehart and Winston, Inc., New York, pp. 3–91.

Mason, J.W. (1975) A historical view of the stress field. *Journal of Human Stress,* **1**, 22–36.

Mason, J.W. and Brady, J.V. (1956) Plasma 17-hydroxycorticosteroid changes related to reserpine effects on emotional behaviour. *Science,* **124**, 983–984.

Mason, J.W., Giller, E.L., Kosten, T.R., Ostroff, R.B. and Podd, L. (1986) Urinary free-cortisol levels in posttraumatic stress disorder patients. *Journal of Nervous and Mental Disease,* **174**, 145–149.

Masterson, F.A. and Crawford, M. (1982) The defense motivation system: A theory of avoidance behaviour. *The Behavioural and Brain Sciences,* **5**, 661–696.

Mather, J.G. (1981) Wheel-running activity: a new interpretation. *Mammal Review*, **11**, 41–51.

Mayr, E. (1974) Behaviour programs and evolutionary strategies. *American Scientist*, **62**, 650–659.

Meaney, M.J., Bhatnagar, S., Diorio, J., Larocque, S., Francis, D., O'Donnell, D., Shanks, N., Sharma, S., Smythe, J. and Viau, V. (1993) Molecular basis for the development of individual differences in the hypothalamic–pituitary–adrenal stress response. *Cellular and Molecular Neurobiology*, **13**, 321–347.

Melzack, R. and Wall, P. (1984) *The Challenge of Pain*. Penguin Books, Harmondsworth.

Micco, D.J. and McEwen, B.S. (1980) Glucocorticoids, the hippocampus and behaviour: interactive relation between task activation and steroid hormone binding specificity. *Journal of Comparative and Physiological Psychology*, **94**, 624–633.

Micco, D.J., McEwen, B.S. and Shein, W. (1979) Modulation of behavioural inhibition in appetitive extinction following manipulation of adrenal steroids in rats: Implications for involvement of the hippocampus. *Journal of Comparative and Physiological Psychology*, **93**, 323–329.

Michael, R.P. and Gibbons, J.L. (1963) Interrelationships between the endocrine system and neuropsychiatry. *International Review of Neurobiology*, **5**, 243–302.

Micheau, J., Destrade, C. and Soumireu-Mourat, B. (1981) Intraventricular corticosterone injection facilitates memory of an appetitive discriminative task in mice. *Behavioural and Neural Biology*, **31**, 100–104.

Micheau, J., Destrade, C. and Soumireu-Mourat, B. (1985) Time-dependent effects of posttraining intrahippocampal injections of cortcosterone on retention of appetitive learning tasks in mice. *European Journal of Pharmacology*, **106**, 39–46.

Miczek, K.A. (1980) The neurochemistry of defensive behaviour and fear. *Behavioural and Brain Sciences*, **3**, 313–314.

Miczek, K.A., Thompson, M.L. and Shuster, L. (1982) Opioid-like analgesia in defeated mice, *Science*, **215**, 1520–1522.

Miczek, K.A., DeBold, J.F. and Thompson, M.L. (1984) Pharmacological, hormonal and behavioural manipulations in the analysis of aggressive behaviour. In *Ethopharmacological Aggression Research* (eds K.A. Miczek, M.R. Kruk and B. Olivier), Alan R. Liss, New York, 1–26.

Mikulaj, L. and Mitro, A. (1973) Endocrine functions during adaptation to stress. *Advances in Experimental Medicine and Biology*, **33**, 631–638.

Miller, N.E. (1959) Liberalization of basic S-R concepts: Extensions to conflict behaviour, motivation and social learning. In *Psychology: A Study of a Science*, Vol. 2 (ed. S. Koch), McGraw-Hill, New York, pp. 196–292.

Miller, R.E. and Caul, W.F. (1973) Effect of adrenocorticotropic hormone on appetitive discrimination learning in the rat. *Physiology and Behaviour*, **10**, 141–143.

Miller, R.E. and Ogawa, N. (1962) The effect of adrenocorticotrophic hormone (ACTH) on avoidance conditioning in the adrenalectomized rat. *Journal of Comparative and Physiological Psychology*, **55**, 211–213.

Milner, P.M. (1961) The application of physiology to learning theory. In *Current Trends in Psychological Theory*, University of Pittsburgh Press, Pittsburgh, pp. 111–133.

Minor, T.R., Chang, W-C. and Winslow, J.L. (1994a) Stress and adenosine: I. Effect of methylxanthine and amphetamine stimulants on learned helplessness in rats. *Behavioural Neuroscience*, **108**, 254–264.

Minor, T.R., Winslow, J.L. and Chang, W-C. (1994b) Stress and adenosine: II. Adenosine analogs mimic the effect of inescapable shock on shuttle-escape performance in rats. *Behavioural Neuroscience*, **108**, 265–276.

Mirsky, I.A., Miller, R. and Stein, M. (1953) Relation of adrenocortical activity and adaptive behaviour. *Psychosomatic Medicine*, **15**, 574–588.

Mitchell, J.B. and Stewart, J. (1990) Facilitation of sexual behaviours in the male rat in the presence of stimuli previously paired with systemic injections of morphine. *Pharmacology Biochemistry and Behaviour*, **35**, 367–372.

Mitev, Y., Almeida, O.F.X. and Patchev, V. (1993) Pituitary–adrenal function and hypothalamic beta-endorphin release *in vitro* following food deprivation. *Brain Research Bulletin*, **30**, 7–10.

Mittleman, G., Jones, G.H. and Robbins, T.W. (1988) The relationship between schedule-induced polydipsia and pituitary–adrenal activity: pharmacological and behavioural manipulations. *Behavioural Brain Research*, **28**, 315–324.

Moberg, G.P. (1985) Biological response to stress: key to assessment of animal well-being. In: *Animal Stress* (ed. G.P. Moberg), American Physiological Society, Bethesda, pp. 27–49.

Moltz, H. (1965) Contemporary instinct theory and the fixed action pattern. *Psychological Review*, **72**, 27–47.

Moore, B.R. (1973) The role of directed Pavlovian reactions in simple instrumental learning in the pigeon. In *Constraints on Learning* (eds R.A. Hinde and J. Stevenson-Hinde), Academic Press, London, pp. 159–188.

Morley, J.E. (1989) Neuropeptide Y: A new stress hormone? In *Frontiers of Stress Research* (eds H. Weiner, I. Florin, R. Murison and D. Hellhammer), Hans Huber, Toronto, pp. 286–301.

Morris, D. (1966) Abnormal rituals in stress situations. *Philosophical Transactions of the Royal Society* (London) **251B**, 327–330.

Motta, M., Fraschini, F. and Martini, L. (1969) 'Short' feedback mechanisms in the control of anterior pituitary function. In *Frontiers in Neuroendocrinology, 1969* (eds W.F. Ganong and L. Martini), Oxford University Press, New York, pp. 211–253.

Motta, M., Piva, F. and Martini, L. (1970) The role of 'short' feedback mechanisms in the regulation of adrenocorticotropin secretion. In *Pituitary, Adrenal and the Brain (Progress in Brain Research Vol. 32)* (eds D. de Wied and J.A.W.M. Weijnen), Elsevier, Amsterdam. pp. 25–32.

Munck, A., Guyre, P.M. and Holbrook, N.J. (1984) Physiological functions of glucocorticoids in stress and their relation to pharmacological actions. *Endocrine Reviews*, **5**, 25–44.

Murison, R. and Overmier, J.B. (1993) Parallelism among stress effects on ulcer, immunosuppression and analgesia: Commonality of mechanisms? *Journal of Physiology (Paris)*, **87**, 253–259.

Murphy, J.V. and Miller, R.E. (1955) The effect of adrenocorticotrophic hormone (ACTH) on avoidance conditioning in the rat. *Journal of Comparative and Physiological Psychology*, **48**, 47–49.

Myers, J.H. and Krebs, C.J. (1974) Population cycles in rodents. *Scientific American*, **230**(6), 38–46.

Natelson, B.H., Tapp, W.N., Adamus, J.E., Mittler, J.C. and Levin, B.E. (1981) Humoral indices of stress in rats. *Physiology and Behaviour*, **26**, 1049–1054.

Natelson, B.H., Creighton, D., McCarty, R., Tapp, W.N., Pitman, D. and Ottenweller, J.E. (1987) Adrenal hormonal indices of stress in laboratory rats. *Physiology and Behaviour*, **39**, 117–125.

Natelson, B.H., Ottenweller, J.E., Cook, J.A., Pitman, D., McCarty, R. and Tapp, W.N. (1988) Effect of stressor intensity on habituation of the adrenocortical stress response. *Physiology and Behaviour*, **43**, 41–46.

Nemeroff, C.B. (1988) The role of corticotropin-releasing factor in the pathogenesis of major depression. *Pharmacopsychiatry,* **21**, 76–82.

Nicolaidis, S. and Rowland, N. (1975) Systemic versus oral and gastrointestinal metering of fluid intake. In *Control Mechanisms of Drinking* (eds G. Peters, J.T. Fitzsimons and L. Peters-Haefeli), Springer-Verlag, Berlin, pp. 14–21.

Novak, M.A. and Suomi, S.J. (1988) Psychological well-being of primates in captivity. *American Psychologist,* **43**, 765–773.

Oakley, D.A. (1979) Cerebral cortex and adaptive behaviour. In *Brain, Behaviour and Evolution* (eds D.A. Oakley and H.C. Plotkin), Methuen, London, pp. 154–188.

Oakley, D.A. (1983) Learning capacity outside neocortex in animals and man: Implications for therapy after brain-injury. In *Animal Models of Human Behaviour* (ed. G.C.L. Davey), John Wiley, Chichester, pp. 247–266.

Oatley, K. (1992) *Best Laid Schemes: The Psychology of Emotions*. Cambridge University Press.

Oatley, K. and Dickinson, A. (1970) Air drinking and the measurement of thirst. *Animal Behaviour,* **18**, 259–265.

Obrist, P.A. (1976) The cardiovascular–behavioural interaction—as it appears today. *Psychopharmacology,* **13**, 95–107.

Obrist, P.A., Howard, J.L., Lawler, J.E., Galosy, R.A., Meyers, K.A. and Gaebelein, C.J. (1974a) The cardiac–somatic interaction. In *Cardiovascular Psychophysiology* (eds P.A. Obrist, A.H. Black, J. Brener and L.V. DiCara), Aldine Publishing Company, Chicago, pp. 136–162.

Obrist, P.A., Lawler, J.E. and Gaebelein, C.J. (1974b) A psychobiological perspective on the cardiovascular system. In *Limbic and Autonomic Nervous Systems Research* (ed. L.V. DiCara), Plenum, New York, pp. 311–334.

O'Connor, P. and Chipkin, R.E. (1984) Comparisons between warm and cold water swim stress in mice. *Life Sciences,* **35**, 631–639.

Ödberg, F.O. (1978) Moderator comments. In *1st World Congress on Ethology Applied to Zootechnics*, Editorial Garsi, Madrid, pp. 475–480.

Ödberg, F.O. (1986) The jumping sterotypy in the bank vole (*Clethrionomys glareolus*). *Biology of Behaviour,* **11**, 130–143.

Ödberg, F.O. (1987) Behavioural responses to stress in farm animals. In *Biology of Stress in Farm Animals: An Integrative Approach* (eds P.R. Wiepkema and P.W.M. Van Adrichem), Martinus Nijhoff, Dordrecht, pp. 135–150.

Ödberg, F.O. (1989) Behavioural coping in chronic stress conditions. In *Ethoexperimental Approaches to the Study of Behaviour* (eds R.J. Blanchard, P.F. Brain, D.C. Blanchard and S. Parmigiani), Kluwer Academic Publishers, Dordrecht, pp. 229–238.

Ödberg, F.O. (1993) Future research directions. In *Stereotypic Animal Behaviour—Fundamentals and Applications to Welfare* (eds A.B. Lawrence and J. Rushen), CAB International, Wallingford, pp. 173–191.

Oitzel, M.S. and De Kloet, E.R. (1992) Selective corticosteroid antagonists modulate specific aspects of spatial orientation learning. *Behavioural Neuroscience,* **106**, 62–71.

O'Keefe, J. and Nadel, L. (1978) *The Hippocampus as a Cognitive Map*. The Clarendon Press, Oxford.

O'Keefe, J. and Nadel, L. (1979) Multiple book review of *The Hippocampus as a Cognitive Map*. *Behavioural and Brain Sciences*, **2**, 487–533.

Olton, D.S., Becker, J.T. and Handelmann, G.E. (1979) Hippocampus, space and memory. *The Behavioural and Brain Sciences*, **2**, 313–365.

Ottenweller, J.E., Natelson, B.H., Pitman, D.L. and Drastal, S.D. (1989) Adrenocortical and behavioural responses to repeated stressors: Toward an animal model of chronic stress and stress-related mental illness. *Biological Psychiatry*, **26**, 829–841.

Overmier, J.B. and Murison, R. (1989) Poststress effects of danger and safety signals on gastric ulceration in rats. *Behavioural Neuroscience*, **103**, 1296–1301.

Overmier, J.B., Patterson, J. and Wielkiewicz, R.M. (1980) Environmental contingencies as sources of stress in animals. In *Coping and Health* (eds S. Levine and H. Ursin), Plenum, New York, 1–38.

Overmier, J.B., Murison, R., Skoglund, E.J. and Ursin, H. (1985) Safety signals can mimic responses in reducing the ulcerogenic effects of prior shock. *Physiological Psychology*, **13**, 243–247.

Overmier, J.B., Murison, R., Ursin, H. and Skoglund, E.J. (1987) Quality of poststressor rest influences the ulcerative process. *Behavioural Neuroscience*, **101**, 246–253.

Pagano, R.P. and Lovely, R.H. (1972) Diurnal cycle and ACTH facilitation of shuttlebox avoidance. *Physiology and Behaviour*, **8**, 721–723.

Palkovits, M. (1987) Organization of the stress response at the anatomical level. In: *Progress in Brain Research*, Vol. 72 (eds E.R. de Kloet, V.M. Wiegant and D. de Wied), Elsevier, Amsterdam, pp. 47–55.

Panskepp, J. (1990) A role for affective neuroscience in understanding stress: The case of separation distress circuitry. In *Psychobiology of Stress* (eds S. Puglisi and A. Oliverio), Kluwer, Dordrecht, pp. 41–57.

Paré, W.P. (1976) Activity-stress ulcer in the rat: Frequency and chronicity. *Physiology and Behaviour*, **16**, 699–704.

Paré, W.P. (1989a) 'Behavioural despair' test predicts stress ulcer in WKY rats. *Physiology and Behaviour*, **46**, 483–487.

Paré, W.P. (1989b) Stress ulcer susceptibility and depression in Wistar Kyoto (WKY) rats. *Physiology and Behaviour*, **46**, 993–998.

Paré, W.P. and Redei, E. (1993) Depressive behaviour and stress ulcer in Wistar Kyoto rats. *Journal of Physiology (Paris)*, **87**, 229–238.

Parrott, R.F. and Matthews, S.G. (1991) Enhanced stress hormone release in dehydrated sheep: Implications for welfare? In *Applied Animal Behaviour: Past, Present and Future* (eds M.C. Appleby, R.I. Horrell, J.C. Petherick and S.M. Rutter), Universities Federation for Animal Welfare, Potters Bar, pp. 136–137.

Pelchat, M.L., Grill, H.J., Rozin, P. and Jacobs, J. (1983) Quality of acquired responses to tastes by *Rattus norvegicus* depends on type of associated discomfort. *Journal of Comparative Psychology*, **97**, 140–153.

Petri, H.L. and Mishkin, M. (1994) Behaviourism, cognitivism and the neuropsychology of memory. *American Scientist*, **82**, 30–37.

Pfaff, D.W. (1980) *Estrogens and Brain Function*. Springer-Verlag, Heidelberg.

Phillips, K. (1989) Psychophysiological consequences of behavioural choice in aversive situations. In *Stress, Personal Control and Health* (eds A. Steptoe and A. Appels), John Wiley, Chichester, pp. 239–256.

Plotsky, P.M. (1987) Facilitation of immunoreactive corticotropin-releasing factor secretion into the hypophysial–portal circulation after activation of catecholaminergic pathways or central norepinephrine injection. *Endocrinology*, **121**, 924–930.

Plotsky, P.M. (1988) Hypophysiotropic regulation of stress induced ACTH secretion. In *Mechanisms of Physical and Emotional Stress* (eds G.P. Chrousos, D.L. Loriaux and P.W. Gold), Plenum, New York, pp. 65–81.

Plotsky, P.M. (1991) Neural coding of stimulus-induced ACTH secretion. In *Stress—Neurobiology and Neuroendocrinology* (eds M.R. Brown, G.F. Koob and C. Rivier), Marcel Dekker, New York, pp. 137–150.

Plotsky, P.M., Cunningham, E.T. and Widmaier, E.P. (1989) Catecholaminergic modulation of corticotropin-releasing factor and adrenocorticotropin secretion. *Endocrine Reviews*, **10**, 437–458.

Pohorecky, L.A. and Brick, J. (1987) Characteristics of the interaction of ethanol and stress. In *Stress and Addiction* (eds E. Gottheil, K.A. Druley, S. Pashko and S.P. Weinstein), Brunner/Mazel Publishers, New York, pp. 75–100.

Poole, T.B. (1992) The nature and evolution of behavioural needs in mammals. *Animal Welfare*, **1**, 203–220.

Potegal, M. (1979) The reinforcing value of several types of aggressive behaviour: A review. *Aggressive Behaviour*, **5**, 353–373.

Powell, D.A., Gibbs, C.M., Maxwell, B. and Levine-Bryce, D. (1993) On the generality of conditioned bradycardia in rabbits: Assessment of CS and US modality. *Animal Learning and Behaviour*, **21**, 303–313.

Powers, W. (1973) *Behaviour: The Control of Perception*. Wildwood House, London.

Prince, C.R. and Anisman, H. (1990) Situation specific effects of stressor controllability on plasma corticosterone changes in mice. *Pharmacology, Biochemistry and Behaviour*, **37**, 613–621.

Rabin, D., Gold, P.W., Margioris, A.N. and Chrousos, G.P. (1988) Stress and reproduction: Physiologic and pathophysiologic interactions between the stress and reproductive axes. In *Mechanisms of Physical and Emotional Stress* (eds G.P. Chrousos, D.L. Loriaux and P.W. Gold), Plenum, New York, pp. 377–387.

Rachlin, H. (1976) *Behaviour and Learning*. W.H. Freeman, San Francisco.

Randrup, A. and Munkvad, I. (1970) Biochemical, anatomical and physiological investigations of stereotyped behaviour induced by amphetamines. In *Amphetamines and Related Compounds* (eds E. Costa and S. Garanttini), Raven Press, New York, pp. 695–713.

Ratner, A., Yelvington, D.B. and Rosenthal, M. (1989) Prolactin and corticosterone response to repeated footshock stress in male rats. *Psychoneuroendocrinology*, **14**, 393–396.

Rawlins, J.N.P. (1985) Associations across time: The hippocampus as a temporary memory store. *The Behavioural and Brain Sciences*, **8**, 479–496.

Reisine, T. (1989) Molecular mechanisms controlling ACTH release. In *Frontiers of Stress Research* (eds H. Weiner, I. Florin, R. Murison and D. Hellhammer), Hans Huber, Toronto, pp. 240–249.

Richter, C.P. (1957) On the phenomenon of sudden death in animals and man. *Psychosomatic Medicine*, **19**, 191–198.

Ridley, R.M. (1994) The psychology of perseverative and stereotyped behaviour. *Progress in Neurobiology*, **44**, 221–231.

Ridley, R.M., Baker, H.F. and Haystead, T.A.J. (1981) Perseverative behaviour after amphetamine; Dissociation of response tendency from reward association. *Psychopharmacology*, **75**, 283–286.

Ritchie, J.C. and Nemeroff, C.B. (1991) Stress, the hypothalamic–pituitary–adrenal axis and depression. In *Stress, Neuropeptides and Systemic Disease* (eds J.A. McCubbin, P.G. Kaufmann and C.B. Nemeroff), Academic Press, San Diego, pp. 181–197.

Rivier, C. (1989) Involvement of endogenous corticotropin-releasing factor (CRF) in modulating ACTH and LH secretion function during exposure to stress, alcohol or cocaine in the rat. In *Molecular Biology of Stress* (eds S. Breznitz and O. Zinder), Alan R. Liss, New York, pp. 31–47.

Rivier, C. (1991a) Role of interleukins in the stress response. In *Stress Revisited 1. Neuroendocrinology of Stress* (eds G. Jasmin and M. Cantin), Karger, Basel, pp. 63–79.

Rivier, C. (1991b) Neuroendocrine mechanisms of anterior pituitary regulation in the rat exposed to stress. In *Stress—Neurobiology and Neuroendocrinology* (eds M.R. Brown, G.F. Koob and C. Rivier), Marcel Dekker, New York, pp. 119–136.

Robbins, T.W. and Sahakian, B.J. (1983) Behavioural effects of psychomotor stimulant drugs: Clinical and neuropsychological implications. In *Stimulants: Neurochemical, Behavioural and Clinical Perspectives* (ed. I. Creese), Raven Press, New York, pp. 301–338.

Robbins, T.W., Mittleman, G., O'Brien, J. and Winn, P. (1990) The neuropsychological significance of stereotypy induced by stimulant drugs. In *Neurobiology of Stereotyped Behaviour* (eds S.J. Cooper and C.T. Dourish), Clarendon Press, Oxford, pp. 25–63.

Robinson, D. (1992) *Neurobiology* (part of course SD206). The Open University, Milton Keynes.

Robinson, T.E. and Berridge, K.C. (1993) The neural basis of drug craving: an incentive–sensitization theory of addiction. *Brain Research Reviews*, **18**, 247–291.

Rodgers, R.J. (1989) Ethoexperimental analysis of 'stress' analgesia. In *Ethoexperimental Approaches to the Study of Behavoiur* (eds R.J. Blanchard, P.F. Brain, D.C. Blanchard and S. Parmigiani), Kluwer Academic Publishers, Dordrecht, pp. 245–264.

Rodgers, R.J. and Randall, J.I. (1987a) Defensive analgesia in rats and mice. *The Psychological Record, 37*, 335–347.

Rodgers, R.J. and Randall, J.I. (1987b) On the mechanisms and adaptive significance of intrinsic analgesia systems. *Reviews in the Neurosciences, 1*, 185–200.

Rodgers, R.J. and Randall, J.I. (1988) Environmentally induced analgesia: situational factors, mechanisms and significance. In *Endorphins, Opiates and Behavioural Processes* (eds R.J. Rodgers and S.J. Cooper), Wiley, Chichester, pp. 107–142.

Roitblat, H.L. (1991) Cognitive action theory as a control architecture. In *From Animals to Animats* (eds J-A. Meyer and S.W. Wilson), The MIT Press, Cambridge, pp. 444–450.

Rose, R.M., Jenkins, C.D., Hurst, M., Kreger, B.E., Barrett, J. and Hall, R.P. (1982) Endocrine activity in air traffic controllers at work. III. Relationship to physical and psychiatric morbidity. *Psychoneuroendocrinology, 7*, 125–134.

Rosellini, R.A. and Wildman, D.R. (1989) Prior exposure to stress reduces the diversity of exploratory behaviour of novel objects in the rat (*Rattus norvegicus*). *Journal of Comparative and Physiologial Psychology*, **103**, 339–346.

Rosenfeld, P., van Eekelen, J.A.M., Levine, S. and de Kloet, E.R. (1993) Ontogeny of corticosteroid receptors in the brain. *Cellular and Molecular Neurobiology*, **13**, 295–319.

Roth, K.A., Katz, R.J., Sibel, M., Mefford, I.N., Barchas, J.D. and Carroll, B.J. (1981) Central epinergic inhibition of corticosterone release in rat. *Life Sciences*, **28**, 2389–2394.

Rovensky, J., Palkovic, M., Vigas, M., Smondrk, J. and Jezova, D. (1981) Plasma concentration of hormones and lipoproteins after hyperthermic bath in man. *Advances in Physiological Science*, **35**, 155–162.

Rushen, J. (1986) Some problems with the physiological concept of 'stress'. *Australian Veterinary Journal*, **63**, 359–361.

Rushen, J. (1993) The 'coping' hypothesis of stereotypic behaviour. *Animal Behaviour*, **45**, 613–615.

Rushen, J. and Ladewig, J. (1991) Stress-induced analgesia and endogenous opioids help pigs cope with stress. In *Applied Animal Behaviour: Past, Present and Future* (eds M.C. Appleby, R.I. Horrell, J.C. Petherick and S.M. Rutter), Universities Federation for Animal Welfare, Potters Bar, pp. 138–139.

Rushen, J., De Passillé, A-M. and Schouten, W. (1990) Stereotypic behaviour, endogenous opioids and postfeeding hypoalgesia in pigs. *Physiology and Behaviour*, **48**, 91–96.

Rushen, J., Lawrence, A.B. and Terlouw, E.M.C. (1993) The motivational basis of stereotypies. In *Stereotypic Animal Behaviour—Fundamentals and Applications to Welfare* (eds A.B. Lawrence and J. Rushen), CAB International, Wallingford, pp. 41–64.

Sachar, E.J. (1970) Psychological factors relating to activation and inhibition of the adrenocortical stress response in man: A review. In *Pituitary, Adrenal and the Brain*, Vol. 32, Progress in Brain Research (eds D. de Wied and J.A.W.M. Weijnen), Elsevier, Amsterdam, pp. 316–324.

Sakellaris, P.C. and Vernikos-Dannellis, J. (1975) Increased rate of response of the pituitary–adrenal system in rats adapted to chronic stress. *Endocrinology*, **97**, 597–602.

Salamone, J.D. (1994) The involvement of nucleus accumbens dopamine in appetitive and aversive motivation. *Behavioural Brain Research*, **61**, 117–133.

Sandi, C. and Rose, S.P.R. (1994a) Corticosterone enhances long-term retention in one day old chicks trained in a weak passive avoidance learning paradigm. *Brain Research*, **647**, 106–112.

Sandi, C. and Rose, S.P.R. (1994b) Corticosteroid receptor antagonists are amnestic for passive avoidance learning in day-old chicks. *European Journal of Neuroscience*, **6**, 1292–1297.

Santiago, J.V., Clarke, W.L., Shah, S.D. and Cryer, P.E. (1980) Epinephrine, norepinephrine, glucagon, and growth hormone release in association with physiological decrements in the plasma glucose concentration in normal and diabetic man. *Journal of Clinical Endocrinology and Metabolism*, **51**, 877–883.

Sapolsky, R.M. (1988) Individual differences and the stress response: Studies of a wild primate. In *Mechanisms of Physical and Emotional Stress* (eds G.P. Chrousos, D.L. Loriaux and P.W. Gold), Plenum, New York, pp. 399–411.

Sapolsky, R.M. (1990) Stress in the wild. *Scientific American*, **262**(1), 106–113.

Sapolsky, R.M. (1991) Effects of stress and glucocorticoids on hippocampal neuronal survival. In *Stress—Neurobiology and Neuroendocrinology* (eds

M.R. Brown, G.F. Koob and C. Rivier), Marcel Dekker, New York, pp. 293–322.

Sapolsky, R.M. (1992) Neuroendocrinology of the stress response. In *Behavioural Endocrinology* (eds J.B. Becker, S.M. Breedlove and D. Crews), The MIT Press, Cambridge, pp. 287–324.

Sapolsky, R.M. (1994) *Why Zebras don't get Ulcers*. W.H. Freeman, New York.

Sapolsky, R.M., Krey, L.C. and McEwen, B.S. (1984) Glucocorticoid-sensitive hippocampal neurons are involved in terminating the adrenocortical stress response. *Proceedings of the National Academy of Sciences, USA*, **81**, 6174–6177.

Savory, C.J. and Maros, K. (1993) Influence of degree of food restriction, age and time of day on behaviour of broiler breeder chickens. *Behavioural Processes*, **29**, 179–190.

Sawchenko, P.E. (1991) A tale of three peptides: corticotropin-releasing factor-, oxytocin-, and vasopressin-containing pathways mediating integrated hypothalamic responses to stress. In *Stress, Neuropeptides and Systemic Disease* (eds J.A. McCubbin, P.G. Kaufmann and C.B. Nemeroff), Academic Press, San Diego, pp. 3–17.

Scanes, C.G., Merrill, G.F., Ford, R., Mauser, P. and Horowitz, C. (1980) Effects of stress (hypoglycemia, endotoxin and ether) on the peripheral circulating concentrations of corticosterone in the domestic fowl (*Gallus domesticus*). *Comparative Biochemistry and Physiology*, **66C**, 183–186.

Schacter, S. and Singer, J.E. (1962) Cognitive, social and physiological determinants of emotional state. *Psychological Review*, **69**, 379–399.

Schatzberg, A.F., Rothschild, A.J., Langlais, P.J., Bird, E.D. and Cole, J.O. (1985) A corticosteroid/dopamine hypothesis for psychotic depression and related states. *Journal of Psychiatric Research*, **19**, 57–64.

Scheel-Krüger, J. and Randrup, A. (1968) Pharmacological evidence for a cholinergic mechanism in brain involved in a special stereotyped behavior of reserpinized rats. *British Journal of Pharmacology*, **34**, 217P–218P.

Scheel-Krüger, J. and Willner, P. (1991) The mesolimbic system: Principles of operation. In *The Mesolimbic Dopamine System: From Motivation to Action* (eds P. Willner and J. Scheel-Krüger), John Wiley, Chichester, pp. 559–597.

Schneiderman, N. (1974) The relationship between learned and unlearned cardiovascular responses. In *Cardiovascular Psychophysiology* (eds P.A. Obrist, A.H. Black, J. Brener and L.V. DiCara), Aldine Publishing Company, Chicago, pp. 190–210.

Schneiderman, N. and McCabe, P.M. (1985) Biobehavioural responses to stressors. In *Stress and Coping* (eds T.M. Field, P.M. McCabe and N. Schneiderman), Lawrence Erlbaum, Hillsdale, pp. 13–61.

Schneirla, T.C. (1959) An evolutionary and developmental theory of biphasic processes underlying approach and withdrawal. In *Nebraska Symposium on Motivation* (ed. M.R. Jones), University of Nebraska Press, Lincoln, pp. 1–42.

Schouten, W.G.P. and Wiepkema, P.R. (1991) Coping styles of tethered sows. *Behavioural Processes*, **25**, 125–132.

Schuurman, T. (1980) Hormonal correlates of agonistic behaviour in adult male rats. In *Progress in Brain Research*, Vol. 53, *Adaptive Capabilities of the Nervous System* (eds P.S. McConnell, G.J. Boer, H.J. Romijn, N.E. Van de Poll and M.A. Corner), Elsevier/North-Holland Biomedical Press, Amsterdam, pp. 415–420.

Schuurman, T. (1981) Endocrine processes underlying victory and defeat in the male rat. Doctoral thesis, University of Groningen.

Schwartz, R., Sackler, A.M. and Weltman, A.S. (1976) Some adrenal correlates of aggression in isolated female mice. *Aggressive Behaviour,* **2**, 1–9.

Segal, D.S. and Schuckit, M.A. (1983) Animal models of stimulant-induced psychosis. In *Stimulants: Neurochemical, Behavioural and Clinical Perspectives* (ed. I. Creese), Raven Press, New York, pp. 131–167.

Seligman, M. (1975) *Helplessness.* W.H. Freeman, San Francisco.

Selye, H. (1973) The evolution of the stress concept. *American Scientist,* **61**, 692–699.

Shallice, T. (1972) Dual functions of consciousness. *Psychological Review,* **79**, 383–393.

Shavit, Y. and Martin, F.C. (1987) Opiates, stress and immunity: Animal studies. *Annals of Behavioural Medicine,* **9**, 11–20.

Siegel, H.S. (1980) Physiological stress in birds. *Bioscience,* **30**, 529–534.

Sigg, E.B., Day, C. and Colombo, C. (1966) Endocrine factors in isolation-induced aggressiveness in rodents. *Endocrinology,* **78**, 679–684.

Simon, H.A. (1967) Motivational and emotional controls of cognition. *Psychological Review,* **74**, 29–39.

Simonov, P.V. (1986) *The Emotional Brain.* Plenum, New York.

Singer, R., Harker, C.T., Vander, A.J. and Kluger, M.J. (1986) Hyperthermia induced by open-field stress is blocked by salicylate. *Physiology and Behaviour,* **36**, 1179–1182.

Smelik, P.G. (1970) Adrenocortical feedback control of pituitary–adrenal activity. In *Pituitary, Adrenal and the Brain,* Vol. 32, Progress in Brain Research (eds D. de Wied and J.A.W.M. Weijnen), Elsevier, Amsterdam, pp. 21–24.

Smelik, P.G. (1984) Factors determining the pattern of stress responses. In *Stress—The Role of Catecholamines and Other Neurotransmitters,* Vol. 1 (eds E. Usdin, R. Kvetnansky and J. Axelrod), Gordon and Breach Science Publishers, New York, pp. 17–25.

Smelik, P.G. and Papikonomou, E. (1973) Steroid feedback mechanisms in pituitary–adrenal function. In *Progress in Brain Research,* Vol. 39, *Drug Effects on Neuroendocrine Regulation* (eds E. Zimmermann, W.H. Gispen, B.H. Marks and D. de Wied), Elsevier, Amsterdam, pp. 99–109.

Smelik, P.G., Tilders, F.J.H. and Berkenbosch, F. (1989) Participation of adrenaline and vasopressin in the stress response. In *Frontiers of Stress Research,* (eds H. Weiner, I. Florin, R. Murison and D. Hellhammer), Hans Huber, Toronto, pp. 94–99.

Smith, E.M., Meyer, W.J. and Blalock, J. (1982) Virus-induced corticosterone in hypophysectomized mice: A possible lymphoid adrenal axis. *Science,* **218**, 1311–1312.

Smith, G.P. (1973) Adrenal hormones and emotional behaviour. In *Progress in Physiological Psychology,* Vol. 5 (eds E. Stellar and J.M. Sprague), Academic Press, New York, pp. 299–351.

Smith, M.A. and Nemeroff, C.B. (1988) Preclinical and clinical evidence for the involvement of corticotropin-releasing factor in the pathogenesis of depression. In *Mechanisms of Physical and Emotional Stress* (eds G.P. Chrousos, D.L. Loriaux and P.W. Gold), Plenum, New York, pp. 479–487.

Smotherman, W.P. and Levine, S. (1978) ACTH effects on response suppression and plasma corticosterone in the mouse. *Physiology and Behaviour,* **20**, 503–507.

Smotherman, W.P., Hennessy, J.W. and Levine, S. (1976) Plasma corticosterone levels during recovery from LiCl produced taste aversions. *Behavioural Biology,* **16**, 401–412.

Stalmans, W. and Laloux, M. (1979) Glucocorticoids and hepatic glycogen metabolism. In *Glucocorticoid Hormone Action* (eds J.D. Baxter and G.G. Rousseau), Springer-Verlag, Berlin, pp. 518–533.

Steffens, A.B., van der Gugten, J., Godeke, J., Luiten, P.G.M. and Strubbe, J.H. (1986) Meal-induced increases in parasympathetic and sympathetic activity elicit simultaneous rises in plasma insulin and free fatty acids. *Physiology and Behaviour,* **37**, 119–122.

Stewart, J., de Wit, H. and Eikelboom, R. (1984) Role of unconditioned and conditioned drug effects in the self-administration of opiates and stimulants. *Psychological Review,* **91**, 251–268.

Stewart, M. (1991) *Animal Physiology.* Hodder and Stoughton, Sevenoaks.

Stolk, J.M., Conner, R.L., Levine, S. and Barchas, J.D. (1974) Brain norepinephrine metabolism and shock-induced fighting behaviour in rats: Differential effects of shock and fighting on the neurochemical response to a common footshock stimulus. *The Journal of Pharmacology and Experimental Therapeutics,* **190**, 193–209.

Stone, E.A. (1982) Noradrenergic function during stress and depression: An alternative view. *The Behavioural and Brain Sciences,* **5**, 122.

Sudakov, K.V. (1980) Systems approach to the problem of emotional stress. In *Catecholamines and Stress: Recent Advances* (eds E. Usdin, R. Kvetnansky and I.J. Kopin), Elsevier/North-Holland, New York, pp. 579–581.

Sumova, A. and Jakoubek, B. (1989) Analgesia and impact induced by anticipation stress: involvement of the endogenous opioid peptide system. *Brain Research,* **503**, 273–280.

Sutton, L.C., Fleshner, M., Mazzeo, R., Maier, S.F. and Watkins, L.R. (1994) A permissive role of corticosterone in an opioid form of stress-induced analgesia: blockade of opiate analgesia is not due to stress-induced hormone release. *Brain Research,* **663**, 19–29.

Swenson, R.M. and Vogel, W.H. (1983) Plasma catecholamine and corticosterone as well as brain catecholamine changes during coping in rats exposed to stressful footshock. *Pharmacology Biochemistry and Behaviour,* **18**, 689–693.

Szafarczyk, A., Malaval, F., Laurent, A., Gibaud, R. and Assenmacher, I. (1987) Further evidence for a central stimulatory action of catecholamines on adrenocorticotropin release in the rat. *Endocrinology,* **121**, 883–892.

Taborsky, G.J. and Porte, D. (1991) Stress-induced hyperglycemia and its relation to diabetes mellitus. In *Stress—Neurobiology and Neuroendocrinology* (eds M.R. Brown, G.F. Koob and C. Rivier), Marcel Dekker, New York, pp. 519–548.

Taché, Y. (1991) Effect of stress on gastric ulcer formation. In *Stress—Neurobiology and Neuroendocrinology* (eds M.R. Brown, G.F. Koob and C. Rivier), Marcel Dekker, New York, pp. 549–564.

Taché, Y., Stephens, R.L. and Ishikawa, T. (1989) Stress-induced alterations of gastrointestinal function: Involvement of brain CRF and TRH. In *Frontiers of Stress Research* (eds H. Weiner, I. Florin, R. Murison and D. Hellhammer), Hans Huber, Toronto, pp. 265–275.

Takahashi, L.K. and Kalin, N.H. (1989) Role of corticotropin-releasing factor in mediating the expression of defensive behaviour. In *Ethoexperimental Approaches to the Study of Behaviour* (eds R.J. Blanchard, P.F. Brain, D.C. Blanchard and S. Parmigiani), Kluwer Academic Publishers, Dordrecht, pp. 580–594.

Tazi, A., Dantzer, R., Mormède, P. and LeMoal, M. (1986) Pituitary–adrenal correlates of schedule-induced polydipsia and wheel running in rats. *Behavioural Brain Research*, **19**, 249–256.

Tazi, A., Dantzer, R. and LeMoal, M. (1987a) Prediction and control of food rewards modulate endogenous pain inhibitory systems. *Behavioural Brain Research*, **23**, 197–204.

Tazi, A., Dantzer, R., Le Moal, M., Rivier, J., Vale, W. and Koob, G.F. (1987b) Corticotropin-releasing factor antagonist blocks stress-induced fighting in rats. *Regulatory Peptides*, **18**, 37–42.

Tazi, A., Dantzer, R., Crestani, F. and Le Moal, M. (1988) Interleukin-1 induces conditioned taste aversion in rats: a possible explanation for its pituitary-adrenal stimulating activity. *Brain Research*, **473**, 369–371.

Teitelbaum, P. and Derks, P. (1958) The effect of amphetamine on forced drinking in the rat. *Journal of Comparative and Physiological Psychology*, **51**, 801–810.

Teitelbaum, P., Pellis, S.M. and DeVietti, T.L. (1990) Disintegration into stereotypy induced by drugs or brain damage: a microdescriptive behavioural analysis. In *Neurobiology of Stereotyped Behaviour* (eds S.J. Cooper and C.T. Dourish), Clarendon Press, Oxford, pp. 169–199.

Terlouw, E.M.C., Lawrence, A.B. and Illius, A.W. (1991a) Influences of feeding level and physical restriction on development of stereotypies in sows. *Animal Behaviour*, **42**, 981–991.

Terlouw, E.M.C., Lawrence, A.B., Ladewig, J., De Passille, A.M., Rushen, J. and Schouten, W.G.P. (1991b) Relationship between plasma cortisol and stereotypic activities in pigs. *Behavioural Processes*, **25**, 133–153.

Terman, G.W., Shavit, Y., Lewis, J.W., Cannon, J.T. and Liebeskind, J.C. (1984) Intrinsic mechanisms of pain inhibition: Activation by stress. *Science*, **226**, 1270–1277.

Thierry, B., Steru, L., Chermat, R. and Simon, P. (1984) Searching–waiting strategy: A candidate for an evolutionary model of depression? *Behavioural and Neural Biology*, **41**, 180–189.

Thompson, R.F. (1975) *Introduction to Physiological Psychology*. Harper and Row, New York.

Tilders, F.J.H. and Berkenbosch, F. (1986) CRF and catacholamines; their place in the central and peripheral regulation of the stress response. *Acta Endocrinologica*, **276** (Suppl.), 63–75.

Timberlake, W. (1993) Behaviour systems and reinforcement: An integrative approach. *Journal of the Experimental Analysis of Behaviour*, **60**, 105–128.

Tinbergen, N. (1969) *The Study of Instinct*. Clarendon Press, Oxford.

Toates, F.M. (1971) The effect of pretraining on schedule induced polydipsia. *Psychonomic Science*, **23**, 219–220.

Toates, F. (1974) Computer stimulation and the homeostatic control of behaviour. In *Motivational Control Systems Analysis* (ed. D.J. McFarland), Academic Press, London, pp. 407–426.

Toates, F. (1975) *Control Theory in Biology and Experimental Psychology*. Hutchinson Educational, London.

Toates, F.M. (1979) Water and energy in the interaction of thirst and hunger. In *Chemical Influences on Behaviour* (eds K. Brown and S.J. Cooper), Academic Press, London, pp. 135–200.

Toates, F. (1983) Exploration as a motivational system—a cognitive–incentive model. In *Exploration in Animals and Humans* (eds J. Archer and L. Birke), VanNostrand, Wokingham, pp. 55–71.

Toates, F. (1986) *Motivational Systems.* Cambridge University Press.

Toates, F. (1987) The relevance of models of motivation and learning to animal welfare. In *Biology of Stress in Farm Animals: An Integrative Approach* (eds P.R. Wiepkema and P.W.M. Van Adrichem), Martinus Nijhoff, Dordrecht, pp. 153-186.

Toates, F.M. (1988) Motivation and emotion from a biological perspective. In *Cognitive Perspectives on Emotion and Motivation* (eds V. Hamilton, G.H. Bower and N.H. Frijda), Kluwer Academic, Dordrecht, pp. 3–35.

Toates, F. (1990) Biological perspectives. In *Introduction to Psychology* (ed. I. Roth), Lawrence Erlbaum, Hove, pp. 191–249.

Toates, F. (1992) *Control of Behaviour* (part of course *Biology, Brain and Behaviour*), The Open University, Milton Keynes.

Toates, F. (1994a) Hierarchies of control—changing weightings of levels. In *Perceptual Control Theory* (eds M.A. Rodrigues and M.H. Lee), The University of Wales, Aberystwyth, pp. 71–86.

Toates, F. (1994b) What is cognitive and what is *not* cognitive. In *From Animals to Animats 3* (eds D. Cliff, P. Husbands, J-A. Meyer and S.W. Wilson), The MIT Press, Cambridge, pp. 102–107.

Toates, F. (1994c) Comparing motivational systems—an incentive motivation perspective. In *Appetite—Neural and Behavioural Bases* (eds C.R. Legg and D. Booth), Oxford University Press, Oxford, pp. 305–327.

Toates, F. (1995a) Animal motivation and cognition. In *Comparative Approaches to Cognitive Science* (eds H. Roitblat and J-A. Meyer), The MIT Press, Cambridge, in press.

Toates, F. (1995b) Cognition and evolution—An organization of action perspective. *Behavioural Processes,* in press.

Toates, F. and Jensen, P. (1991) Ethological and psychological models of motivation—towards a synthesis. In *From Animals to Animats* (eds J-A. Meyer and S. Wilson), MIT Press, Cambridge, pp. 194–205.

Toates, F. and Slack, I. (1990) Behaviourism and its consequences. In *Introduction to Psychology* (ed. I. Roth), Lawrence Erlbaum, Hove, pp. 250–313.

Trowill, J.A., Panskepp, J. and Gandelman, R. (1969) An incentive model of rewarding brain stimulation. *Psychological Review,* **76**, 264–281.

Turnbull, A.V., Dow, R.C., Hopkins, S.J., White, A., Fink, G. and Rothwell, N.J. (1994) Mechanisms of activation of the pituitary–adrenal axis by tissue injury in the rat. *Psychoneuroendocrinology,* **19**, 165–178.

Udelsman, R., Harwood, J.P., Millan, M.A., Chrousos, G.P., Goldstein, D.S., Zimlichman, R., Catt, K.J. and Aguilera, G. (1986) Functional corticotropin releasing factor receptors in the primate peripheral sympathetic nervous system. *Nature,* **319**, 147–150.

Ursin, H. (1988) Expectancy and activation: An attempt to systematize stress theory. In *Neurobiological Approaches to Human Disease* (eds D. Hellhammer, I. Florin and H. Weiner), Hans Huber, Toronto, pp. 313–334.

Ursin, H. and Murison, R. (1986) Ethical issues in stress research: Facts, fiction and rational decisions. *Acta Physiologica Scandinavica,* **128** (Suppl. 554), 234–242.

Uvnäs-Moberg, K. and Winberg, J. (1989) Role for sensory stimulation in energy economy of mother and infant with particular regard to the gastrointestinal endocrine system. In *Textbook of Gastroenterology and Nutrition in Infancy,* 2nd edn (ed. E. Lebenthal), Raven Press, New York, pp. 53–62.

Valenstein, E.S. (1969) Discussion. *Annals of the New York Academy of Sciences,* **157**, 1117–1119.

Valentino, R.J. (1988) CRH effects on central noradrenergic neurons: relationship to stress. In *Mechanisms of Physical and Emotional Stress* (eds G.P. Chrousos, D.L. Loriaux and P.W. Gold), Plenum, New York, pp. 47–64.

Van de Kar, L.D., Richardson-Morton, K.D. and Ritterhouse, P.A. (1991) Stress: Neuroendocrine and pharmacological mechanisms. In *Stress Revisited 1. Neuroendocrinology of Stress* (eds G. Jasmin and M. Cantin), Karger, Basel, pp. 133–173.

Vander, A.J., Sherman, J.H. and Luciano, D.S. (1994) *Human Physiology.* McGraw-Hill, New York.

Van Wimersma Greidanus, T.B. (1970) Effects of steroids on extinction of an avoidance response in rats. A structure–activity relationship study. In *Pituitary, Adrenal and the Brain. Progress in Brain Research* (Vol.32), (eds D. De Wied and J.A.W.M. Weijnen), Elsevier, Amsterdam, pp. 185–191.

Van Wimersma Greidanus, T.B. and de Wied, D. (1969) Effects of intracerebral implantation of corticosteroids on extinction of an avoidance response in rats. *Physiology and Behaviour,* **4**, 365–370.

Van Wimersma Greidanus, T.B. and De Wied, D. (1971) Effects of systemic and intracerebral administration of two opposite acting ACTH-related peptides on extinction of conditioned avoidance behaviour. *Neuroendocrinology,* **7**, 291–301.

Veith, R.C. (1991) Sympathetic nervous system function in depression and panic disorder. In *Stress—Neurobiology and Neuroendocrinology* (eds M.R. Brown, G.F. Koob and C. Rivier), Marcel Dekker, New York, pp. 395–435.

Velhuis, H.D., De Kloet, E.R., Van Zoest, I. and Bohus, B. (1982) Adrenalectomy reduces exploratory activity in the rat: a specific role of corticosterone. *Hormones and Behaviour,* **16**, 191–198.

Vingerhoets, J.J.M. (1985) The role of the parasympathetic division of the autonomic nervous system in stress and the emotions. *International Journal of Psychosomatics,* **32**, 28–33.

Walters, E.T., Carew, T.J. and Kandel, E.R. (1981) Associative learning in *Aplysia:* Evidence for conditioned fear in an invertebrate. *Science,* **211**, 504–506.

Watkins, L.R. and Mayer, D.J. (1982) Organization of endogenous opiate and nonopiate pain control systems. *Science,* **216**, 1185–1192.

Weijnen, J.A.W.M. and Slangen, J.L. (1970) Effects of ACTH-analogues on extinction of conditioned behaviour. In *Pituitary, Adrenal and the Brain*, Vol. 32, Progress in Brain Research (eds D. de Wied and J.A.W.M. Weijnen), Elsevier, Amsterdam, pp. 221–235.

Weinberg, J., Erskine, M. and Levine, S. (1979) Shock-induced fighting attenuates the effects of preshock experience in rats. *Physiology and Behaviour,* **25**, 9–16.

Weiner, H. (1991a) From simplicity to complexity (1950–1990): The case of peptic ulceration—II. Animal studies. *Psychosomatic Medicine,* **53**, 491–516.

Weiner, H. (1991b) From simplicity to complexity (1950–1990): The case of peptic ulceration—I. Human studies. *Psychosomatic Medicine,* **53**, 467–490.

Weiner, H. (1992) *Perturbing the Organism—The Biology of Stressful Experience.* The University of Chicago Press, Chicago.

Weingarten, H.P. (1984) Meal initiation controlled by learned cues: basic behavioural properties. *Appetite,* **5**, 147–158.

Weiss, J.M. (1968) Effects of coping responses on stress. *Journal of Comparative and Physiological Psychology,* **65**, 251–260.

Weiss, J.M. (1970) Somatic effects of predictable and unpredictable shock. *Psychosomatic Medicine,* **32**, 397–408.

Weiss, J.M. (1971) Effects of coping behaviour in different warning signal conditions on stress pathology in rats. *Journal of Comparative and Physiological Psychology,* **77**, 1–13.

Weiss, J.M. and Simson, P.G. (1985) Neurochemical mechanisms underlying stress-induced depression. In *Stress and Coping* (eds T.M. Field, P.M. McCabe and N. Schneiderman), Lawrence Erlbaum, Hillsdale, pp. 93–116.

Weiss, J.M. and Simpson, P.E. (1988) Neurochemical and electrophysiological events underlying stress-induced depression in an animal model. In *Mechanisms of Physical and Emotional Stress* (eds G.P. Chrousos, D.L. Loriaux and P.W. Gold), Plenum, New York, pp. 425–440.

Weiss, J.M., McEwen, B.S., Teresa, M., Silva, A. and Kalkut, M.F. (1969) Pituitary–adrenal influences on fear responding. *Science,* **163**, 197–199.

Weiss, J.M., McEwen, B.S., Silva, M.T. and Kalkut, M. (1970) Pituitary–adrenal alterations and fear responding. *American Journal of Physiology,* **218**, 864–868.

Weiss, J.M., Pohorecky, L.A., Salman, S. and Gruenthal, M. (1976) Attenuation of gastric lesions by psychological aspects of aggression in rats. *Journal of Comparative and Physiological Psychology,* **90**, 252–259.

Weiss, J.M., Glazer, H.I., Pohorecky, L.A., Bailey, W.H. and Schneider, L.H. (1979) Coping behaviour and stress-induced behavioural depression: studies of the role of brain catecholamines. In *The Psychobiology of the Depressive Disorders—Implications for the Effects of Stress* (ed. R.A. Depue), Academic Press, New York, pp. 125–160.

Weiss, J.M., Goodman, P.A., Losito, B.G., Corrigan, S., Charry, J.M. and Bailey, W.H. (1981) Behavioural depression produced by an uncontrollable stressor: Relationship to norepinephrine, dopamine and serotonin levels in various regions of rat brain. *Brain Research Reviews,* **3**, 167–205.

Weiss, J.M., Simson, P.G. and Simson P.E. (1989) Neurochemical basis of stress-induced depression. In *Frontiers of Stress Research* (eds H. Weiner, I. Florin, R. Murison and D. Hellhammer), Hans Huber, Toronto, pp. 37–50.

Wemelsfelder, F. (1990) Boredom and laboratory animal welfare. In *The Experimental Animal in Biomedical Research,* Vol. 1 (eds B.E. Rollin and M.L. Kesel), CRC Press, Boca Raton, pp. 243–272.

Wemelsfelder, F. (1993) The concept of animal boredom and its relationship to stereotyped behaviour. In *Stereotypic Animal Behaviour—Fundamentals and Applications to Welfare* (eds A.B. Lawrence and J. Rushen), CAB International, Wallingford, pp. 65–95.

Wertheim, G.A., Conner, R.L. and Levine, S. (1967) Adrenocortical influences on free-operant avoidance behaviour. *Journal of the Experimental Analysis of Behaviour,* **10**, 555–563.

White, N.M. (1989) Reward or reinforcement: What's the difference? *Neuroscience and Biobehavioural Reviews,* **13**, 181–186.

Wiepkema, P.R. (1985) Abnormal behaviours in farm animals: Ethological implications. *Netherlands Journal of Zoology,* **35**, 279–299.

Wiepkema, P.R. (1987) Behavioural aspects of stress. In *Biology of Stress in Farm Animals: An Integrative Approach* (eds P.R. Wiepkema and P.W.M. Van Adrichem), Martinus Nijhoff, Dordrecht.

Wiepkema, P.R. (1990) Stress: ethological implications. In *Psychobiology of Stress* (eds S. Puglisi and A. Oliverio), Kluwer, Dordrecht, pp. 1–13.

Wiepkema, P.R. and Koolhaas, J.M. (1992) The emotional brain. *Animal Welfare,* **1**, 13–18.

Wiepkema, P.R. and Koolhaas, J.M. (1993) Stress and animal welfare. *Animal Welfare,* **2**, 195–218.

Wiepkema, P.R. and Schouten, W.G.P. (1992) Stereotypies in sows during chronic stress. *Psychotherapy and Psychosomatics,* **57**, 194–199.

Wiepkema, P.R. and Van Adrichem, P.W.M. (1987), *Biology of Stress in Farm Animals: An integrative Approach.* Martinus Nijhoff, Dordrecht.

Wiersma, A., Bohus, B. and Koolhaas, J.M. (1993) Corticotropin-releasing hormone microinfusion in the central amygdala diminishes a cardiac parasympathetic outflow under stress-free conditions. *Brain Research,* **625**, 219–227.

Wiertelak, E.P., Maier, S.F. and Watkins, L.R. (1992) Cholecystokinin antianalgesia: Safety cues abolish morphine analgesia. *Science,* **256**, 830–833.

Wilkinson, C.W., Shinsako, J. and Dallman, M.F. (1982) Rapid decreases in adrenal and plasma corticosterone concentrations after drinking are not mediated by changes in plasma adrenocorticotropin concentration. *Endocrinology,* **110**, 1599–1606.

Williams, J.L., Worland, P.D. and Smith, M.G. (1990) Defeat-induced hypoalgesia in the rat: Effects of conditioned odors, naltrexone and extinction. *Journal of Experimental Psychology: Animal Behaviour Processes,* **16**, 345–357.

Williams, R. (1989) *The Trusting Heart.* Times Books, New York.

Williams, R.B. (1991) A relook at personality types and coronary heart disease. *Progress in Cardiology,* **4**, 91–97.

Williams, R.B. and Eichelman, B. (1971) Social setting: Influence on the physiological response to electric shock in the rat. *Science,* **174**, 613–614.

Willner, P. (1985) *Depression—A Psychobiological Synthesis.* John Wiley, Chichester.

Willner, P., Ahlenius, S., Muscat, R. and Scheel-Krüger, J. (1991) The mesolimbic dopamine system. In *The Mesolimbic Dopamine System: From Motivation to Action* (eds P. Willner and J. Scheel-Krüger), John Wiley, Chichester, pp. 3–15.

Wise, R.A. (1994) A brief history of the anhedonia hypothesis. In *Appetite—Neural and Behavioural Bases* (eds C.R. Legg and D.A. Booth), Oxford University Press, Oxford, pp. 243–263.

Woods, S.C. (1991) The eating paradox: How we tolerate food. *Psychological Review,* **98**, 488–505.

Wright, L. (1988) The Type A behaviour pattern and coronary artery disease. *American Psychologist,* **43**, 2–14.

Yates, F.E. (1967) Physiological control of adrenal cortical hormone secretion. In *The Adrenal Cortex* (ed. A.B. Eisenstein), Little, Brown and Company, Boston, pp. 133–183.

Yates, F.E. and Maran, J.W. (1974) The physiology of the mammalian hypothalamo-adrenohypophysial–adrenal glucocorticoid system—a new hypothesis. In *Chronobiological Aspects of Endocrinology* (eds J. Aschoff, F. Caresa and F. Halberg), F.K. Schattuer, Stuttgart, pp. 351–377.

Yates, F.E. and Urquhart, J. (1962) Control of plasma concentrations of adrenocortical hormones. *Physiological Reviews,* **42**, 359–443.

Yehuda, R. and Antelman, S.M. (1993) Criteria for rationally evaluating animal models of posttraumatic stress disorder. *Biological Psychiatry,* **33**, 479–486.

Yehuda, R., Giller, E.L., Southwick, S.M., Lowy, M.T. and Mason, J.W. (1991) Hypothalamic–pituitary–adrenal dysfunction in posttraumatic stress disorder. *Biological Psychiatry,* **30**, 1031–1048.

Young, P.T. (1966) Hedonic organization and regulation of behaviour. *Psychological Review,* **73**, 59–86.

Zhuikov, A.Y. (1993) Avoidance learning and aggression in guppies. *Animal Behaviour,* **45**, 825–826.

Index

Note: Page references in *italics* refer to Figures; those in **bold** refer to Tables

Index compiled by Annette Musker